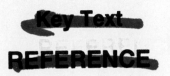

Key Text

REFERENCE

Radiotherapy: Principles to Practice

For Churchill Livingstone

Publisher: Mary Law
Project Editor: Dinah Thom
Senior Project Controller: Neil A. Dickson
Project Controller: Nicky S. Carrodus
Indexer: Liza Weinkove
Sales Promotion Executive: Maria O'Connor

Radiotherapy:
Principles to Practice

A manual for quality in treatment delivery

Sue E. Griffiths HDCR DHSM BEd(Hons) FCR
Superintendent Radiographer, Cookridge Hospital,
Yorkshire Regional Centre for Cancer Treatment, Leeds

Chris A. Short HDCR DHSM
Clinical Superintendent Radiographer, Cookridge Hospital,
Yorkshire Regional Centre for Cancer Treatment, Leeds

Educational Adviser
Christine S. Jackson MPhil TDCR DipAdEd
Principal Lecturer and Course Leader BSc(Hons), Therapeutic Radiography,
University of Derby

Foreword by
Dan Ash FRCP FRCR
Consultant in Clinical Oncology, Cookridge Hospital, Yorkshire
Regional Centre for Cancer Treatment, Leeds;
Honorary Senior Lecturer, Leeds University

CHURCHILL LIVINGSTONE
EDINBURGH LONDON MADRID MELBOURNE NEW YORK AND TOKYO 1994

CHURCHILL LIVINGSTONE
Medical Division of Pearson Professional Ltd

Distributed in the United States of America by Churchill
Livingstone Inc., 650 Avenue of the Americas, New York,
N.Y. 10011, and by associated companies, branches and
representatives throughout the world.

First published 1994
  Reprinted 1995

ISBN 0-443-04783-9

British Library Cataloguing in Publication Data
A catalogue record for this book is available from the British
Library.

Library of Congress Cataloging in Publication Data
A catalog record for this book is available from the Library
of Congress.

The
publisher's
policy is to use
**paper manufactured
from sustainable forests**

Produced by Longman Singapore Publishers (Pte) Ltd.
Printed in Singapore

Contents

Foreword

Although radiotherapy has been used in the treatment of cancer for nearly 100 years it is only in the last 30 to 40 years that it has become widely used and consistently effective in the cure of cancer. As late as the mid-1960s most dose distributions were prepared by hand and there were few treatment simulators and even fewer quality assurance programmes to confirm the accuracy of treatment. Treatments were often simple and guided by skin marks that were placed on the patient using knowledge of surface anatomy. It was often difficult to precisely determine the site of the tumour and thus, by today's standards, most of the links in the data acquistion–treatment-planning–treatment-delivery chain were relatively weak. The last 20 years have seen major changes in all aspects of treatment, planning and delivery. These have had an impact on all those involved in the treatment of cancer by radiation, and in particular on the radiographers who are ultimately responsible for ensuring that the prescribed treatment is accurately and reproducibly delivered to the patient at each treatment session. Radiographers are increasingly involved in the development of new treatment techniques and in the evaluation and assessment of new technology applied to treatment. There is now a need for them to be familiar with the role of computers in radiotherapy, particularly in relation to treatment verification systems and computer control of treatment.

As treatment techniques become more complex it is increasingly important that appropriate quality assurance measures are developed to ensure that what is planned is what is actually delivered. Radiographers have a key role in developing quality assurance programmes at the treatment machine–patient interface and the authors of this book have been very active in these developments.

This book brings together for the first time all the complex and interrelated factors which are important in ensuring a high quality of treatment delivery. It reflects the very high degree of professionalism that has been developed in therapeutic radiography over the last few years. It will be of particular value to students training in therapeutic radiography and will also include much valuable information for staff already trained who wish to be brought up to date on current concepts and developments. As we increasingly work in multidisciplinary teams there is also much of value in this book for both clinicians and physicists who, with radiographers, form an integral part of the treatment planning and delivery team.

1993   Dan Ash

Preface

The purpose of this book is to set out the broad principles of technical practice in radiotherapy. All of the subject material is concerned with the safe use of radiation for patients receiving treatment. It is our aim to present topics in a way which will enable the reader to apply theory and principles to techniques that he or she may encounter. The book is designed to fill a gap in the literature on the practical aspects of radiotherapy and to bring current quality assurance issues into focus with each topic.

Peripheral topics and those on which detailed literature already exists, are mentioned only where they have relevance to quality assurance or to link the theory to practice. Literature on these subjects is listed as background reading at relevant points in the text.

The format of the book has been designed for its use as a practical manual for students or for staff wishing to refresh their knowledge, either in conjunction with a training course or independently. We begin by outlining basic concepts underpinning the radiation treatment of patients, then moving on to the important features of radiation beams and the way in which equipment is used to treat patients. After looking at planning principles, we move to treatment practice for various sites of the body, giving details of various setting-up techniques and their relative strengths and weaknesses. Finally, some new technology and treatments which are at the forefront of present developments in radiotherapy practice are discussed. The book concludes with a section on management, skills and training issues in radiotherapy departments.

This book is intended to give a grounding to those new to the subject, and to stimulate an enquiring attitude of mind in those who are more familiar with radiotherapy practice. Qualified readers are asked to bear with the authors' wish to start with simple outlines of the process, where introductions to various quality assurance concepts are used to set the scene for later chapters.

1993   S.G.
                                                                      C.S.

Acknowledgements

The grateful thanks of the authors are extended to: Christine Jackson, University of Derby, for checking the manuscript for educational relevance and style; Peter Jones, Medical Physics Department, St. George's Hospital, Lincoln, for checking the manuscript on teletherapy equipment and dosimetry; Dan Ash, Consultant in Radiotherapy and Oncology, Cookridge Hospital, Leeds, for the foreword and for checking the text on brachytherapy; Roger Taylor, Consultant in Radiotherapy and Oncology, Cookridge Hospital, Leeds, for checking the text on paediatric treatments and total body irradiation; Andrew Morgan, Medical Physics Department, Cookridge Hospital, Leeds, for producing isodose charts for illustrations and for checking the text on treatment planning and whole-body electron work; George Pitchford, Medical Physics Department, Cookridge Hospital, Leeds, for checking the text on TBI and advice on electron physics; Davinia Honess (MRC) for checking the text on radiobiology; Ian Driver, Radioisotope Department, Cookridge Hospital, Leeds, for checking the text on unsealed sources.

Diagrams were kindly supplied by: Jane Garrud, Medical Illustrator, Cookridge Hospital, Leeds (also using work from the illustration department of the Yorkshire Regional Cancer Organisation); Stuart McNee, Beatson Oncology Centre, Glasgow; Peter Williams, Christie Hospital, Manchester; Philips Medical Systems; Varian Oncology Systems; Nucletron, Simed bv; Sue Pickering, Airedale General Hospital, as well as the following Cookridge staff: Gillian Quinn, John Tuohy, Bryan Dixon, Heidi Probst, Alex Smith, Judith Clinkard, Anthony Flynn, Ian Driver.

1

About radiotherapy

OUTLINE OF THE RADIOTHERAPY PROCESS

What is radiotherapy?

Radiotherapy is the treatment of disease, primarily malignant tumours, using electromagnetic and particle radiations. The radiation may be applied as beams from the outside of the body, a process known as external beam radiotherapy, or by introducing radioactive 'sources' into body cavities, which is called intracavitary or intraluminal radiotherapy. Sources may be implanted into tissue to give interstitial radiotherapy. Occasionally radioactive fluids are introduced into the body either via a vein or into a cavity. The type of treatment used depends partly on the body site requiring treatment. These types of radiotherapy treatment are practised in most radiotherapy departments and most will be described later in detail.

What are the aims of radiotherapy?

Radiotherapy is usually prescribed according to the intention, radical or palliative, required for each patient.

Radical radiotherapy

Treatment intended to cure the patient of his or her disease is known as radical radiotherapy. In such patients the area to be treated includes the tumour and any areas where there is a known risk of microscopic disease being present. The treatment may involve administering radiation beams from a number of directions and sometimes combines more than one type of radiotherapy. The radiation dose given is so high that

1

some side-effects are unavoidable, but these are accepted as an inevitable part of attempted cure.

Palliative radiotherapy

The purpose of palliative radiotherapy is to relieve the distressing symptoms of advanced disease as, for example, in most lung cancers. These treatments are simple compared with radical treatments, and are executed over a shorter time. Palliative treatment is kept to a low dosage to give minimal side-effects.

However, there is a grey area between the two aims, when palliative treatments are given in a radical style. This is used in head and neck tumours where high doses of radiation are necessary to achieve symptom relief, but where it is important to avoid organs such as the eye, and this cannot be achieved with a simple treatment technique.

How is radiotherapy administered?

Radiotherapy machines which produce radiation have features which show where the radiation will be emitted, allowing the patient to be aligned correctly for tumour irradiation. The most common way of indicating where the radiation will be is a light beam mimicking the shape of the radiation beam used for external beam radiotherapy. Often, marks on the surface of the patient are required to indicate where the radiation beam should be applied to treat a tumour at the surface or deep in the body. In another form of radiotherapy called brachytherapy, a guide tube into which radioactive sources will be driven, is introduced into body cavities or tissue.

Radiotherapy treatment is prescribed by a radiotherapist. Each course of treatment usually consists of several doses or fractions, each given on a particular date. Typically, radiotherapy is delivered as one fraction each weekday. Before patients commence treatment, the tissue to be treated is localised and the appropriate treatment schedule calculated. This is referred to as 'radiotherapy planning'. The bulk of this book will be devoted to theory and practices involved in the use of external beam treatments, but a brief outline is necessary at this point.

One or more radiation beams or fields are directed at a tumour on or within a patient. The patient first undergoes various planning procedures, during which the tissue to be treated is accurately localised. Then the number of beams and the type of beam to be used are selected, together with a level of radiation dose. The selected treatment method will require the use of a treatment machine with suitable radiation beams, technological features and accessories to ensure that the treatment is practically viable. A suitable method of 'setting up' the patient to receive treatment, which is the task of the radiographer, is the final requirement for success.

Precision in ensuring that the planned treatment is accurately given to the tumour, is the basis of the profession and practice of therapeutic radiography.

Radiotherapy treatment options

There are various radiotherapy treatment options available for patients with malignant disease. A patient may be treated by one modality, or by using combinations of two or more options. Other adjuvant treatments such as chemotherapy may be combined with radiotherapy. Chemotherapy will only be mentioned where it dictates protocols for radiotherapy treatment given in combination with drug regimes. Radioisotope therapy is outside the scope of this book.

The majority of radiotherapy treatments use external beams of X-rays produced at various energies by a range of treatment machines. Electron beams are also used in many departments. Other machines, including those utilising radioactive isotopes as the source of gamma rays, are also used for specific purposes. Other types of external beam particle radiation may be used but this is infrequent as there are very few facilities.

How does radiotherapy work?

If a tumour is exposed to enough radiation, exponential cell kill results in eradication of the tumour. Adjacent normal tissue cells will also be killed especially those which divide frequently, such as gut mucosa cells. If treatment is planned so that the tumour receives a higher radiation dose than surrounding normal tissue, and the dose is spread out so that the normal tissue can recover, the tumour may be locally eradicated without serious normal tissue damage.

Some of the organs in the body are easily and permanently damaged by radiation, and a relatively low dose will impair their function. They are often referred to as critical organs. The eye, the spinal cord and the kidney are the most sensitive, and their radiation dosage must be kept to a minimum. Organs such as the gut and the lungs are easily damaged, but it is usually possible to avoid irradiating the whole organ and minimise reaction.

The response of different tumour types to a particular dose of radiation varies, so that higher or lower doses are required to cure different diseases. Often the doses which are prescribed are on the limit for normal tissue tolerance, and a 5% increase in dose may result in unacceptable damage. Similarly, a 5% decrease in dose may mean tumour control is less likely. It is a difficult challenge to plan and deliver treatment of the target tissue to within a few percent of the expected dose consistently, because we are treating a patient rather than an immobile uniformly shaped phantom. Quality assurance procedures, a very important part of practice, are built into each method to ensure that each course of treatment fulfils, as closely as possible, the required prescription.

In curing the tumour, normal tissue damage must be minimised by ensuring that the treatment plan, prescription and treatment delivery are appropriate, together with adequate patient monitoring. This requirement links all the main subjects related to radiotherapy practice: anatomy and physiology, oncology, radiobiology, radiation physics and equipment (dosimetry and correct equipment function and usage), radiation protection (of the patient's normal tissue), radiotherapy planning and technique (ensuring that the target tissue is irradiated) and patient care (ensuring that appropriate care and support are given, including care of reactions).

What is the role of the radiographer?

Radiographers are solely responsible for carrying out the prescribed radiation treatment. They have a major role to play in ensuring that accurate and appropriate planning and treatment techniques are used, and in developing and improving practice.

In addition, radiographers monitor side-effects by means of conversation with patients, referring them for examination when necessary. This ensures that treatment is only continued where it is safe to do so. For example, where large volumes of gut are treated, diarrhoea and nausea may necessitate a break in treatment for the gut to recover. It is the responsibility of the radiographer to gain information from the patient and take appropriate action. Radiographers also help to give moral support to patients, and detect individual needs for support from a counselling service.

SOME RADIOBIOLOGICAL TERMS AND CONCEPTS

Radiation dose

There are various ways of defining radiation dose. The dose prescribed for and received by the patient, defines the required dose of energy actually absorbed by the patient, at the tumour site, from the radiation beam. The SI unit of absorbed dose is the gray (Gy). The potential of each radiation beam to deliver energy under specified treatment conditions is determined from detailed measurements made under simulated treatment conditions. This measured potential is also expressed in grays, so that treatment machine output may be expressed as grays per minute and be used in computing the dosimetric effect of each treatment.

The effect of radiation on the tissues

Radiosensitive and radioresistant tumours

Some tumours are eradicated by relatively low radiation doses and are said to be radiosensitive. Some require very high doses and are said to be radioresistant.

Biological effect of radiation, fractionation and tolerance dose

The biological effect on tissue of an absorbed radiation dose varies with the type of radiation, its particular pattern of energy release to tissue and the constituent processes. It also varies with biological factors. Discussions of the biological effects of doses, given in grays, relate to photon or electron radiation only, therefore discussions in this book relate only to these except where other particle beams are specifically under consideration (see Ch. 5).

Fractionation of treatment allows recovery of normal cells (Fig. 1.1) while depleting the number of surviving tumour cells.

The total dose tolerated, or tolerance dose, depends on the dose per fraction (and the dose rate), the sensitivity of the tissues and the amount of recovery which can take place between fractions. With a given tumour and radiation type, the biological effect is influenced by three main interdependent factors:

• total dose delivered
• time over which the dose was delivered
• volume irradiated.

Fractionation and overall time. The dose that can be tolerated by normal tissue in the treatment zone varies with the total time over which the dose is given. A dose can be delivered to a particular area over a few weeks which is larger than could be given in 1 week or 1 day. The dose which can be tolerated is finite, within a maximum period of 7 or 8 weeks; for example using 2 Gy daily fractions to a total of 50–70 Gy. No advantage would be gained by spreading treatment out further; in fact treatment would then become less effective. Many departments successfully use higher fraction sizes over a 4-week treatment period.

For a given volume, the size of each fraction dose and the time interval between fractions alters the biological effect. There is similarly a dose rate effect, which is important in brachytherapy work and total body treatments where different dose rates are used. The higher the fraction dose, or, in brachytherapy the higher the dose rate, the greater the late damage potential. Conventional fractionated courses consist of once-daily doses given 5 days per week, usually Monday to Friday, with a recovery period at the weekend. Other types of fractionation are increasingly used for specific purposes.

Complications can arise in any regime if the patient misses treatment on several days, due to illness, severe reaction, machine breakdown or

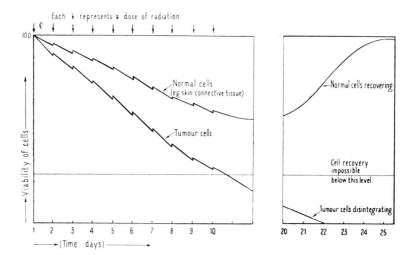

Figure 1.1 Diagrammatic representation of the effect of fractionated radiotherapy on cell viability. (Reproduced from Walter et al 1982.)

servicing, Bank Holidays etc., leading to an over-all treatment period which is significantly longer than intended. Some extra dose may occasionally be given, but this does not fully compensate for the effect of the breaks. There is evidence that patients having treatment for head and neck tumours are at a survival disadvantage if the treatment duration is lengthened (Barton et al 1992). Once some cells are killed the cell kinetics change and there is a potential for very rapid repopulation (Dische & Saunders 1992).

Volume irradiated. In general, the smaller the volume to be treated the higher the total dose which may be tolerated, but the dose fraction-ation schedule used also affects the normal tissue tolerance. A single dose of 20 Gy may be given to a 2 cm diameter area of skin, using low energy X-rays, over a period of a few minutes. This dose would not be tolerated by a larger volume of tissue, and would therefore be divided into sev-eral daily fractions.

Patient and biological factors. The type of tissue treated, poor dietary or fluid intake or concomi-tant drug treatment, may affect the level of dose tolerated. The effect on treatment outcome of various drugs which change the response of tissue to radiation is an area of current study.

Normal tissue tolerance dose levels

A quantity of normal tissue is inevitably irradi-ated during radiotherapy. Continuing practice and associated research and clinical trials fre-quently change perceptions of acceptable dose levels for normal tissue. Therefore it is difficult to define the highest doses tolerated by particular organs, but examples of currently accepted levels using 2 Gy daily fractions (Dobbs et al 1991) are:

Whole brain	50–55 Gy; damage to op-tic nerve beyond this
Spinal cord (10 cm at neck level)	44 Gy
Brachial plexus	50 Gy threshold for neur-itis, arm function loss
Whole lungs	20 Gy, 25–30 Gy leads to pneumonitis

Part lung	40–50 Gy; irreversible fi-brosis, at and beyond this level
Pericardium	40 Gy
Whole liver	20–30 Gy (up to half liver – higher dose tolerated)
Thyroid gland	30 Gy before functional problems occur
Skin	55 Gy; alopecia reversible at this level, permanent above
Parotid gland	10 Gy; temporary dryness 40 Gy; prolonged dryness
Both kidneys	20 Gy
Up to one-third each kidney	40–50 Gy

Sterility and cataract formation occur after relat-ively low doses (ICRP 1990):

Ovary	2–6 Gy; permanent steril-ity
Testes	3–4 Gy; permanent steril-ity
Lens	5–10 Gy cataract forma-tion

Other fractionation regimes

Less than 5 fractions per week. There are various reasons why different types of lowered weekly fractionation regimes may be used, which in-clude:

- fewer visits and less travelling time for patients
- shortage of treatment machine availability and consequent design of regimes to use minimal machine time for long courses
- clinical indications.

Once-, twice- or three times weekly treatments may be given, where a relatively higher dose per fraction is used but is tolerated because of the gap between each fraction. The use of resource-saving policies allows more patients to be offered treatment with a given number of staff and machines; however, the potential for late radia-tion damage increases with high fraction doses.

Treatments may occasionally be given once per week, for example, for very sensitive tumours such as skin lymphomas; to the spleen to reduce white cell counts in chronic leukaemias, or for palliation to contain the growth of a slow-growing tumour, e.g. an advanced breast mass.

Hyperfractionation. Shortening the treatment course duration but giving a high number of small fractions may improve control for tumours with a fast cell-doubling time such as 5 days. Such regimes may result in more acute injury but an unchanged potential for late damage.

Twice- or three times daily fractions, with a 6-hour gap between the exposures, may be given. This is called hyperfractionation, and allows a larger dose per day to be given by allowing recovery for the normal tissue between doses. The 6-hour gap allows approximately five cell division times of one-and-a-quarter hours between treatments for tissues such as gut and lung endothelium. For example twice-daily fractions are given for paediatric total body irradiation (TBI), to maximise the dose given and allow recovery of the lung between fractions (see Ch. 22).

A Medical Research Council trial is underway for a treatment course where 36 fractions are given in 12 days (Continuous Hyperfractionated Accelerated Radiotherapy Treatment, or CHART regime), with a control arm using conventional fractionation (36 fractions at five daily each week). In the CHART arm, three fractions at 6-hourly intervals are given on each of 12 consecutive days, so that the overall treatment time is shortened from 7 weeks to less than 2 weeks.

Oxygen effect

The size of a tumour influences the total dose and fractionation which is required for tumour eradication. This effect is related to the number of cells in the tumour mass, and the number of cells which are well oxygenated. The response of cells to radiation is thought to vary with their oxygenation (Fig. 1.2).

Good oxygenation increases the chance of radiation damage to cells. Cells are less susceptible to radiation damage if they are hypoxic, as are many of the cells within a large cell mass where there is no organised blood supply. Tumour cells therefore tend to be less well oxygenated than normal tissue, and hence less sensitive to radiation. The magnitude of the difference in response

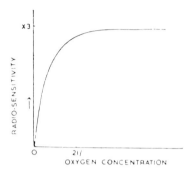

Figure 1.2. Oxygen effect. (Reproduced from Walter et al 1982.)

is called the oxygen enhancement ratio (OER). The OER is reduced at very low dose rates, and also with some particle radiations such as neutron therapy.

During the treatment course, outer, oxygenated cells in the tumour mass are damaged, die and break down so that the next layer of cells becomes oxygenated, etc. In this way the cell mass reduces with each fraction, until all the mass is destroyed at the end of the course. This process, together with a need for a recovery period between doses for normal tissue (which receives a sublethal dose at each fraction), influences the dose and fractionation needs. Patients with low haemoglobin levels are usually transfused prior to treatment to improve cell oxygenation in the tumour-bearing zone.

Cell doubling time. A further factor complicating this process is the rate at which the tumour cells are proliferating. This is variable and tumour-specific, certain histological types proliferating at faster rates than others. If the number of cells doubles (cell doubling time being regarded as one division of all cells in the mass) within the time interval between two fractions, treatment may fail, depending on the radiosensitivity of the tumour and type of radiation used, i.e. on the damage produced by each fraction. For tumours where the cell doubling rate is fast, hyperfractionation may be used to attempt tumour control.

Radiobiological dose rate effects

Radiotherapy can be delivered at varying dose rates. At low dose rate, tumours are eradicated by high doses of radiation delivered in a single continuous fraction, with good normal tissue recovery. Radiotherapy dose regimes and the concept of tissue tolerance doses have evolved from the historical use of radium sources, where the dose rate was low. The dose which a given volume of a certain type of tissue could tolerate in a given time was established in part using radium dose rates. At the range of dose rates normally used in external beam therapy, to deliver a similar dose to the same tumours, without severely damaging normal tissues, would take several weeks of fractionated radiotherapy.

Treatment machines used in external beam radiotherapy normally employ a high dose rate e.g. 2.5 Gy/minute. This may be lowered under certain controlled circumstances to a rate more equivalent to that used in low dose rate brachytherapy applications e.g. 1 Gy/hour. The radiobiological effect, that is the effect of the dose on the tissues, from the same dose given at the two dose rate examples, is different (Fig. 1.3). Low dose rate regimes are used in brachytherapy and in total body irradiation. Higher dose rate treatments using teletherapy are established, but regimes continue to evolve especially in brachytherapy, with increasing knowledge and practice. There are many different dose regimes which produce similar results, but all fall within established tissue tolerance limits. Dose rate issues are discussed further in Chapter 6, and detailed by Sutton (1986) and Steel et al (1990).

Effect of dose rate on cellular processes

The differing radiobiological effects arise from variations, with differing dose rates, in the processes which modify the response of tissue to radiation (Boxes 1.1 and 1.2). Mammalian cells sustain less radiation damage at low dose rate.

Box 1.1   During exposure at low dose rates, order of 0.6 Gy/hour

- Some repair of sublethal damage to cells in normal tissue, giving increased resistance to sustained radiation damage
- Cell proliferation can take place, so repopulation decreases damage to rapidly proliferating tumour or normal tissue
- Cells accumulate in the G2 stage of the cell cycle (Fig. 1.4), when they are most sensitive to radiation, which increases the radiosensitivity of the tumour but also that of normal tissue
- Oxygen enhancement ratio reduced
- Tumour reoxygenation can take place so cells become more sensitive to radiation

---

Box 1.2   During exposure at high dose rate, few Gy/minute

- No cell repair/recovery
- No cell proliferation or repopulation
- No effect on cell cycle
- No reoxygenation or reduced oxygen enhancement ratio

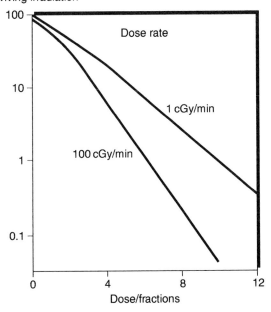

% of cell population surviving irradiation

Figure 1.3   Effect of two different dose rates on cell survival for a particular dose-range. (After Dixon 1982.)

Acute and late radiation effects

Permanent cell damage is expressed when the cell attempts to divide. Acute radiation effects are seen in tissues which divide and repopulate

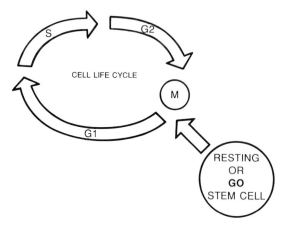

Figure 1.4 Stages in the cell division cycle. S – synthesis of DNA, M – mitosis, G1 – initial resting phase, G2 – second resting phase.

frequently, thus damage is expressed early. Late effects occur in highly differentiated tissue, such as nervous tissue which does not frequently divide, but does so only in response to a stimulus produced by cell death in the tissue. Therefore damage is expressed after a time interval of weeks or years. Radioresistant tumours are difficult to treat without incurring permanent damage to adjacent normal tissue by exceeding the dose tolerance. Permanent damage may take the form of a fistula or an ulcerated area of skin, or paralysis effects occurring some months after treatment due to spinal cord damage.

When doses are within tolerance levels, acute radiation reactions in normal tissue occur concurrently with tumour destruction and will subsequently heal with minimal long-term or late effects. The therapeutic effect relies on differing responses and healing ability for tumour cells and normal tissue, both for early and late damage. The differences between the two vary with tumour histology. Susceptibility to damage from higher fraction sizes varies between early- and late-reacting tissues. This is an important factor taken into account when fraction sizes are varied.

Relative biological effect (RBE) of different types of radiation

Energy absorption in tissue occurs as a result of interaction processes between the radiation and tissue constituents. The interaction processes vary with the energy and type of radiation. Irradiation with photons, electrons, neutrons or protons produces varying patterns of dose absorption. The number of interactions per centimetre of tissue travelled, vary with the nature of the radiation, and thus the energy absorption per centimetre, or the linear energy transfer (LET), varies also.

The biological effect is changed depending on the OER and the radiosensitivity variation with radiation type. This will be further discussed in Chapter 21.

THE SAFE USE OF RADIATION FOR PATIENTS RECEIVING TREATMENT

The 1987 Ionising Radiation Regulations include the ALARA principle: during the course of a medical examination or treatment by radiation, the dose to the patient should be as low as reasonably achievable.

The dose received outside the site targeted for treatment should be minimised, critical organs being excluded from the high dose zone when possible. If treatment is not achieved as intended, organs and uninvolved tissue adjacent to the target volume will be irradiated inadvertently. The consequences of this may be extremely serious, or damaging to the long-term function of organs. Spinal cord damage or the loss of vision reduce the value of treatment.

Treatment-related morbidity (permanent normal tissue damage) is the most important radiation safety issue for the patient. The degree of morbidity depends crucially on technical factors, on precision in treatment delivery and on dosimetry factors. In 33% of patients treated radically, the treatment fails to control local disease. Where the treatment fails, the radiotherapy process and related stress and inconvenience to the patient have been inflicted with little benefit and at great cost to the patient, his/her family and the healthcare system.

Prerequisites for safe and effective treatment include the use of optimal methods of tumour staging, of localisation and of treatment planning and dosimetry, as well as accurate treatment methods and appropriate fractionation. Other related issues are the education and training and thus the quality and skills of staff, appropriate identification of patients and associated record-keeping and organisation and systems of work.

REFERENCES AND FURTHER READING

Barton M B, Keane T J, Gadalla T, Maki E 1992 The effect of treatment time and treatment interruption on tumour control following radical radiotherapy of laryngeal cancer. Radiotherapy and Oncology 23: 137–143

Bleehen N M 1988 Radiobiology in radiotherapy. Croom Helm Springer, London

Dische S, Saunders M I 1992 Clinical fractionation studies. In: Peckham M, Pinedo R, Veronesi U (eds) Oxford textbook of oncology. Oxford University Press, Oxford

Dixon 1982 In: Joslin C A (ed) Cancer topics and radiotherapy. Pitman, London

Dobbs J, Barrett A, Ash D 1991 Practical radiotherapy planning, 2nd edn. Arnold, London

Saunders M I, Dische S, Grosch E J et al 1991 Experience with CHART. International Journal of Radiation Oncology, Biology, Physics 21: 871–878

Steel G G, Kelland L R, Peacock J H 1990 The radiobiological basis for low dose rate radiotherapy. Brachytherapy 2, Nucletron, Leersum

Sutton M L 1986 Some clinical aspects of radiobiology. In: Hope-Stone H F (ed) Radiotherapy in clinical practice. Butterworths, London

Tepper J E (ed) 1992 Seminars in radiation oncology, fractionation in radiation therapy. W B Saunders, Pennsylvania

Walter J, Miller H, Bomford C K 1982 A short textbook of radiotherapy, 4th edn. Churchill Livingstone, Edinburgh, p 178, 180.

Radiotherapy practice: the tools

2

High energy X-ray beams

In most radiotherapy departments X-rays are produced by linear accelerators (linacs) (Fig. 2.1). The method of X-ray production is outside the scope of this book, but is widely documented (Green 1986). It is important for radiographers to be conversant with the method of X-ray generation as they are required to monitor the linac's performance during clinical work.

TREATMENT ENERGIES

The range of energies employed in treatment delivery varies from 4 MV to a maximum of 25 MV; commonly only beams of up to 10 MV are used. Many papers have been written which discuss the optimal energy for the irradiation of various tumour sites within the body.

Typical X-ray energies for the treatment of head and neck or breast are 4–6 MV. For tumours sited deeper in the body, e.g. pelvic tumours, energies of 8–10 MV (Laughlin et al 1986) are appropriate. Energies above 10 MV are less

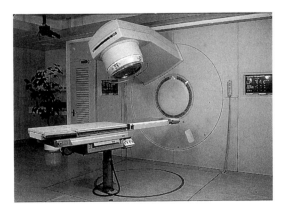

Figure 2.1   A linear accelerator. (Courtesy of Philips Medical Systems.)

common but can be used for pelvic and lung tumours.

CLINICAL ADVANTAGES

High energy X-ray beams offer two main advantages to clinical practice.

The dose absorbed is not dependent upon tissue type

The predominant interaction process of the X-ray beam with the body tissue is the Compton process (Walter et al 1982).

Skin-sparing and the build-up effect

The dose absorbed builds up in the first few centimetres of tissue, and results in the skin receiving a relatively low dose. Hence the skin is

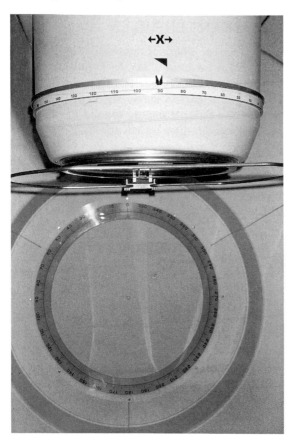

Figure 2.2 Illuminated gantry scale not obscured by a patient in the treatment position.

spared the maximum absorbed dose which is delivered below the skin surface, contrasting with orthovoltage and superficial beams (see Ch. 4). This effect occurs because interactions produce a predominantly foward scatter at high energies (Meredith & Massey 1968).

The relationship between beam energy and depth of maximum absorbed dose

Maximum absorbed dose is delivered at a depth, in centimetres, of one-quarter of the beam energy in MV, e.g at 6 MV the maximum absorbed dose is delivered at 1.5 cm tissue depth.

In practice this means that a treatment beam can be directed at the lens of the eye to treat deeper tissue but will spare the anterior chamber. Where the skin has folds which extend down to the depth of maximum absorbed dose, the skin will receive the same dose as the tissue at that depth, thus skin folds of the abdomen and the axilla often get very sore whilst the rest of the surrounding skin shows little reaction.

The build-up effect must be considered during the planning process. Skin-sparing considered detrimental to the treatment outcome can be reversed by adding a tissue-equivalent bolus of an appropriate thickness (see Ch. 8).

FUNDAMENTAL DESIGN FEATURES

The methods of treatment delivery described in the second section of this book have developed because of the design and range of movements available on the current generation of linacs.

Isocentric mounting

The linac is mounted to permit rotation of the gantry through 360°, so that treatment fields may be directed at the patient from any angle within the circle. The position of the gantry is indicated by a protractor-type scale which should be visible during all routine treatment positions, and well illuminated to enable it to be read in the dark (Fig. 2.2).

The centre of the circle described by the rotation of the gantry is known as the isocentre (Fig. 2.3). All rotational movements of the machine are about this point. The linac is specially

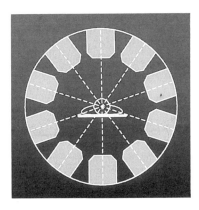

Figure 2.3 The isocentric rotation of the gantry. (Courtesy of Philips Medical Systems.)

constructed to enable the isocentre to be contained within a very small volume of a few cubic millimetres for all movements of the gantry.

Isocentre height

The height of the isocentre from the floor affects the ease with which patients can be accurately positioned, and is governed by the design and shape of the gantry arm and the treatment head. The higher the isocentre the harder it is to see the field light on the patient's skin. Furthermore, if the isocentre is high it is difficult to locate treatment accessories in the treatment head, which is also high (Fig. 2.4).

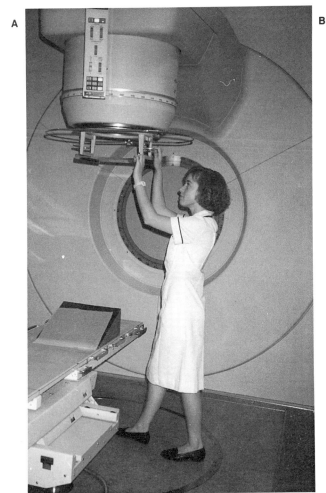

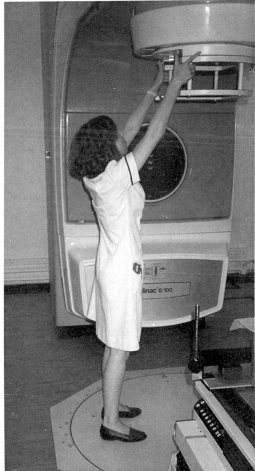

Figure 2.4 Comparison of two linacs demonstrating the difficulties of locating accessories in a high treatment head. The head height of the linac shown in **A** is 13.5 cm lower than that of the linac shown in **B**.

Rotation of the collimators

For the greatest flexibility in treatment field positioning, the collimators must rotate through 360°. The position of the collimators should be indicated by an analogue scale (Fig. 2.5) encircling the treatment head. Computer-controlled and verified linacs will also provide a digital readout.

The axis of rotation is the central axis of the radiation beam, which intersects the isocentre at 100 cm focus–skin distance (f.s.d.), i.e. the isocentre is 100 cm away from the X-ray target. This distance allows enough room between the patient and the treatment head to permit a wide range of treatment techniques, whilst ensuring that the treatment head height can be reached easily by the radiographers.

Rotation of the couch

The couch rotates about the isocentre on a turntable, and the scale indicating the position of the couch runs around the edge of the turntable. Convention dictates that the turntable indicates zero when the couch is in the normal treatment position.

A couch rotation of up to 110° from zero will enable most techniques to be achieved. A restricted couch rotation of only 90° from zero will render some treatments impossible.

Position of the lasers

Lasers mounted on the walls and the ceiling define the isocentre at the lateral and anterior quadrants. Additional lasers may include a sagittal and backpointing laser (see Ch. 9).

SHAPING THE RADIATION BEAM

To permit the treatment of areas of different sizes within the patient, it is essential that the size and shape of the useful beam can be altered. The patient must be protected from any part of the radiation beam not required for the treatment plan. The beam is shaped by two sets of collimators: primary and secondary.

Primary collimation

The primary collimator comprises a large block of lead or heavy alloy with a conical aperture through which the useful beam travels to the secondary collimation (Fig. 2.6).

Shape of the radiation beam after primary collimation

The radiation is effectively emitted from a point on the target radially, and predominantly in a

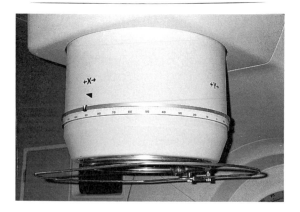

Figure 2.5 Analogue diaphragm scales, clearly visible for most setups.

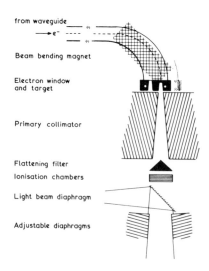

from waveguide

e⁻

Beam bending magnet

Electron window and target

Primary collimator

Flattening filter

Ionisation chambers

Light beam diaphragm

Adjustable diaphragms

Figure 2.6 Schematic diagram of linac head showing primary and secondary collimators. (Reproduced from Walter et al 1982.)

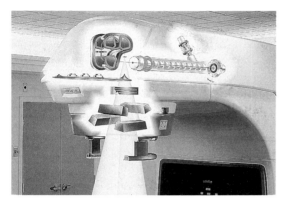

Figure 2.7 Diagram showing the shape of the X-ray beam after primary and secondary collimation. (Courtesy of Varian Oncology Systems.)

forward direction (Fig. 2.7). The sides of the aperture are angled and positioned so that they run parallel with the direction of the X-rays at the edge of the beam, so a cone-shaped beam is produced, with a circular cross-section.

Secondary collimation

The secondary collimation is provided by two pairs of lead collimators of sufficient thickness to absorb most of the primary beam. They are conventionally moved in pairs symmetrically about the central axis of the beam to permit variably sized treatment fields. However, modern linacs have the facilities to move the collimators in an asymmetric manner.

Construction of secondary collimators

The detail of collimator construction varies (Walter et al 1982). The single thick block collimators (Fig. 2.8) are the most commonly used, but they result in one pair of field edges being better defined than the other. This is demonstrable on machine check films (Fig. 2.9). Usually any rectangle or square from 1 cm × 1 cm to 40 cm × 40 cm at

 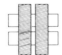 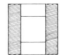

Figure 2.8 The position and movements of the secondary collimators of a linac. (Reproduced from Walter et al 1982.)

the isocentre, i.e. 100 cm f.s.d., is possible.

It is important to note that very large fields may sometimes have rounded corners caused by the primary collimation.

Shape and movement of the secondary collimators. A sharply defined edge is always ensured as the collimators are designed in such a way that their inner faces defining the beam are always aligned with the angle of the X-rays at the edge of the beam they define. A small focal spot ensures the linac has a sharply defined edge, even at 100 cm f.s.d., ensuring a sharp cut-off of radiation at the field edge.

Why have a sharp edge?

It is necessary to have a sharp edge so that only the tissue intended to be treated is irradiated. Also areas may be treated which are next to critical organs such as the eye. The penumbra (dose gradient at the field edge) is wider on teletherapy units (see Ch. 3) than on linacs, making linacs the machine of choice for radical work.

Interestingly at very high X-ray energies, e.g. 16 MV, the effective penumbra in tissue widens (Laughlin et al 1986) because of the increased range of travel of scatter from the beam edges. Therefore the application of higher energy beams is limited to tumour sites and functions where a less sharp edge is acceptable.

Defining the field length and width

The cross-sectional area of the radiation beam is referred to as the treatment field. The field size is defined by the field length, i.e. along the patient, and the field width, i.e. across the patient, measured in centimetres at the treatment f.s.d.

Linac field size readouts

The field size is set by the secondary collimators of the linac. These are calibrated to show the field size in centimetres at 100 cm f.s.d.

Historically the field size of each collimator was indicated on the treatment head and controlled by a switch mounted next to the readout, making

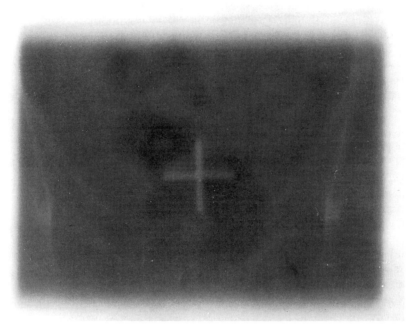

Figure 2.9 A check film demonstrating the difference in field edge sharpness of each pair of collimators.

the orientation and dimensions of the field easy to visualise and obvious from the readouts on the treatment head.

This arrangement has now been superseded by remote digital readouts of the collimators, with control switches mounted on the handset. This has necessitated the labelling of each collimator of the radiation field. Commonly X and Y are used, where X is the field axis across the wedge and Y is the field axis along the wedge (see Fig. 2.5). Unfortunately this labelling is not consistent throughout all linacs, being reversed from one manufacturer to another. This complicates their use, as the radiographer has to mentally switch the orientations on moving from one unit to another.

Setting field sizes

As the field axis readouts are distant from the treatment head, it is vital that the axes are clearly labelled, so that the field size being set using the remote readouts can be easily related to the axes on the treatment head. This labelling helps to ensure the field is correctly orientated on the patient. Furthermore if an internal wedge system is used, the wedge orientation should also be clearly marked on the treatment head so that the field can be correctly aligned with the wedge.

Extended f.s.d. treatments

At a distance from the source which is greater than the isocentric distance, the field size is increased due to the divergent shape of the beam (see Fig. 15.2). The patient may be treated at a greater distance away from the machine if a suitable range of couch movements or other practical arrangements are available. The field sizes indicated by the treatment machine are then incorrect, but true field size may be calculated using a simple formula:

$$\text{Required collimator setting} = \frac{\text{Required field size}}{\text{Treatment distance}} \times 100$$

ASYMMETRIC AND INDEPENDENT COLLIMATORS

Conventionally the collimators move symmetrically about the beam axis, but modern linacs have the additional facility to move the collimators independently of the field centre. This is effected in one of two ways, but the same result is achieved in both cases. Each system has advantages in different set-ups, so some linacs provide both functions.

In practice, if only one pair of collimators are able to move in this way the range of use is greatly restricted.

Asymmetric collimators. The jaws move as a pair independently of the central axis.

Independent collimators. Each one of the collimators moves separately, and can be positioned at different distances from the central axis thereby creating an asymmetric field.

Operation of asymmetric collimators

To ensure that treatment fields are offset by the correct amount in the correct direction, it is important that a clear system of communication is developed. This should ensure that a clear and unambiguous field geometry instruction is given, which ideally should relate to the patient's anatomy: for example the field is offset 2 cm to the patient's right.

The system nomenclature for inputing this into the linac control system can operate on a graph axis as in Figure 2.10. For example: when the collimators are symmetrical about the field centre the collimator offset readout will be zero. As the collimators are offset towards the thick

end of the wedge, the offset readout will indicate the number of centimetres travelled from the symmetric position. Counting down, 99 on the offset readout indicates a 1 cm offset towards the thick end of the wedge, 98 indicates 2 cm etc. When the collimators are offset towards the thin end of the wedge, then the offset readout indicates the true measurement in centimetres.

Asymmetric collimators in clinical practice

It is important to note that as the collimators are still moving in pairs the field size remains constant. The usual method of operation is to first set the collimators to the required field size, then to move the preset field size in an asymmetric manner.

Operation of independent collimators

As either collimator of a pair can be moved separately, any movement of one collimator alters the field size, since the other collimator remains in its original position. The method of specifying collimator position must be different from that of asymmetric collimators. Each collimator is labelled separately, for example, Y1 and Y2 and X1 and X2. The collimators can then be identified on the treatment head, and their distance in centimetres from the central axis can be set.

For example, a symmetric field size 6 cm × 6 cm could be described:

> Collimators   X1 = 3 cm
> X2 = 3 cm
> Y1 = 3 cm
> Y2 = 3 cm

If the field was offset:

> Collimators   X1 = 1 cm
> X2 = 5 cm
> Y1 = 3 cm
> Y2 = 3 cm

The collimator positions must then be related to the patient. It is more difficult to annotate the position of the independent collimators in an unambiguous manner. One possible method is to relate the position of each collimator to the anatomy of the patient in the form of a diagram (Fig. 2.11).

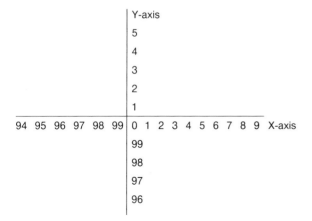

Figure 2.10 The graph axes for defining the position of the asymmetric collimators.

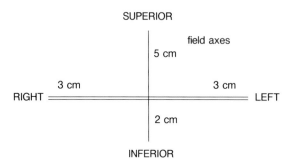

Figure 2.11 A method for defining the position of independent jaws in relation to patient anatomy.

Practical uses of asymmetric and independent collimators

Some of the ingenious uses are described in Chapters 17, 19 and 23. Usage must take into consideration that the different beam edges will have different penumbras. One collimator can be positioned on the central axis, thus one beam edge has no divergence and can be used in matching fields at field junction edges (Chs 17 and 19).

In many radiotherapy centres, linacs with asymmetric or independent jaws have treatment verification systems. Correct data input for the position of the jaws requires considerable expertise.

VISUALISING THE RADIATION BEAM

The area of radiation available after secondary collimation is made visible to the eye by a light beam which is positioned in the treatment head, so as to simulate the radiation beam as closely as possible. There are several methods used to create a coincident light field but the most common employs a radiotranslucent foil mirror. This reflects light from a bulb situated to the side of the radiation beam (Fig. 2.12).

Cross-wires

A pair of fine cross-wires defines the centre of the radiation beam in the light field (Fig. 2.13). This allows fields to be aligned on the patient by the field centre, instead of by the edges. This is

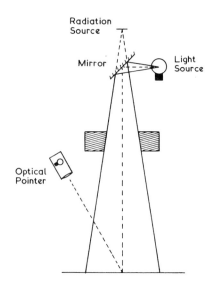

Figure 2.12 Schematic diagram of the field-defining light and rangefinder. (Reproduced from Walter et al 1982.)

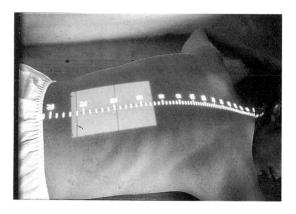

Figure 2.13 The field light, cross-wires and rangefinder. The scale is easy to read, with sufficient graduations to permit the accurate setting of f.s.d.

particularly useful where isocentric treatments are set up using a tattoo.

Rangefinder

The rangefinder is a numerical scale, projected from the treatment head or gantry arm, which indicates the distance in centimetres from the target to a surface. Typically the scale indicates the treatment distance where it crosses the central axis cross-wires (Fig. 2.13). The range of distances measurable should be 80–150 cm f.s.d., to allow for treatment at extended f.s.d. and to permit most tumour–skin distances to be measured.

Rangefinders should be positioned so that they are not projected through, and thus distorted by, the lead platform as this leads to inaccuracies in setting the treatment distance.

Important features of beam definition in practice

To facilitate accurate treatment delivery for all treatment set-ups the beam defining system needs to meet the following criteria:

• The coincidence of the radiation beam with the light beam and the rangefinder; accuracy must be at normal treatment distance to within 2 mm.
• The light beam must be bright enough to be clear at extended f.s.d. with the lead tray in situ.
• The cross-wires must be thin but clear so they can be seen on a dark surface.
• The rangefinder must have wide spacing between the numbers and sufficient graduations to permit accurate rangefinder settings across the scale.

These features must be considered during the equipment selection process (see Ch. 24).

QUALITY ASSURANCE

A linac is a complex piece of equipment. Safe and accurate radiotherapy demands a well-defined and consistent performance. Monitoring this is the purpose of the quality assurance programme.

The specification

The requirements of a linac are defined by a multidisciplinary equipment selection committee, which should involve radiographers and physicists. These requirements form the department specification. During the selection process the department specification will be compared against the equipment manufacturers' specifications.

The specification should include the standards documented by the British Standards Institute in document number BS 5724, the detail of which is derived from recommendations of the International Electrotechnical Commission (IEC).

Acceptance and commissioning tests

After installation the linac undergoes extensive testing (see Ch. 7) known as commissioning tests. The testing includes: data acquisition, ensuring the linac meets the required purchase specification (acceptance tests), and defining a baseline standard for the future quality assurance programme (IPSM 1988).

It is impossible for the linac to meet the performance specification perfectly and indeed there will be some variation in its performance over its useful life. Therefore a clinically acceptable tolerance must be agreed for each measurement performed.

Constancy checks

The performance of the linac is then compared at regular intervals with the baseline standard established. These checks are known as constancy checks and are the basis of the quality assurance programme.

The quality assurance programme

The quality assurance programme sets out the planned tests, their frequency and performance tolerances. Yearly and monthly checks are usually carried out by the medical physics department, as documented in the IPSM Report number 54. This Report defines the minimum possible schedule to ensure a safe linac.

These checks should also be carried out after major breakdown, and any parameters whose performance gives cause for concern should be tested more frequently.

Monthly checks

Typically carried out as part of routine service, monthly checks include:

Cookridge Hospital

Varian 2

Daily Quality Assurance Tests

Week commencing _____

	Test	Mon	Tue	Wed	Thur	Fri	Sat	Sun
D1	**Rangefinder**							
	Tol: +/-2mm @ 100cm							
D2	**Optical Field Size**							
	Tol: +/-2mm on 10x10cm							
D3	**Crosswires**							
	Tol: within 2mm circle - full coll. rot.							
D4	**Optical Field Alignment**							
	Tol: +/-2mm at each collimator angle							
D5	**Isocentric Lasers**							
	Tol: indicate isocentre within +/-2mm in X,Y,Z							
	Signature							

V2DQA93

Figure 2.14 An example of a quality assurance log sheet.

- repeat by an independent person of the daily checks
- the relation between the indicated isocentre and the centre of rotation of the collimators and the gantry
- alignment of the radiation beam with the light beam
- flatness of the radiation beam
- beam energy check.

Daily checks

Daily checks are the responsibility of the radiographers and thus will be discussed in detail. The process of ensuring that the linac is performing within the defined tolerances from day to day is defined in the daily checks.

It is important to note that these checks may not identify some mechanical problems, which may occur during clinical use. Therefore it is of paramount importance that the radiographer constantly monitors the linac during treatment procedures, and that any unexplained changes are investigated immediately.

Documentation

Each linac should have a clear set of instructions describing the agreed checks. This should be supplemented by a log sheet/book (Fig. 2.14), in which each check should be identified, acceptable tolerances documented and space provided for daily comments and a full signature.

Mechanical checks and equipment used

The mechanical checks are designed to ensure that the field-defining system is operating within defined tolerances. They are carried out using a test object, a 'T' bar and a platform which can be moved in the vertical plane. These checks should be carried out prior to the machine calibration check as any inaccuracies in the mechanical checks render the calibration void.

The platform (Fig. 2.15) is a safety measure; fine adjustments to the height of the test object can be carried out manually to prevent damage to the linac head.

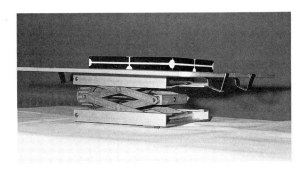

Figure 2.15 Platform with the facility for small height adjustments to be carried out without risk of damage to the treatment head.

The test object permits the position of the central axis, the edges of the light beam and the position of the lasers in relation to the isocentre to be visually checked, using a test pattern showing the field size, the central axis and the acceptable limits (Fig. 2.16).

The 'T' bar. The length of the 'T' bar is the exact distance from the face of the linac head to the isocentre (Fig. 2.17).

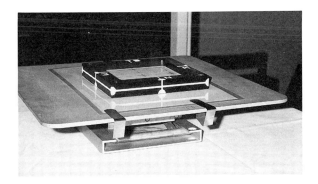

Figure 2.16 The test object.

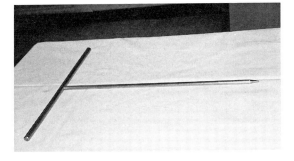

Figure 2.17 The 'T' bar.

The procedure for mechanical checks

The tests are carried out with the gantry, diaphragms and floor rotation set at 0° and the field size set to 10 cm × 10 cm.

Accuracy of the rangefinder. *Tolerance*: the rangefinder must indicate the target-to-isocentre distance on the beam axis to within 2 mm. *Method*: set the test table to the isocentre using the 'T' bar. Check that the rangefinder indicates between 99.8 and 100.2 cm.

Accuracy of the optical field size. *Tolerance*: with an indicated field size of 10 cm × 10 cm the dimensions of the optical light beam should correspond to the indicated field size to within 2 mm. *Method*: with the test table set at 100 cm f.s.d. ensure that the measurement of the field light along the field axis falls between 9.8 cm and 10.2 cm. These limits are etched on to the test pattern.

Accuracy of the cross-wires. *Tolerance*: the cross-wires must indicate the centre of rotation to within 2 mm. *Method*: set the test table at 100 cm f.s.d. and observe the travel of the cross-wires whilst rotating the diaphragms through their full range. The central cross-wires must describe a circle of diameter less than 2 mm, i.e. the circle described by the cross-wires must be within the circle on the test table.

Alignment of the field light with the central axis. *Tolerance*: the alignment of the optical field with respect to the central axis must be correct to within 2 mm. *Method*: with the central axis of the beam correctly aligned on the test table, rotate the collimators to each quadrant and check that

the central axis-to-field edge measurement falls between 4.8 and 5.2 cm.

Accuracy of the lasers. *Tolerance*: the lasers must define the isocentre to within 2 mm. *Method*: with the test table set at 100 cm f.s.d. and the central axis in the correct position, check that the lateral and sagittal lasers indicate the respective isocentric planes to within 2 mm. Move the gantry to check the top cross in a similar way.

Output checks

Output checks (calibration) are carried out for each modality and energy to be used in clinical practice before commencing clinical use. The theory behind the measurement of output at megavoltage (Greening 1985) photon energies is outside the scope of this book.

Equipment required includes:

1. water phantom of minimum size 20 cm × 20 cm × 10 cm
2. ion chamber positioned at the required depth in the phantom
3. suitable meter, e.g. Ionex etc., and connecting cable.

Or an integral ion chamber and meter, e.g. a Keighley (Fig. 2.18).

In addition a barometer and thermometer are required for measurement of ambient temperature and pressure.

The method is as follows:

• Set 10 cm × 10 cm field on the collimators of the linac.
• Position the phantom with the ion chamber in situ, so that the central axis of the radiation beam is centred on the ion chamber. NB: the phantom should be kept in the treatment room or at the same temperature as the treatment room.
• Set the anterior face of the phantom to 100 cm f.s.d.
• Place thermometer in the room.
• Reset meter and set 100 monitor units.
• At the end of the exposure, note reading.
• Repeat exposure three times, noting the meter readings each time.

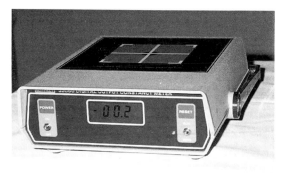

Figure 2.18 A Keighley constancy meter with integral ion chamber.

Calculation of the output is as follows:

- Take an average of these readings.
- Apply corrections for ambient temperature and pressure, plus quality and exposure to absorbed dose factors to arrive at an output which should be unity.

- The tolerance for the measurement of output is plus or minus 3%.

When all the checks described are complete and are found to be within the required tolerance the linac is ready for clinical use.

REFERENCES AND FURTHER READING

Greene D 1986 Linear accelerators for radiation therapy. Hilger, Bristol

Institute of Physical Sciences in Medicine 1988 Commissioning and quality assurance of linear accelerators. IPSM, York

Laughlin J S, Mohan R, Kutcher G 1986 Choice of optimum megavoltage for accelerators for photon beam treatment. International Journal of Radiation Oncology, Biology and Physics 12: 1551–1557

Meredith W J, Massey J B 1968 Fundamental physics of radiology. Wright, Bristol

Walter J, Miller H, Bomford C K 1982 A short textbook of radiotherapy, 4th edn. Churchill Livingstone, Edinburgh

3

Gamma ray beams used in external beam therapy

Gamma rays interact with tissue in the same way as X-ray beams of equivalent energy but their method of production is different.

Gamma rays are emitted as part of the process of radioactive decay of a radioisotope (Meredith & Massey 1968). They represent excess energy resulting from changes in the atom after emission of a particle. Unlike X-rays, gamma rays are emitted at discrete energies, one or more energy emissions making up the useful beam. It is essential that the particle emissions from the source do not contribute to the dose delivered to the patient. In the case of cobalt-60 the beta emission is absorbed by the source capsule.

REQUIREMENTS FOR RADIOISOTOPES USED IN EXTERNAL BEAM THERAPY

The requirements of gamma ray beams used for external beam therapy are dictated by the need for:

- treatment times to be acceptably short
- treatment at adequate source-to-skin distances, ideally a minimum of 80 cm (see Ch. 2)
- a clinically acceptable penumbra
- a decay process which does not result in the emission of potentially hazardous radioactive gases (Meredith & Massey 1968).

These requirements affect the choice of radioactive source, and indeed in modern radiotherapy only cobalt-60, with a half-life of 5.26 years and a beam energy which can be equated to a 2 MV linac, is usually considered to be useful.

Properties of radioactive sources used for external beam therapy

- A combination of high energy and high gamma ray emission, to permit a useful treatment distance.
- A long half-life to reduce the need for expensive source changes.
- A small effective source size, to minimise penumbra, achieved by a high specific activity.

THE PENUMBRA AND ITS EFFECT ON TREATMENT DELIVERY

The penumbra is the dose gradient produced outside the useful radiation beam. There are two components, the transmission and the geometric penumbra.

Transmission penumbra. This is the dose received outside of the useful beam, as a result of transmission through the secondary collimators. This is common to linacs and gamma ray units. On gamma ray units it is a small component of the total penumbra.

Geometric penumbra. The geometric penumbra results from the effective area of the radiation source (Fig. 3.1). Linacs typically have a very small effective source size, approximately 2 mm, and have a very small geometric penumbra. However, a gamma ray beam has an effective source size of approximately 17 mm (Walter et al 1982), which gives rise to a large penumbra.

Implications of a large penumbra for treatment delivery

The continuing move towards accurate tumour shaping and minimising the dose to normal tissues, reduces the value of external beam source machines for radical treatment delivery. Therefore the role of cobalt-60 source machines is primarily the treatment delivery for palliation to anatomical areas where less well-defined treatment beams are acceptable.

Treatment machines using cobalt-60 as an external gamma beam treatment source

As a result of the requirements mentioned above, modern treatment machines (Fig. 3.2) containing cobalt-60 are usually isocentrically mounted (see Ch. 2) with a source-to-skin distance of 80 cm. However, some high source activity machines may use a source-to-skin distance of 100 cm, thereby facilitating the use of most techniques which are normally only achievable on a linac (providing that the cobalt-60 penumbra is considered to be acceptable for the treatment types).

SHAPING THE RADIATION BEAM

As gamma rays emanate in all directions the shielding is of equal thickness all around the

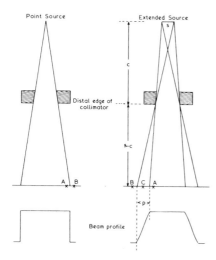

Figure 3.1 The effect of source size on penumbra. (Reproduced from Walter et al 1982.)

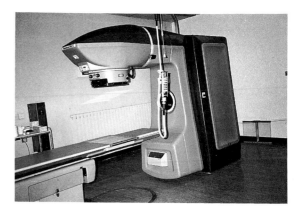

Figure 3.2 An isocentrally mounted cobalt-60 external beam machine.

source. Furthermore, the housing must be of sufficient thickness to reduce the emissions to the required limit (Regulations for the Use of Ionising Radiations 1985) to ensure the safety of radiographers and patients.

Primary collimation

The primary collimation is a conical hole in the source shielding through which the useful beam is emitted (Fig. 3.3). Some units have a source which is driven into the exposed position and returned to the safe position by a motor or pneumatics, while others have a stationary source and motorised shutter. Thus the components for radiation production are much easier to maintain than those of a linac (Van der Giessen 1991).

Secondary collimation

For most treatment machines that use a cobalt-60 source, the collimation and field definition are similar to those described in Chapter 2. The penumbra of the beam is reduced if the collimator-to-patient distance is reduced. The penumbra can be reduced if an interleaved collimation system is used. In practice the treatment distance is typically 80 cm, which means that the anterior face of the collimator is some distance from the patient. Therefore the practical solution to achieve a small penumbra is to reduce the collimator-to-patient distance when it is consid-

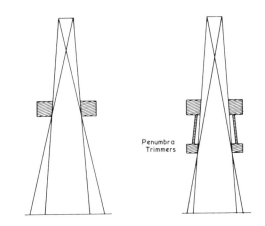

Figure 3.4 The reduction in penumbra with the addition of penumbra trimmers. (Reproduced from Walter et al 1982.)

ered necessary for the treatment technique. This is achieved using penumbra trimmers (Fig. 3.4).

Penumbra trimmers

Penumbra trimmers are heavy metal blocks which can be mounted on to the treatment head so that the inner faces of the blocks are parallel with the divergent gamma ray beam. They serve to reduce the patient-to-collimator distance, thus reducing the geometric penumbra.

Practical restrictions

The penumbra trimmers reduce the clearance around the treatment head and thus can only be

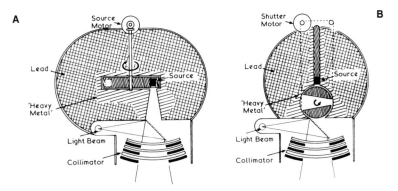

Figure 3.3 Schematic diagram of treatment head components. **A** Moving source. **B** Fixed source. (Reproduced from Walter et al 1982.)

used for a restricted number of treatment techniques. For many isocentric treatments it is impossible to fit this device, particularly if the treatment machine is in a lateral or posterior oblique position, where the structure of the treatment couch restricts the available space.

VISUALISING THE RADIATION BEAM

Modern, isocentrally mounted gamma beam machines are fitted with the same radiation field-defining system as a linac, discussed in detail in Chapter 2.

Alternative method for measuring the treatment distance

Historically, gamma beam source machines were designed to be used at only a single treatment distance; thus the rangefinder was preceded by a pair of light spots or arrows which were emitted from light sources mounted on either side of the treatment head. The spots converged at the treatment distance, so when the two spots were coincident the patient was at the right distance from the machine.

If this system was used on an isocentrically mounted treatment machine, setting the patient to the required distance from the machine at distances other than the treatment distance was difficult and inaccurate.

PRACTICAL IMPLICATIONS OF ADDITIONAL RADIATION PROTECTION PROCEDURES

Use of a radioactive source for treatment delivery presents a greater risk of exposure to radiation for the radiographers than electrically produced X-rays. The main hazard is the possibility that the source may stick in the treatment position.

The local rules required by the Guidance notes (1985) for the protection of persons against ionising radiations arising from medical and dental use require a documented procedure for getting the patient out of the treatment room and returning the source to the safe position. All users need to be familiar with this procedure.

The detailed method of manually returning the source to the safe position varies with each treatment machine manufacturer. Typically a manual pump, or ramrod is used. The primary duty of the radiographers in this situation is to minimise the dose to the patient and to themselves.

A further potential source of radioactive exposure results from the possibility of a source leaking some of its contents. (This possibility is remote due to the careful construction and sealing of the source capsule.) Regular wipe tests of all surfaces of the treatment machine are carried out. Surfaces are wiped with a damp cloth and the dust collected is tested for radioactive emissions using a detector such as a Geiger counter.

The frequency of testing for both of the above procedures is covered in the IPSM Report 54.

SHORT DISTANCE EXTERNAL BEAM SOURCE MACHINES

In the past several different radionuclides have been used for gamma beam treatment machines. The main alternative to cobalt-60 was caesium-137. As the latter radioisotope has a relatively low gamma ray emission, unacceptably large source sizes would be needed to permit reasonable treatment times at the same treatment distance as cobalt-60. Therefore caesium-137 was used at a much shorter source-to-skin distance (s.s.d.). Typically 20–40 cms s.s.d. was used. Because of the relatively low energy, 0.662 MeV, of the gamma rays emitted the machines were designed for the treatment of head and neck lesions. Some short s.s.d. head and neck units used cobalt-60 but caesium-137 was the source of choice.

The majority of these machines are now obsolete but a few remain which are used for palliation and for boosts to the tumour site in intact breast treatment.

Collimation

The method of collimation may involve adjustable collimators or applicators. Applicators, and the short s.s.d., often restrict the positioning of the treatment head and the field sizes available. When collimators are used, a device is required for setting the correct treatment distance. This can be a simple telescopic stick which is moved into the central axis of the beam on an arm. When the correct distance is set, the device is folded away out of the treatment beam.

QUALITY ASSURANCE

Most of the quality assurance tests outlined in Chapter 2 are applicable to gamma beam units. Several differences in the quality assurance programme are of importance and these are discussed below.

The source

Every source installed in a gamma beam machine must be accompanied by the source supplier's test/calibration certificate. This certificate will include details of the source activity. The initial calibration checks should be compared with the certificate to ensure that the results are consistent.

Output measurements

As the radioactive decay of a gamma ray beam is predictable it is possible to measure output in seconds, therefore there are no ionisation chambers situated in the treatment head. It is of great importance that the timers employed to measure treatment time are accurate and remain so throughout the life of the gamma beam machine. Thus there are three main components to the monthly output checks on a gamma beam machine:

1. to test the accuracy of the treatment timers and check the source transit time
2. to cross-check the calculated new outputs
3. to ensure that if the source moves it is in the correct position during treatment exposures.

The equipment used and the method employed for calibration checks are essentially the same as those used for a linac (see Ch. 2) and will not be described again.

Changes in output factors

As the source decays, the number of seconds required to deliver 1 gray must increase. Because the source decays in a predictable manner it is possible to calculate the output changes mathematically; however it is wise to confirm these with calibration checks.

Typically output factors are revised every 3 months for cobalt-60 sources and once per annum for caesium-137 sources.

Daily mechanical checks

The daily mechanical checks carried out on a gamma ray machine are almost identical to those of a linac. There is, however, one difference, arising from the design of the field-defining light. On some gamma beam machines the field-defining light does not move round with the collimators and, therefore, it is not possible to demonstrate misalignment of the light beam by rotating the collimators.

COBALT-60 EXTERNAL BEAM MACHINES VERSUS LINACS

The role of the cobalt-60 treatment machine in the radiotherapy department is increasingly difficult to define. In countries where the cost of maintenance of linacs is prohibitive then cobalt-60 units still play an important part in the provision of radiotherapy. Many papers which evaluate cost show cobalt-60 machines to be cheap to run compared with single energy and modality linacs. However, this has to be offset against technical, and other, disadvantages.

- Cobalt-60 machines have no asymmetric or independent jaws, which are important for many radical treatment techniques.
- The relatively low machine output and slower machine movements give rise to a much lower patient throughput. Typically a cobalt-60 machine can only achieve 70% of the exposures per day possible on a low energy linac.
- Cobalt-60 machines have a large penumbra.
- The cost of new sources is high and the cost of disposing of spent sources has recently risen.

Thus, if finance, accessibility of parts and restricted maintenance are a high priority then a cobalt-60 unit will be the machine of choice.

However if complex treatment techniques and high patient throughput are required, a single energy linac must be preferable.

REFERENCES AND FURTHER READING

Institute of Physical Sciences in Medicine 1988 Commissioning and quality assurance of linear accelerators. IPSM, York

HMSO 1985 The code of practice for the protection of persons against ionising radiations arising from medical and dental use. HMSO, London

Meredith W J, Massey J B 1968 Fundamental physics of radiology. Wright, Bristol

Van der Giessen P H 1991 A comparison of maintenance of cobalt machines and linear accelerators. Radiotherapy and Oncology 20: 64–65

Walter J, Miller H, Bomford C K 1982 A short textbook of radiotherapy, 4th edn. Churchill Livingstone, Edinburgh

4

Orthovoltage and superficial X-rays

BACKGROUND

The energy range of X-rays known as 'orthovoltage' is 200–500 kV and the superficial X-ray energy range is 50–150 kV. An X-ray beam in these energy ranges has two components to its description:

- X-ray tube accelerating voltage
- filtration.

Historically, superficial and orthovoltage X-rays were the only electrically-produced beams available for radiotherapy treatment. However, the advent of high energy linac beams with advantageous beam characteristics has drastically reduced the role of these units in radical treatment delivery.

Superficial X-rays

The role of superficial X-rays has been less affected by the introduction of high energy X-ray beams, although some tumour sites traditionally treated by superficial X-rays are now managed using electrons. Thus most radiotherapy centres still have superficial X-ray equipment (Fig. 4.1).

Orthovoltage X-rays

Many radiotherapy centres no longer have orthovoltage equipment (Fig. 4.2), and those that do are likely to have a multienergy machine which also generates X-rays across the superficial range.

33

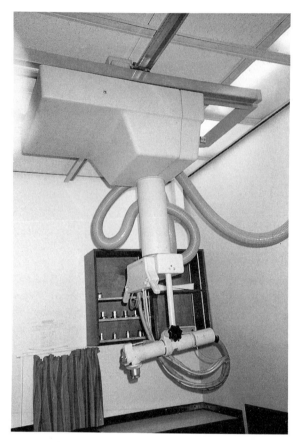

Figure 4.1 A superficial X-ray tube on a diagnostic X-ray tube mounting to permit easier tube positioning.

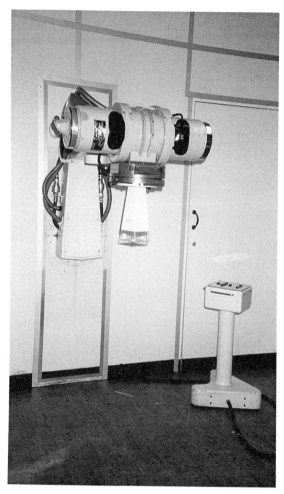

Figure 4.2 An orthovoltage machine with a single treatment energy of 250 kV.

PROPERTIES

Superficial and orthovoltage X-ray beams have no skin-sparing properties and wide penumbras, and beam characteristics which do not permit the modification of beam profiles possible at megavoltage energies (Meredith & Massey 1968). It is not therefore possible to produce the high dose, homogeneous treatment volumes which are achieved using multiple, wedged fields at megavoltage. Furthermore the interactions of X-ray beams in this energy range, resulting in energy deposition in the tissue, are very dependent upon atomic number. In practice this leads to dose inhomogeneities which are particularly significant when there is bone in the treated volume (Walter et al 1982).

Lack of skin-sparing

Superficial X-rays

In the case of superficial X-rays, the function is to treat tumours on the skin surface, the lack of skin-sparing is ideal. When the depth–dose data is compared with electrons the fall-off in dose with depth is much slower for X-rays, thus structures underlying the treated volume receive a higher dose. For the majority of anatomical sites this is not clinically significant, therefore, because of the relatively low cost, superficial X-rays are the treatment of choice. However when tissue such as cartilage, with a poor blood supply and a high risk of radiation damage, underlies the treated area, the sharp fall-off of the electron beam is advantageous (see Ch. 5).

Orthovoltage X-rays

In the case of orthovoltage X-rays, where tumours at depth were treated, the lack of skin-sparing effect resulted in considerable skin damage to the patient, which gave radiotherapy its image of 'burning' the skin. To keep the skin dose within tolerable limits, deep-seated tumours were treated with multifields positioned around the body surface. This resulted in a high integral dose as well as in sore skin. Comparison of the depth–dose data and skin doses of orthovoltage X-rays with megavoltage X-rays clearly demonstrates the advantage of megavoltage beams for the treatment of tumours at depth in the body. Thus treatment with orthovoltage X-rays has become outmoded.

PRODUCTION

Low energy X-ray beams are produced using a specialised X-ray tube (Fig. 4.3) (Walter et al 1982). The design of radiotherapy X-ray tubes is based on the need to provide a stable beam for long, low dose rate exposures. This is quite the opposite case to diagnostic tubes where very short, high dose rate exposures are required.

The need for a large symmetric beam for radiotherapy affects the design of the X-ray tube target. A compromise is achieved, where the effective focal spot and hence the geometric

penumbra (see Ch. 3) is acceptable, but the beam is symmetric over a large field size.

Filtration

At this energy range the desired beam characteristics are achieved by filtering the beam. The filtration required for each treatment energy will be different (Walter et al 1982). A multienergy treatment machine will have a series of filters, each of which is interlocked to the appropriate treatment energies.

CONTAINING AND DEFINING THE BEAM

The target design of the X-ray tube results in the majority of the X-rays emerging in the direction of the useful beam. The anode design and the tube housing reduce the intensity of any unwanted X-rays to an acceptable level. The primary collimator of the beam is a block of heavy metal containing a conical hole.

Secondary collimation

Low energy X-rays are collimated with applicators. A selection of applicators needs to be available, covering a wide range of field sizes; however, costs will limit the number purchased by radiotherapy departments.

Function of applicators

The function of the applicators is to collimate the

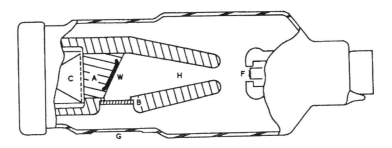

Figure 4.3   A 250 keV tube showing: A – anode, W – target, C – oil cooling spray, H – anode hood and B – beryllium window. F – filament and G – thin window are also shown. (Reproduced from Walter et al 1982.)

beam, define the field size and the treatment f.s.d. The applicators are a fixed length and the aperture at the treatment end defines the treatment field.

At orthovoltage energies, the lower 5 cm of the applicator (Fig. 4.4) is made of perspex with the central axis of the field etched on to the base in contact with the patient. This aids accurate positioning of the applicator. At superficial energies the applicator (Fig. 4.5) is open-ended; the last 1 cm of the applicator can be made of thick glass to aid accurate field positioning. Typically the treatment f.s.d. is 50 cm for orthovoltage X-rays and 10–30 cm for superficial X-rays.

Applicator design

Details of the design of applicators vary with the manufacturers, but they may be straight-sided or divergent. Straight-sided applicators are often used at superficial energies (Fig. 4.5) where the weight of the applicator is not significant.

As the treatment distance is greater for orthovoltage energies, the weight of orthovoltage applicators is considerable. Divergent applicators (Fig. 4.4) are commonly used but there is little advantage in terms of weight from this design; however it is less bulky to carry.

Care and storage of applicators

All applicators are susceptible to damage. Their

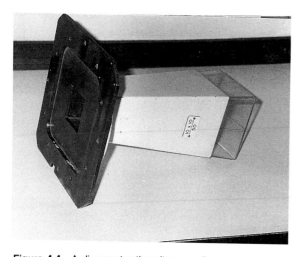

Figure 4.4 A divergent orthovoltage applicator.

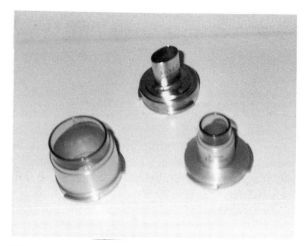

Figure 4.5 Straight-sided superficial applicators.

position in the beam and the condition of the collimating sides of applicators greatly affect their performance. Storage racks should be custom-made at an appropriate lifting height to minimise the handling risks.

Applicators which are inadvertently dropped or damaged must be immediately removed from clinical use until appropriate repairs and mechanical and X-ray tests have been carried out, to ensure the applicator is fit for clinical use.

Additional field shaping

Additional field shaping is simple at the superficial and orthovoltage energy range. Almost any field shape or size can be achieved with a lead cut-out which rests on the patient's skin. The thickness of lead required for the cut-out is dependent on the energy of the X-ray beam: at 100 k V the lead thickness is 1 mm and at 250 kV the lead thickness is 2 mm. The lead may be covered in wax to absorb any secondary electrons produced in the lead.

BEAM DATA AND DOSE CALCULATION

The majority of treatments delivered at this energy are single fields and therefore dose calculation is simple. Data provided for dose calculation will include depth–dose data and outputs for each applicator. Typically the dose will be prescribed as an applied dose. The required time or monitor units may then be calculated, using the output and the applied dose.

Outputs for lead cut-outs

The large influence on the output of backscatter, at orthovoltage and superficial energy ranges (Walter et al 1982), necessitates output adjustments whenever a lead cut-out is used. The amount of backscatter depends upon the energy of the beam and the shape of the field; however, the output may be corrected by calculation or direct measurement.

QUALITY ASSURANCE

Quality assurance can be divided into mechanical and X-ray checks of the applicators and X-ray checks of the output and energy. The checks required to confirm the accuracy of the alignment of applicators are well documented (Walter et al 1982). Quarterly energy and filtration checks are recommended. These can be achieved by the measurement of the half-value layer (Walter et al 1982). Finally daily output checks are recommended for machines with a high output. These are usually carried out by the radiographers using the method described in Chapter 2.

REFERENCES AND FURTHER READING

Meredith W J, Massey J B 1968 Fundamental physics of radiology. Wright, Bristol

Walter J, Miller H, Bomford C K 1982 A short textbook of radiotherapy, 4th edn. Churchill Livingstone, Edinburgh

CHAPTER CONTENTS

Various particle beams are used in external beam radiotherapy. In certain situations, a therapeutic advantage over photon or electron beams may be gained by using other particle beams (Fig. 5.1). Before considering this further, the features of the more commonly used electron beam and its production in the high energy linac are described.

% of cell population surviving irradiation

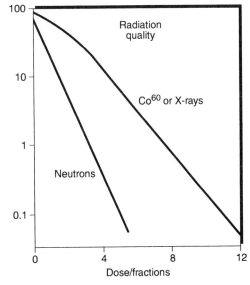

Dose/fractions

Figure 5.1 Particle beams (neutrons) have a larger cell kill than photon beams, i.e a higher therapeutic effect. (After Dixon 1982.)

ELECTRONS

The majority of clinical electron beams are produced by dual modality linacs which also provide photon beams. The range of electron energies available is dependent upon the maximum accelerating voltage of the linac. Typically the lowest electron energy provided by a linac is approximately 4 MeV and a range of energies can be produced up to the maximum available energy. There is some flexibility in the choice of electron energies. The manufacturer's specification will include the number of electron energies available and the possible energy range, the purchaser may then select the required operating energies prior to commissioning.

Describing the electron beam

The energy of electron beams relates to the accelerating voltage of the linac or betatron. However, the energy ascribed to a given electron beam has a nominal value based on the depth–dose characteristics, where the energy of the electron beam in MeV is approximately 2.5 times the depth in centimetres of the 50% isodose curve. This definition may not always be used in all radiotherapy departments, and electron beam energies may be labelled differently in each department.

Properties

The interaction processes involved in the deposition of energy in tissue, and the pattern of energy deposition, are entirely different from those occurring with photons (Klevenhagen 1985). The electron isodose curves have features that make electron beams the modality of choice for some treatments.

The complex physics associated with electron dose distribution is well documented (Klevenhagen 1985). However, a brief description of the dose deposition characteristics of electron beams in tissue will help to clarify their role in clinical radiotherapy.

In water or tissue, electron depth–dose curves (Fig. 5.2) demonstrate a plateau of relatively even dose and a sharp dose fall-off beyond the 80% isodose curve. The size of the plateau and the rapidity of dose fall-off is energy- and linac-dependent. Thus in practice, a homogeneous dose can be delivered by a single beam to a defined depth of tissue with little dose received beyond that depth.

The scatter paths of the electrons in the tissue are not primarily in a forward direction, thus at depth a significant dose is deposited outside the defined field. This is clearly demonstrated by an electron isodose chart (Fig. 5.3), where the isodoses are seen to balloon outside the delineated field. The extent of this ballooning is dependent upon the scattering system employed by the linac and upon the energy of the beam.

The dose received outside the area delineated on the skin may become important when two fields are abutted, or electron fields are close to vital structures such as the eye.

Production

Treatment electrons are produced by a linac when the X-ray target is removed from the end of the flight tube. Due to inefficiencies in X-ray production, the intensity of the electron stream required to produce an X-ray beam is much too high for electron beam treatment, therefore the gun current is automatically reduced by the linac when the electron mode is set.

This narrow stream of electrons is spread over the maximum electron field size, typically 25 cm × 25 cm at 95 cm f.s.d., by scattering foils (Klevenhagen 1985). The majority of modern linacs scatter the electrons with a series of scattering foils to give an even distribution over the required field.

Containing and defining the electron beam

Initially the electron beam is collimated by the primary collimator in the same way as the X-ray beam. The required electron field size is then achieved by a combination of the linac secondary collimators and the electron applicators. The detail of the collimation of the field depends upon the scattering system employed by the linac.

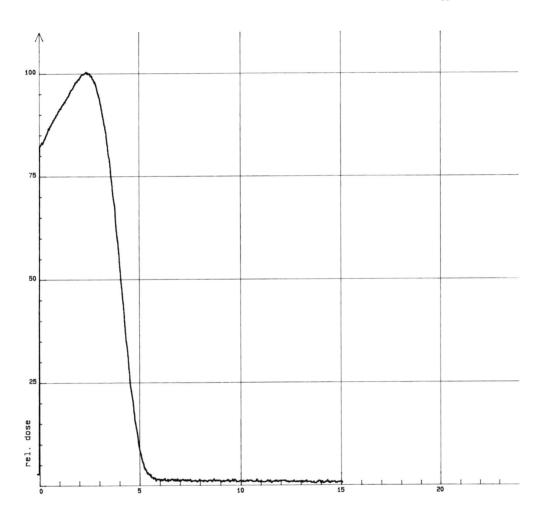

Figure 5.2 Depth–dose curve for electrons.

As electrons are readily scattered by air, the electron applicators are required to collimate the beam between the patient and the linac head to achieve better field definition. As with X-rays, the field-defining light delineates the 50% isodose curve.

The treatment distance is defined by the length of the applicator, and for most electron treat-ments it is usual for the face of the applicator to be in contact with the patient's skin.

Electron applicators

Electron applicators are available in circles, squares and rectangles, over field sizes ranging from 6 cm × 6 cm to 25 cm × 25 cm for normal f.s.d. The required size is finally defined by an

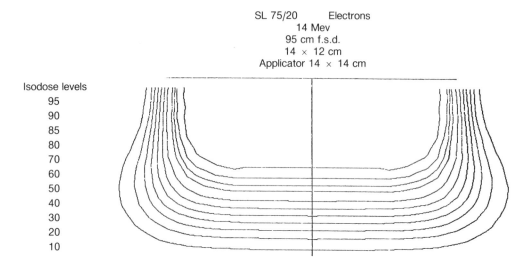

SL 75/20   Electrons
14 Mev
95 cm f.s.d.
14 × 12 cm
Applicator 14 × 14 cm

Isodose levels
95
90
85
80
70
60
50
40
30
20
10

Figure 5.3   Isodose chart for electrons.

end frame incorporated into the treatment end of the applicator. A range of applicators is usually purchased which, in conjunction with the end frames, encompasses all required field sizes.

Universal electron applicators are available that can collimate the electron beam to any size up to the maximum available in the same way as normal X-ray collimators. However, the size of the universal applicator makes it difficult to set up fields in awkward anatomical sites, and the weight presents a handling hazard.

Two types of electron applicators are in current clinical use: closed- and open-sided.

Closed-sided electron applicators

The older style electron applicators have closed-in sides to within 3 cm of the treatment distance (Fig. 5.4). They are used in conjunction with a single scattering foil in the head. The single scattering foil in itself does not produce a flat electron beam, therefore the electron beam flatness is further refined by altering the field size on the secondary collimators of the linac so that some of the electron beam bombards the sides of the electron applicator. The interaction of the electron beam with the sides of the electron applicator causes more electrons of a lower energy to be produced at the edges of the beam.

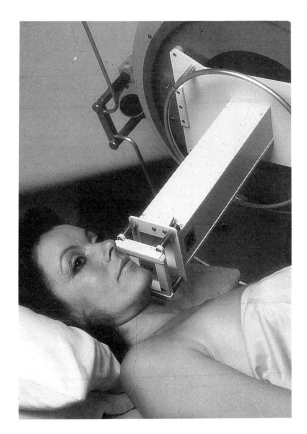

Figure 5.4   Closed-sided electron applicator. (Courtesy of Philips Medical Systems.)

Thus the flatness of the electron beam can be fine-tuned at commissioning by altering the field size on the secondary collimators of the linac. In routine use the required field size is automatically set when the applicator is located in the linac head and, once it has been defined, remains unchanged.

Open-sided electron applicators

The open-sided electron applicator is used in conjunction with a dual foil scattering system. As previously described, the initial collimation of the electron beam is provided by the secondary collimation of the linac. However, when electron beams are produced by dual scattering foils, the resultant beam is sufficiently flat to meet the required standard. Therefore the applicators act only as penumbra trimmers between the treatment head and the patient. Thus the structure of the electron applicator is essentially a set of penumbra trimmers joined by rigid columns (Fig. 5.5) (Box 5.1).

Box 5.1 Open-sided electron applicators

Advantages:
- They are lighter and easier to handle for most electron applicators
- There is a better view of the set-up

Disadvantage:
- The bulky size of the penumbra trimmers limits the positioning of the applicator in close proximity to the skin, particularly when treating posterior neck

---

Short f.s.d. applicators

Sometimes it is necessary to treat a large area around the body using electrons. This can be achieved using arc therapy (Freeman et al 1992). In these circumstances the electron applicator must not touch the skin of the patient, thus short f.s.d. applicators should be available. Typically these have a collimated length of 80 cm.

End frames

The final field shape and size is defined by the

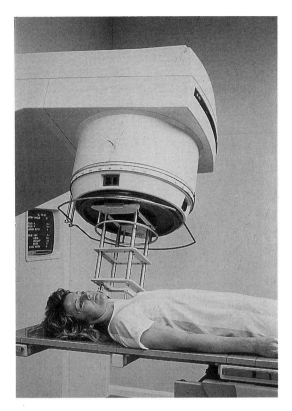

Figure 5.5 Open-sided electron applicator. (Courtesy of Philips Medical Systems.)

end frame (Fig. 5.6). This shape will be smaller than the nominal applicator field size. The end frame is a flat plate of a heavy metal of the correct size to fit into the end of the electron applicator. There are two methods for the production of end frames:

- by machining from a plate of heavy metal, e.g. lead
- by casting from low melting point alloy in special frames provided by the manufacturer. Any shape can be defined in this way including irregular and patient-customised shapes.

Modern linacs provide a coding system to identify the end frame in position and ensure correct selection and orientation.

Field-shaping using lead pieces. Further field-shaping can be achieved by fixing lead pieces to either the patient's skin or to the electron applicator. As a rule of thumb the thickness in

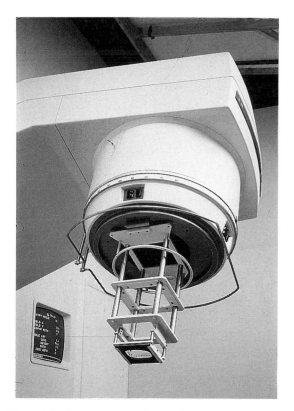

Figure 5.6 A machined end frame. (Courtesy of Philips Medical Systems.)

millimetres, of lead used for shielding, must be at least half the value of the energy of the electron beam. Thus typically electron end frames are manufactured from 1 cm thick lead. For accurate reproducibility of field shapes, customised end frames are preferable to pieces of lead used in an ad hoc fashion.

Storage of electron applicators and end frames

Electron applicators are very expensive and delicate. Accurate treatment delivery depends upon the geometry of the applicator remaining constant. They are susceptible to damage if they are not stored in an appropriate way. Ideally a custom-built hanging rack should be constructed, which stores the applicators and the end frames together. When designing a rack consideration should be given to the height and distance the applicators are to be lifted to transfer them to the treatment head.

To increase efficiency and reduce the risk of error, the rack and the end frames should be clearly labelled.

Beam data and dose calculation

As part of the commissioning process, the performance of the electron beams is measured and data collected which is required for treatment delivery. The data required to permit dose calculation is less complex than for X-rays as the majority of treatments are, in effect, single fields at a fixed f.s.d. There are some exceptions to this such as whole-body electrons or arc therapy which require special planning.

Depth–dose data and output charts

The details of the presentation of electron data for clinical use will vary between departments.

Depth–dose data. Depth–dose data for each electron applicator and electron energy will be provided which can be presented in graph or table form (Table 5.1). Additional information about skin dose with and without bolus may also be documented.

Output. Output charts will include the output for each end frame of each electron applicator at each electron energy. In practice not all of these

Table 5.1 SL75-14 electron beam. Percentage depth–dose data at energies shown. Depths are shown in cm. Field size 10 cm × 10 cm; applicator 10 cm × 10 cm; f.s.d. 97 cm

% Depth– dose	Energy (MeV)					
	4	6	8	10	12	14
100	1.2	1.7	2.2	2.6	2.9	3.0
90	1.5	2.2	2.8	3.5	4.1	4.4
80	1.6	2.4	3.1	3.8	4.5	4.8
70	1.7	2.5	3.2	4.0	4.8	5.1
60	1.8	2.7	3.4	4.3	5.0	5.4
50	1.9	2.8	3.6	4.5	5.2	5.6
40	2.0	2.9	3.7	4.7	5.4	5.9
30	2.1	3.1	3.9	4.9	5.6	6.1
20	2.2	3.2	4.1	5.1	5.9	6.4
10	2.4	3.4	4.3	5.4	6.2	6.9

results need to be documented as the output will be unchanged across a wide range of end frames and applicators, particularly if the open-sided applicators are used. End frames that are custom-made should have a measured output, especially if the field is a very irregular shape making the scatter conditions for the field unpredictable.

Prescription and calculation

The details of the prescription will vary between departments. However the method for selecting the required electron energy will be fundamentally the same.

A treatment depth will be chosen; this may be the skin surface and/or a defined depth beneath it. An electron energy that best delivers a homogeneous dose is selected. To modify the skin dose and the dose at depth, bolus of varying thickness may be applied to the treatment field. The required dose is then prescribed to the selected percentage depth dose, and the skin dose calculated if considered relevant. The applied or 'given' dose is calculated using the equation below:

$$\text{Given dose} = \frac{\text{Dose required at depth}}{\text{Percentage depth dose}} \times 100$$

The number of monitor units required is then calculated from the output and the given dose, as described in Chapter 7.

Air gaps or 'stand-off'

All data collection for electron treatment delivery assumes the end frame to be flat on the phantom surface. Obviously this is often not possible in clinical practice, where electron beams are applied to curved surfaces. An air gap or applicator 'stand-off' will have a considerable effect on the dose delivered. The problem has several components:

- reduced output associated with the increased treatment distance
- reduced effective field size as the high value isodose curves converge
- higher skin dose resulting from the obliquity of electrons scattered from the collimators

- possible increase in percentage depth dose associated with increased f.s.d.

These difficulties are reduced by open-sided applicators where the beam uniformity is maintained up to 5 cm away from the applicator end.

To ensure accurate dose delivery it is vital that radiographers are aware of the effects of air gaps, and a procedure should be documented for the measurement of air gaps and the corrective measures required. Although these procedures may differ depending on the anatomical site being treated, as a minimum, the output should be corrected for the measured air gaps.

QUALITY ASSURANCE

The quality assurance programme for a dual modality linear accelerator will include additional checks and tests required for electrons. The baseline for the constancy checks will have been set at commissioning.

Typically a programme to include the minimum checks (IPSM 1988) required includes:

1. Output factors for end frames checked every 3 months
2. Electron beam energy and applicator fixings checked monthly
3. Electron beam flatness checked weekly
4. Daily output calibration.

Daily output calibration is usually the responsibility of the radiographer. Each energy to be used clinically must be calibrated each day. The output for custom-made end frames may be measured at the same time.

TREATMENT OF TUMOURS USING OTHER PARTICLE BEAMS

Rationale for particle therapy

Different types of radiation have different absorption effects in tissue (see Ch. 1), particle beams being the most damaging (Fig. 5.1). The level of damage inflicted depends on the amount of dose absorbed per unit length of tissue traversed by a beam (Linear energy transfer or LET). Heavier particles have a high LET, i.e. more interactions per unit length than photon or electron beams (Fig. 5.1), so giving up more energy within a small volume of tissue. This gives rise to much greater damage and overcomes some of the problems of cell resistance to damage from conventional beams. The main factors involved are outlined below.

The oxygen effect

Hypoxic cells are relatively radioresistant to conventional radiotherapy. It is proven that the higher LET of neutron beams improves cell kill rates of the hypoxic tumour cells, by a factor specific to the beam (oxygen enchancement ratio, OER, of the beam).

However, tumours are reoxygenated as therapy begins to take effect so the advantage of neutrons is then lost. Mixed beam schedules are particularly useful where there are hypoxic cells but the sequence of application is important. Particle radiation results in a reduced oxygen effect, and is therefore more useful at the start of mixed-beam regimes.

Cell cycle effect

Cells undergoing mitosis are more sensitive to radiation, particularly in the 'S' phase of the cycle, than are cells which are not actively dividing. The difference in sensitivity of dividing and non dividing cells decreases with high LET. Thus slowly proliferating tumours would benefit more from particle therapy than would faster-growing tumours. Thus the effect of the cell cycle on response is reduced.

Relative biological effect (RBE) and high LET beams

The radiobiological advantages of using high LET beams are:

- lower radioresistance of hypoxic tumour cells
- less variation of radiosensitivity around the phases of the cell cycle
- less repair of sublethal cell damage
- shorter overall treatment time gives advantage for rapidly proliferating tumours.

When selecting tumours for particle therapy, consideration must be given to the relative radiosensitivity of the surrounding tissue and the sensitivity of the tumour to conventional radiotherapy. Careful selection of tumours for high LET beam treatments is of paramount importance. There is a need to look at cell assays to assess the proliferation rate in addition to considering histology and site. (Tumour proliferation rates for individual tumours are independent of histology and site.)

Tumours which are not sensitive to X- and gamma rays may be more sensitive to high LET beams and thus may be better treated by them, providing the surrounding tissue will tolerate the local effects. Thus, by using high LET beams, the range of tumours where there is a useful response to radiation of the tumour above that of surrounding tissue is extended.

Fast neutron beams

The beam characteristics of fast neutrons offer no clinical advantage over X-rays. Beams have a large penumbra, less skin-sparing and dose is received along the beam path distal to the target volume. The only biological advantage is the relatively low absorption in bone. However, this is offset by the very high relative absorption in fatty tissue, which gives a poor cosmetic effect after treatment due to tissue wastage and subcutaneous induration. An 8 MV X-ray beam has a similar depth–dose curve to a 66 MeV neutron beam.

Equipment limitations

During the last decade the neutron beams used for various clinical trials varied in energy from 66 MeV to 8 MeV. The equipment varied in versatility and many centres used equipment designed for the laboratory. The problems in clinical use of these facilities included:

- fixed horizontal beam
- poor depth doses
- poor skin-sparing
- poor collimation
- simulation inconsistent

- beam flatness inadequate
- logistics difficult
- frequent equipment breakdown.

However, modern cyclotrons produce high energy beams, incorporate multileaf collimators for reducing treatment volume and provide isocentric mounting.

Light ions

Light ion interactions give a low LET at the surface and greater LET at depth, so that there is the potential for giving dose at the tumour only, thus achieving a dose distribution in tissue which is closer to the clinical ideal than with photons. Protons are the most clinically useful light ions. Helium and carbon ions are also used. Equipment for producing He or C ions is very expensive and therefore limited in availability compared with the lower cost cyclotrons which produce protons.

Proton beams

Compared with photons, protons have several favourable characteristics, leading to increased interest in their use. They can deliver a high dose to a finite area with a very low integral dose because there is virtually no dose to tissue outside the target volume, either at the surface or distally along beam paths.

Properties of proton beams

These include:

- well defined range in tissue
- minimal scattering outside the beam
- good skin-sparing
- high dose to tumour region
- low integral dose
- nondivergent.

The developments made to produce clinically suitable beams on the Clatterbridge cyclotron include beam-flattening systems. The shape of the proton depth–dose curve is literally square, so the beam cuts off at a particular depth.

Other particles in clinical use

Pi-mesons (negative, 'pions')

The production of negative pi-mesons is extremely expensive. Thus the clinical use of these particles is limited by their availability. Their advantage for therapy is that it is possible to deliver a more concentrated dose to the tumour but not to the proximal tissue. Pions, which have a high LET, give a greater build-up of dose at depth than neutrons.

Thermal neutrons

Thermal neutrons, which have high LET and low penetrating power in tissue (associated with an energy of only a few eV) offer the possibility of better localisation of dose within the targeted tissue, i.e. virtually zero dose outside the target tissue. This treatment is achieved by administering Boron-10, in association with suitable compounds, locally to the target tissue, rather than as a neutron beam. At present, several centres are using this treatment technique for brain tumours.

REFERENCES AND FURTHER READING

Bonnett D E, Kacperek A, Sheen M A, Goodall R, Saxton T E, 1993 The 62 MeV proton beam for the treatment of ocular melanoma at Clatterbridge British Journal of Radiology 66: 907–914

Dixon 1982 Radiotherapy Concepts. In Joslin C A F (ed) Cancer topics and Radiotherapy. Pitman, London

Freeman C R, Suissa S G, Shenoun T et al 1992 Clinical experience with a single rotational total skin electron irradiation: technique for cutaneous T-cell lymphoma. Journal of Radiotherapy and Oncology 24: 155–162

Institute of Physical Sciences in Medicine 1988 Commissioning and quality assurance of linear accelerators, IPSM, York

Klevenhagen S C 1985 Physics of electron beams. Adam Hilger, Bristol

6

Brachytherapy equipment and dosimetry principles

INTRODUCTION

Brachytherapy, in the present context, is the application of small sealed sources directly to the body either from within or from near the surface. In this way a relatively high dose can be given to a small volume of tissue within the body, without the radiation incidentally passing through large tracts of tissue which do not require treatment. The sources are positioned central to or evenly spaced throughout the volume of tissue which requires treatment. The inverse square principle is extremely important in brachytherapy. The high dose zone is confined to the immediate tissue surrounding the sources since the dose falls quickly with distance from the sources.

Brachytherapy has not always been in widespread use, except for gynaecological purposes, because of the relatively high exposure to radiation of staff, compared with external beam treatments where staff are outside the room during patient irradiation. There are other safety risks connected with manual source handling. Brachytherapy applications are now, however, rapidly developing due to the introduction of a range of 'afterloading' treatment machines, the use of which has increased the safety and precision of brachytherapy procedures. This chapter deals with the types of equipment and various safety aspects, but first we will look briefly at the broad categories of brachytherapy practice.

Intracavitary and intraluminal radiotherapy

Small source pellets are introduced into a catheter which has been previously inserted into a body cavity or lumen. A high dose is delivered directly to the site of interest within the patient, for example to the uterus, cervix, prostate or oesophagus.

Implants or interstitial radiotherapy

Radioactive sources can also be applied directly to tissue at or near the surface of the body. Surgical techniques are used to insert rigid guide tubes into which radioactive wires are to be introduced after verification of guide positioning.

Intraoperative therapy

Brachytherapy may be delivered during operative procedures. In its broadest sense this includes treatment delivery to patients who have had catheters positioned whilst in the operating theatre and who then receive treatment via those applicators, either whilst still anaesthetised, or in subsequent treatments. To give treatment in the operating theatre, a suitably shielded operating room equipped with a dedicated table, an imaging device, and means of obtaining dose distribution information must be available. Several centres have specially designed brachytherapy suites, incorporating a theatre and associated facilities together with outpatient areas.

Combined modalities

External beam treatment is often used either concurrently or sequentially, in conjunction with brachytherapy, to give a single dose distribution to a tumour.

AFTERLOADING PRINCIPLES AND EQUIPMENT

Afterloading allows the accurate placement of source carriers within the body and their positional verification, before radioactive sources are introduced. Thus an improved dose distribution to the tumour can be obtained via the greater precision in source positioning, without radiation exposure to staff.

Remote afterloading systems

Remote afterloading machines control radioactive sources, which are contained within them and connected applicator systems, via computer keyboards. There are different types of equipment available, using a variety of source types and applicators to achieve different functions. The keyboards themselves, or control systems linked to them, are located outside the treatment room so that the sources are remotely loaded into the applicator (and patient) when required.

Improved radiation safety. The improved radiation protection to staff accrues because of the elimination of all steps in the treatment and pretreatment processes which would have involved the manual preparation, transport or placing within a patient, of active sources.

Using remote afterloading equipment, there is no handling of sources. Patients receiving low dose rate treatment over many hours are made comfortable within special rooms (Fig. 6.1) with protecting walls, and are monitored via closed-circuit TV, intercom and call systems. The sources are automatically withdrawn from the patient into a safe (Fig. 6.2) when the room door is opened, so that there is no dose to nursing staff, or other patients, even during a treatment time as long as 2 days. With manual systems office staff, theatre staff, radiographers, radiotherapists, porters and other patients were potentially exposed.

Basic steps in treatment procedures

Although treatment procedures are dealt with in Chapter 20, it is necessary to outline the main concepts here, so that they can be related to the equipment functions described.

1. To facilitate treatment, catheters or applicators are introduced into a conscious, anaesthetised or sedated patient.
2. Various types of applicators are connected both to the patient and to the machine.
3. The applicator positions are radiographically checked to verify their alignment with each other and to the anatomy.
4. Once the alignment is satisfactory, the source arrangement to give the required dose distribution for a particular patient or tumour

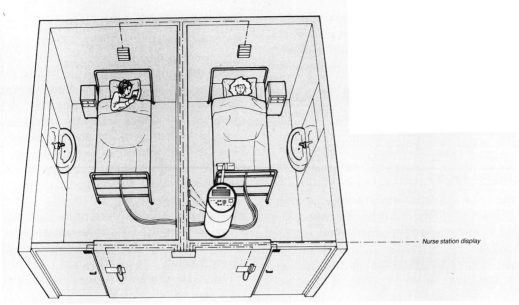

Figure 6.1   The six-channel Selectron-LDR can be used to treat two patients simultaneously, in separate specially designed rooms. Each treatment is independently controlled by separate remote control units. (Courtesy of Nucletron Trading Ltd.)

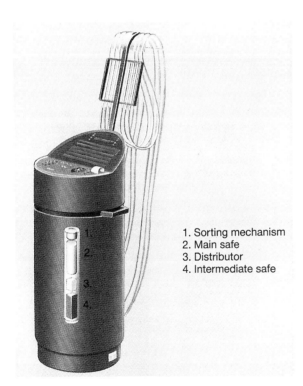

1. Sorting mechanism
2. Main safe
3. Distributor
4. Intermediate safe

Figure 6.2   The LDR/MDR Selectron system, showing source control components and six source transit/applicator channels. (Courtesy of Nucletron Trading Ltd.)

geometry, is determined from films by measurement and calculation. The number and position of active source points can be varied, as can the exposure time during which they are in place.

5. The required source arrangement is programmed independently for each channel. The machine organises its sources to achieve the program, before the command is keyed-in which sends the sources out of the safe and into the applicators.

Source programming

For many applications, standard source configurations together with a range of doses can be used, without individual dosimetry calculations being performed for each patient. Some machines can hold information on 'standard' source configurations and doses within the computer memory, with an automatic correction for dose rate changes due to the decay of the sources.

Programming for the selected treatment can be carried out simply by keying-in a one- or two-digit code number for the standard treatment required, and by checking displays and printouts to verify that the expected values are correct, both for source positions and times. For example, by use of tabulated data and the application of a decay factor, a check may be made that the overall time shown on the machine display corresponds with that expected. Connections are made between the appropriate machine channels and the catheters in the patient, then the sources are driven into the catheter to preprogrammed positions.

Equipment types

Nucletron is a specialist manufacturer of afterloading equipment. The following descriptions of their Selectron remote afterloading units contain technical information derived from their product literature. Other, less commonly used afterloading systems such as the Buchler system, the Cathetron and the Curietron, use modified methods of achieving varied source lengths and positions (high dose rate).

Source types

Sources used within the afterloading units described below may be one of various isotopes, formed into small pellets, ribbons or wire. Some of the units use a combination of 48 spacers and sources in a continuous line, known as a source train (see Fig. 20.1A).

Alternatively, single 'stepping' a source pellet may be used. The pellet moves to a preset 'step' position within an applicator, remains there ('dwells') for a set time, then moves forward to the safe in a stepping fashion, staying for preset times at any desired point. Different step lengths can be selected to allow variations in dose distribution and total length treated (Fig. 6.3).

Selectron-HDR 60Co

The Selectron-HDR is a three-channel, high dose rate system consisting of a treatment unit, in which the cobalt-60 sources are stored within a lead-shielded safe, and a desk-top control unit. The control unit, remote from the treatment room, has a memory for 50 standard source loadings, together with the treatment times. These are automatically corrected for source decay. When the system is programmed for a treatment and the start button activated, source trains loaded with dummy sources are automatically prepared and a check carried out before the active sources are loaded, ready to start treatment. Treatment starts at the completion of active source loading.

The 20 equal activity sources are 1.5 mm × 1.5 mm steel-encapsulated cylinders which form spheres of outer diameter 2.5 mm. Stainless steel nonmagnetic spheres of the same dimensions as the sources are used as spacing devices.

In the Selectron-HDR 60Co, 20 sources are available with activities of 18.5 GBq per source.

Selectron-LDR/MDR 137Cs

The Selectron-LDR/MDR is a three-to-six channel low dose rate system. Each source is a caesium-137 glass bead encapsulated in a stainless steel pellet of outer diameter 2.5 mm. The pellet activities available are 518, 740, 1110 or 1480 megabecquerels (MBq). The source container, transfer and control systems are contained in the same mobile unit (Fig. 6.2). This is designed to take a minimum of floor space in the patient's room. There is a remote control unit available to display treatment time, other data and start/ interrupt buttons, stationed at a convenient

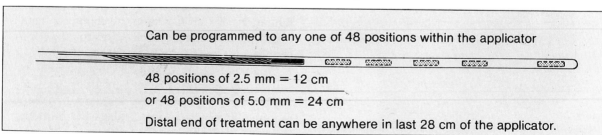

Can be programmed to any one of 48 positions within the applicator

48 positions of 2.5 mm = 12 cm

or 48 positions of 5.0 mm = 24 cm

Distal end of treatment can be anywhere in last 28 cm of the applicator.

Figure 6.3 Dwell positions for the microSelectron. (Courtesy of Nucletron Trading Ltd.)

location outside the treatment room. On activating the start button, prior to source transfer to the applicators, an automatic air check of the channels is performed to detect constrictions or faulty connections.

With a six-channel Selectron unit, two patients can be treated simultaneously, either in the same room with protective screening between them (Fig. 6.1), or in separate rooms.

Although initially developed for low dose rate gynaecological treatments, the Selectron-LDR/MDR is also used for medium dose rate treatments of brain, bronchus, nasopharynx, oesophagus, prostate, rectum and skin tumours, and has many other applications. (The same range of applications at high dose rate are provided by the Selectron-HDR, originally developed for gynaecological treatments.) A large variety of intracavitary and intraluminal applicators is available.

Quality assurance features. From the shielded safe, source trains are pneumatically transferred into the patient's applicator. For both the units so far described, the accuracy of the source positioning is continuously monitored and maintained to within ± 1 mm, using a pneumatic air check patented by Nucletron. If there is power failure alarm is registered, a pneumatic back-up automatically withdraws the sources to the safe and a battery back-up maintains all the treatment data.

microSelectron-LDR/MDR 192Ir/137Cs

The microSelectron-LDR/MDR is an interstitial 15-channel system for low and medium dose rates. It can be connected to either flexible or rigid implants. The microSelectron-LDR/MDR is designed to operate with standard iridium-192 ribbons and wires or special caesium-137 seeds. The commercially available iridium ribbons or wires are cut to the required active and inactive lengths and then adapted for use with the microSelectron. The system can also be used with various applicators.

microSelectron-HDR 192Ir

The microSelectron-HDR is a high dose rate interstitial and intraluminal system. It consists of a treatment unit in which a single miniature iridium source is stored within a shielded safe. The source can be remotely afterloaded into a small diameter catheter (less than 2 mm) for high dose rate intraluminal treatments or interstitial implants. Dose distributions are obtained by programming dwell positions and times for the single source, for each applicator.

Sources. The high activity 370 GBq (10Ci) iridium-192 source is 1.1 mm in diameter with an active length of 3.5 mm. The rigid needles or flexible plastic applicators have an outer diameter of 1.9 mm. An 18-channel indexer automatically guides the source successively through 1 to 18 applicators according to programmed requirements.

Each channel has 48 possible source positions. The step length between source positions may be set at either 2.5 mm or 5 mm to allow different overall lengths to be treated (Fig. 6.3). For example with 2.5 mm steps the maximum treated length is 12 cm (48×2.5 mm). A different distribution of dose along the 12 cm could be obtained by using fewer dwell positions and a step size of 5 mm. Each position can have a different dwell time, programmable up to 999.9 seconds. (If no time is selected, the source does not dwell in that position.)

The system has a control unit with a memory for 50 'standard' treatments. The treatment times are automatically corrected for source decay.

Although initially designed for low or medium breast-preserving treatment, the microSelectron-HDR is also used for treatment of the brain, bile duct, bronchus, endometrium, head and neck, prostate, rectum and vagina, and has many other applications. It was originally designed as a multipurpose HDR afterloading system.

Quality assurance features. An integrated check cable runs out to the distal programmed dwell point to check the system and applicator(s) for constrictions, before the source leaves the safe. This device, patented by Nucletron, helps the therapist to set up or check the programmed source movements in the patient, since it can be used to simulate all programmed source dwell positions under fluoroscopy. The check cable run can be used for measuring skin entry and exit points or visible tumour borders or markers. Battery back-up and software features provide a means to retain source programs and treatment details in the event of power failures, when the source is automatically returned to the safe. After treatment the system returns the source to the safe.

microSelectron-PDR

The microSelectron-PDR is a new variable dose rate system which operates on a pulsed brachy-therapy principle. It enables the equivalent of continuous low dose rate treatments to be given. The stepping source with its variable dwell time, enables the isodoses to be optimised for individual patients, using what is effectively an infinitely variable source strength. A typical pulse length is 10 minutes per hour, increasing to approximately 30 minutes as the iridium-192 source decays. The patient can be disconnected between pulses. Intracavitary, interstitial, intraoperative and intra-luminal treatments are all possible using a single microSelectron-PDR afterloader.

The source activity is in the range 18.5–37 GBq; the diameter is 1.1 mm and length 2.5 mm. Source positions can be programmed in a maximum of 48 different locations within each of 18 catheters. Two different step sizes determine the maximum treatment lengths to either 12 or 24 cm. Treatment times can be programmed from 0 to 999.9 seconds per position per pulse.

User features of Selectron units

For all the Selectron units described, relevant treatment data are shown on the display and automatically printed out (Fig. 6.4) when a control key is turned to the 'treatment' position. The sources are driven out, following system checks, on pressing the start button. Further printouts giving confirmation of exposure times for all channels, details of stops and starts, and any error codes for occurrences causing treatment to stop, are printed out on a real-time basis. A microprocessor controls all the hardware and processing functions, and a self-diagnosis facility gives appropriate warnings of any faults and automatic source withdrawal.

Treatment interruption. Treatment can be interrupted if necessary, when sources are returned to safe positions and treatment timers stopped. Remaining treatment times are indicated and monitored. Sources will not be transferred to applicators if connections are not correctly made. All applicators have fast uncoupling connections. Audible alarms are fitted to alert the user to stoppages caused by the equipment or power faults. (These are particularly useful where low or medium dose rate units are treating patients who are remotely monitored by nursing staff. Some units incorporate audible alarms to indicate the end of the treatment exposure.

Treatment planning system. There is also a special treatment planning system available to plan the many modes of brachytherapy treatment, and to prepare program cards which may be used with the microSelectron systems. A program card carries the source loadings and times required for an individual patient, so that on insertion of the card into the control unit, the particular treatment program is quickly loaded for immediate use.

Machine quality assurance

The various safety features have already been outlined and it follows that safety checks are carried out before and during all use of the equipment. In addition, it is necessary to undertake daily or weekly quality assurance procedures.

Daily checks. For the microSelectrons, various dwell positions are programmed on one channel, and a special quality check scale connected. The source is then transferred to the programmed positions, and the actual source position within the channel/scale (Fig. 6.5) viewed by close-up TV to check continued accuracy.

For the HDR Selectron, a source and time are programmed and a 'treatment' performed to check that the system is operating correctly.

After source changes and at appropriate periods, output calibrations are performed and calculations made to check that treatment times used are correct for the expected doses to be given. Periodical checks include leak and wipe tests to detect possible source contamination of equipment.

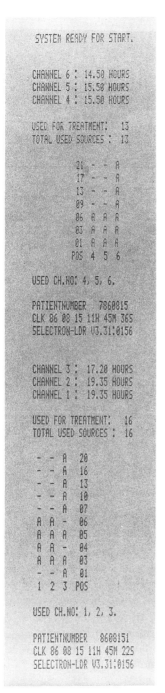

Figure 6.4 HDR printout of source program. (Courtesy of Nucletron Trading Ltd.)

There is a wealth of new literature on the quality assurance of these machines, particularly relating to the minute detail of the source train positions within applicators. References for articles detailing this are given at the end of the chapter.

The following should be checked regularly by a physicist:

- coupling and connection interlocks
- door and other interlocks
- source transport mechanisms
- machine functions
- interrupt and termination functions
- timers
- treatment programming functions and procedures
- all applicators in use
- source positioning accuracy and reproducibility in the range of applicators used
- in vivo dosimetry measurement should be used to verify the accuracy of treatment planning and dose delivery, especially since the system is otherwise totally software-driven and software faults could cause the actuality to be entirely different from the expectation
- autoradiographs of the source positions are required periodically.

Checks which are the responsibility of the radio graphers using the unit. It is advisable to check that the expected source configuration and approximate times are shown on the display/printout when giving treatment, to detect possible error.

Procedures such as interrupts, door interlocks and the exposure monitoring system should be checked daily before clinical use, and all tests and results recorded in a log book. There should be documented procedures for the event of timer failure, failure of the source to return to the safe and power failures.

Dose rate issues in brachytherapy

The dose schedules used for brachytherapy treatments are derived historically from effective regimes established from the practice of using radium. For higher dose rate treatments, adapted doses and fractionation regimes have been and are being developed taking into account the differing radiobiological responses and effects at

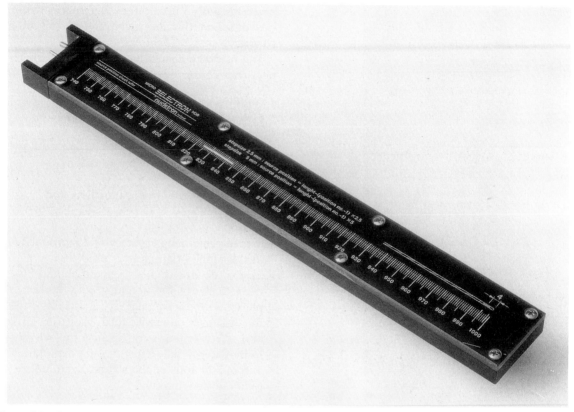

Figure 6.5 Calibration scale attachment for microSelectron. (Courtesy of Nucletron Trading Ltd.)

varied dose rates. The main factors involved are described in Chapter 1 (also by Sutton 1986). High dose rate regimes demand adequate fractionation since the potential for late tissue damage is increased. (The move to high dose rate techniques has been driven by socioeconomic factors and the availability of high technology afterloading systems with a greater geometrical accuracy potential, as well as greater operator safety.)

At low dose rates, a small increase in the dose rate changes the clinical effect, so that the use of a dose rate correction factor is required to adjust given dosages to achieve equal effects. For example, when using the Selectron with caesium at 150–170 cGy/hour at a particular point, a correction factor of 11% is required to reduce the prescribed dose to get a clinical effect equal to that when using 53 cGy/hour. Low dose rate is defined by the ICRU Report 38 to be less than 2

Gy/hour. High dose rate is 12 Gy/hour or more, medium dose rate being the range between the two (ICRU 1985).

Brachytherapy implants provide dose rates down to 1 cGy/hour to tissue outside the target zone. Thus the overall effect is for less radiation damage to be incurred to normal tissue than from higher dose rates, so a high dose, such as 65 Gy, may be given within a week. With conventional fractionation at high dose rate, 6 or 7 weeks would be required to deliver this dose to most sites. Fewer late tissue effects will be seen with the low dose rate treatment.

Isoeffect surfaces. An envelope of tissue surrounding the source(s) has layers receiving equal dose, and therefore equal effects. These may be referred to as isoeffect surfaces, which differ in position for early and late effects. Acute and late isoeffects, and the overall effects of the different dose rates are dose-time dependent. The incidence of radiation-related morbidity increases with dose per fraction and with reductions in fraction numbers. Late tissue effects are more dependent on fraction size than total dose. There is also a volume dependence since damage to a larger tissue volume is less likely to heal. Regimes at high or low dose rate must take into account both the acute and late effects on the tissues irradiated.

A survey of the literature presently available reveals that, overall, the treatment outcomes of low and high dose rate are similar in terms of local control, survival, and local complications. Ideal treatment schemes for higher dose rates have yet to be established.

Using high dose rates

Source types. High dose rate treatment was not possible using radium, owing to the incompatibility between its low specific activity and the clinical need for small sources.

The development of cobalt-60 and iridium-192 sources for medical use made high dose rate techniques possible. Iridium is an extremely dense material (22.5 g/cm^3) so a high activity source of diameter 1.1 mm can be used. Using cobalt-60, applicators can still be small in diameter and in many cases can still be inserted without total anaesthesia. Small high activity sources cannot be safely handled so mechanical and pneumatic machines were developed for their use. Most centres choose cobalt-60 for high dose rate work, since it has a much higher specific activity than caesium-137, and does not require frequent source exchange as does iridium-192 (half-life, 74 days).

Source strength is specified in units of radioactivity. Formerly, the unit of activity was the curie (Ci), but is now superseded by the SI unit equivalent, the becquerel (Bq).

Advantages of high dose rate:

• Short treatment times, a few minutes up to 20 minutes is the norm.
• No major anatomy changes during the short treatment time.
• Rigid, fixed geometry multiapplicator systems may be used, thus allowing dose optimisation because of the stable source arrangement.
• Applicators can be inserted in the treatment room with or without local anaesthetic.
• Good patient acceptance and socioeconomic advantages because treatment can be given on an outpatient basis.
• Less chance of deep vein thromboses, pulmonary emboli, backache and general distress developing during treatment as compared with low dose rate treatment given over several days.
• No requirement for protected patient rooms.
• No overnight nursing staff required.

Clinical weaknesses of high dose rate:

• Fractionation is required, cannot equate with effect of continuous exposure.
• Total dose reduction necessary for tissue tolerance.
• Limited fraction size required to avoid late damage.

Advantages of low dose rate. Some advantages of low dose rate are:

• Equivalence with radium dose rates, so that clinical effects can be well predicted.
• Less damage to normal tissue.
• The dose to adjacent organs may be spread out due to organ movement during the treatment time, thus reducing the risk, for example, of bowel stenosis (lower morbidity).
• Treatment may be given in one or two short-stay episodes as opposed to a longer fractionated course (useful for palliation for elderly and immobile patients).

Dosimetry

The dose rate for any application will depend on source decay relative to a calibration date and on the geometry of sources used. During source calibration, various parameters are measured for each source:

• the air Kerma rate in centigrays per hour (cGy/h) at 1 metre (relates to radiation intensity per square metre, and time)
• the exposure rate in milliroentgens per hour (mR/h) at 1 metre

• the activity in millibecquerels per hour (mBq/h) at 1 metre.

There is some difficulty in taking accurate measurements close to the source because of the very steep dose gradient resulting from the inverse square law. In practice, positioning of measuring chambers to 1 mm accuracy is unlikely to be possible. For example, the dose rate measured at 5 mm will be increased by 55% if the chamber is actually at 4 mm, and out by 31% if the dosemeter is at 6 mm. It is easier to use film than a Farmer dosemeter for achieving accurate measurements.

Measuring a line source at close range is slightly more accurate than measuring a 'point' source.

Isodose distributions. The three dose rates are measured around all sources and source combinations, and patterns of relative dose rates established around each source (Fig. 6.6).

For example, around a cylindrical source concentric isodose rings will occur. The dose rates will decrease with distance from the source. Towards the ends of the source the isodose patterns will change from those seen near the centre. Where two or more sources are present, the isodose patterns for each will overlap and combined isodose lines can be calculated (see

Fig. 20.8). For routine use the known patterns can be applied to various situations by computation, but need to be checked out empirically by taking selected measurements.

Treatment planning and dosimetry calculations are carried out using a grid of reference points around each source. The more complex the implant, the more complex are the dosimetry calculations. These are essentially required in three dimensions, and are obtained by looking at various slices through the implant configuration. For multiple source arrangements, the shielding effect of each source (a few percent) on the overall dose distribution may be taken into account.

Selectron sources. For Selectron source trains each 'source' is made up of one or more identical sources spaced out equally or unequally to produce differing dose rate patterns.

With a stepping source, a further variation is introduced by the potential to vary dwell times, thus effectively increasing the 'activity' of each constituent source. The dose distribution from a given implant can be optimised in this way.

Dosimetry systems

The oldest established system, dictating the ideal geometrical arrangement of sources in order to achieve predictable and uniform dose distributions, is the Manchester system. This evolved through long usage of radium sources, the size, shape and activity of which fell within certain ranges. The system is well documented elsewhere (Paterson 1963).

Typically radium line sources had a nonuniform activity along their length so the Manchester system is suitable for brachytherapy work where the activity distribution is similar to that obtained from radium sources. Implants using iridium wire with uniform activity along its length required the development of a modified set of rules, e.g. the Paris system, because the activity does not equate to radium activity patterns.

Using afterloading sources, patterns suitable for using the Paris system can be obtained with stepping sources to simulate the effect of a wire.

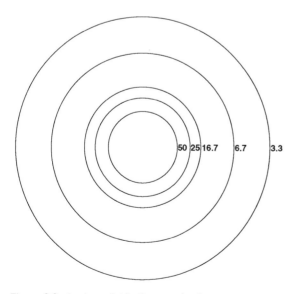

Figure 6.6 Isodose distribution round a line source.

However, the same system using different non-uniform patterns of dwell positions and times, may be used to produce distribution patterns suitable for use with the Manchester system.

Distribution rules for iridium wire/linear source implants (Paris system)

In the Paris system (Ash 1986), dosimetric calculations use the dose distribution at the central, cross-sectional plane of the implant, rather than using a plane outside the sources to define the treated volume as in the Manchester system. Several parallel sources in one plane may be used for a single plane implant. Implants in more than one plane are used for larger or thicker volumes and are called volume implants. The following must apply:

- Active sources must be parallel and straight.
- The separation between the source lines may vary with the length and number of sources from one implant to another. The separation range is 5–20 mm.
- Within one implant the lines should be equidistant.
- Activity should be uniform along the length of each source and identical for each.
- The distribution of sources in the central cross-sectional plane should be a line, equilateral triangles (Fig. 6.7) or squares.
- The active length of the sources must be 25–30% longer than the target volume depending on the number and separation of sources used. This is to account for noncrossing of the ends.

An example of a central plane dose distribution is shown in Figure 20.8. A check autoradiograph of iridium wire is taken to show the actual dosimetric pattern prior to its use. With an afterloaded single-plane implant using a standard

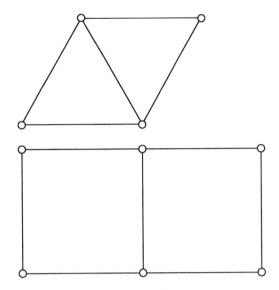

Figure 6.7 Cross-sectional view of source arrangements using equilateral triangles or squares.

geometry template, a similar check autoradiograph (Fig. 6.8) or autoradiographs may be taken by carrying out the exposure program.

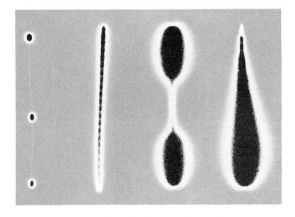

Figure 6.8 Autoradiograph of source for various programs. (Courtesy of Nucletron Trading Ltd.)

REFERENCES AND FURTHER READING

Ash D V 1986 Interstitial therapy. In: Hope-Stone H F (ed) Radiotherapy in clinical practice. Butterworths, London
Baltas D 1991 Quality assurance in HDR brachytherapy. Selectron Brachytherapy Journal 5(3): 149–153

Bridier A, Briot E 1991 Quality control of sources in LDR brachytherapy. Selectron Brachytherapy Journal 5(2): 54–58
Ezzell G A 1991 Quality assurance in HDR brachytherapy:

physical and technical aspects. Selectron Brachytherapy Journal 5(2): 59–62

ICRU 1985 Dose and volume specification for reporting intracavitary therapy in gynaecology. ICRU Report No 38. ICRU, Bethesda

Jones C H 1990 Quality assurance using the Selectron-LDR/MDR and microSelectron-HDR. Selectron Brachytherapy Journal 4(3): 48-52

Joslin C A 1990 Brachytherapy: a clinical dilemma. Interna-

tional Journal of Radiation Biology, Oncology and Physics 19: 801–802

Paterson R 1963 Treatment of malignant disease by radiotherapy, 2nd edn. Arnold, London

Slessinger E D 1990 Selectron LDR quality assurance. Selectron Brachytherapy Journal 4(2): 36–40

Sutton M L 1986 Some clinical aspects of radiobiology. In Hope-Stone H F (ed) Radiotherapy in clinical therapy. Butterworths, London

7

Collection and manipulation of beam data

BACKGROUND

In this chapter the procedures involved in the collection and manipulation of beam data for linacs are examined and descriptions given relating how this data is presented and used in practice. Presentation of data and the theory of dose calculation can be applied to all energies of radiation used in external beam radiotherapy treatment. The content of this chapter is therefore relevant to gamma ray beams, orthovoltage and superficial beams and associated treatment calculations. The measurement of beam performance for electrons is dealt with in Chapter 5.

The commissioning tests for linacs are more complex than those for other radiotherapy equipment but the requirements behind the procedures apply to them all.

Radiation physics is not covered here, but references will be given for relevant theory and documentation. The availability of accurate beam data is a prerequisite for treatment delivery. Beam data is used daily by radiographers for dose calculation and treatment field delineation. The acquisition of this data is not usually within the remit of the radiographer, but a thorough understanding of the information it provides is vital to safe dose calculation and delivery.

The beam data is collected initially as part of the commissioning process, and it is important that sufficient key parameters are checked regularly, particularly after any major alterations in the beam-producing components, so as to ensure that the data as a whole are valid. The frequency of, and procedures associated with, these checks are outlined in the Quality assurance sections of Chapters 2, 3 and 4.

Measurements and doses

Since we are primarily interested in the dose received by body tissue, beam data collection is carried out using a large water-filled container known as a plotting tank. As there is little difference at megavoltage beam energies between the behaviour of water and most body tissues (unlike orthovoltage energies), water is the most suitable medium for this procedure. The dose received by tissue is known as *absorbed dose* and is a measurement of the energy deposited in the body tissue from the radiation beam. The unit of absorbed dose is the gray, which is equivalent to an energy transfer of one joule per kilogram.

In the calculation of treatment dose two quantities are of particular interest: firstly the dose delivered to the tumour volume, known as *tumour dose*, and secondly the maximum dose delivered by each field contributing to the tumour dose, known as *applied* or *given dose*. The terms 'given dose' and 'tumour dose' will be used throughout the text.

THE RADIATION BEAM: ESSENTIAL INFORMATION

The process of treatment calculation, whether it is for a complex multifield plan, or a simple parallel opposed pair (see Ch. 15), may be divided into two main components:

- the distribution of the radiation (see Ch. 14)
- the amount of radiation delivered by the treatment machine under treatment conditions.

The presentation of this data in the radiotherapy department and the way in which it is used will be discussed later in this chapter.

The distribution of radiation is described by isodose charts, central axis depth–dose data, and isodose charts customised to the patient, known as treatment plans (see Ch. 14). The amount of radiation delivered by the treatment machine under treatment conditions is detailed in output charts.

The isodose chart

The isodose chart is a diagrammatic representation of the radiation distribution in a uniform absorber, such as a water-filled plotting tank, where points receiving an equal dose are joined together. These lines of equal dose are known as isodose curves or lines. A series of isodose curves for a beam of radiation are combined to give an isodose chart. The factors affecting the shape and depth of isodoses are well documented (Mould 1981).

For most radiotherapy treatments the isodose chart is a cross-section taken normal to the patient or phantom surface in the middle of the radiation beam (Fig. 7.1). Thus the isodose chart presents the field width on the chart horizontal axis and the depth of tissue on the chart vertical axis (Fig. 7.2). The maximum dose detected during the data acquisition is annotated as 100%. Further isodoses are plotted for different values, as a percentage of this maximum. Annotation of

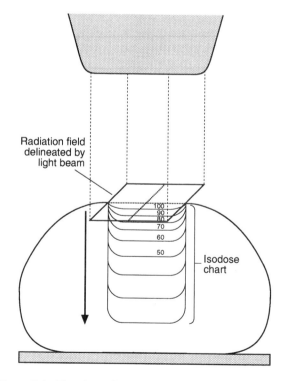

Figure 7.1 The plane of measurement of a central axis isodose chart shown within the patient cross-section.

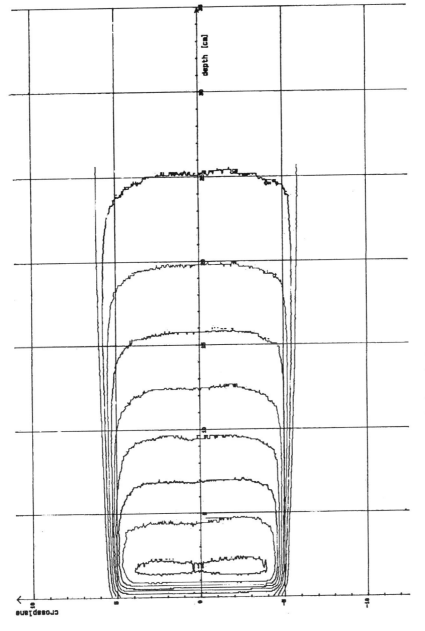

Figure 7.2   10 cm × 10 cm central axis isodose chart.

the dose delivered, at depth, as a percentage, permits the value of each isodose to be fixed in relation to others. Thus if the dose delivered at a certain depth is known it is simple to calculate doses at any other depth within the treatment field.

Several single-field isodose charts are combined in order to give isodose charts for multifield treatments, this being the basis for manual treatment planning (see Ch. 14).

The normal convention is that the edges of the treatment machine field delineation light beam define the 50% isodose curve, therefore the patient receives some radiation outside the area visible to the radiographers. This is only significant for treatment techniques where the treatment fields are close to critical organs.

The information provided by isodose curves is used to select suitable treatment machines and techniques for each treatment site.

Central axis depth–dose curves

A central axis depth-dose curve is a graph show-

ing the radiation delivered, at different depths, on the central axis of the radiation beam, for a defined field size. Again the maximum dose detected is said to be 100%, and all other doses are presented as a percentage of the dose maximum. The relationship between a central axis depth–dose chart and an isodose chart is demonstrated in Figure 7.3. In practice, the information provided by the central axis depth–dose curve alone is adequate for the calculation of the dose received at depth for simple treatment set-ups, such as single fields or parallel opposed pairs.

Treatment plans

A treatment plan is a pictorial representation of the radiation distribution in the patient. It takes into consideration the shape of the patient, the position of the tumour volume and the tissue types treated and critical organs. It is the result of complex planning procedures, detailed in Chapter 14. The treatment plan used in practice is generally a transverse section of the patient in the

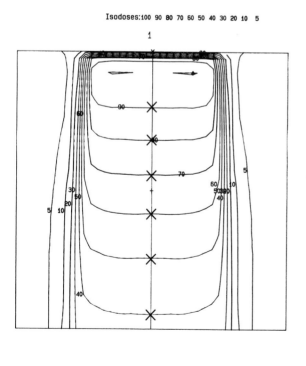
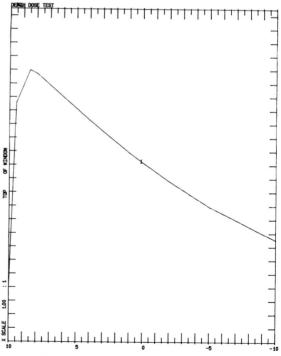

Figure 7.3 Relationship between an isodose chart and a central axis depth–dose chart. The crosses marked on the isodose chart indicate the values plotted to obtain a central axis depth–dose chart.

plane of the central axes of the applied radiation beams (Fig. 7.4). Treatment plans at other sections parallel to this one are often produced to ensure that the dose distribution is homogeneous along the length of the treated volume. Further developments in technology permit tumours to be visualised and treatments planned in three dimensions (see Ch. 23).

Output

The amount of radiation delivered in a given time by the treatment machine under treatment conditions is known as the output. The units in which output is quoted depend on whether the machine is a linac or one containing a radioactive source. A cobalt unit delivers radiation at a predictable rate (which decreases slowly and uniformly with time). Therefore treatment exposures are measured in seconds or minutes. By contrast the radiation delivered by a linac is not inherently predictable and must be monitored by a transmission dosemeter, which measures the amount of radiation delivered.

COLLECTION OF DOSIMETRY DATA

Measurement of the radiation beam during commissioning serves two purposes:

• Collection of beam data to provide sufficient information to accurately predict the outcome of all possible treatment procedures.

Measurements to compare the performance of the radiation beam with that specified by the manufacturer and national and international guidelines (ICRU 1969).

This information provides the basis for subsequent quality assurance checks, as described in Chapters 2, 3 and 4. The same measuring equipment is used for both.

Equipment

Modern commissioning equipment includes a large water tank, the dimensions of which exceed the dimensions of the maximum field size of the linac by 5 cm, and a microprocessor-controlled ion chamber which is capable of three-dimensional movement within the water tank. This equipment permits accurate and relatively quick data collection. Prior to the introduction of the microprocessor, the ion chamber was driven manually or along simple straight lines, and the process of commissioning took considerably longer.

Measurement of beam performance against the specification

To ensure that the radiation beam is fit for clinical use and meets the required specification, measurements of photon energy, beam symmetry and flatness, and output are carried out.

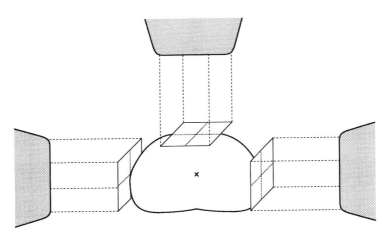

Figure 7.4 Position of fields on a transverse section of the patient.

Photon energy

Radiographers describe linac radiation beams in terms of beam energy. The nominal energy of the radiation beam is equal to the energy of the electron beam incident on the target. The beam specification is further defined in terms of the penetrating power of the X-rays produced (British Institute of Radiology 1983).

Beam symmetry and flatness

To ensure that the dose delivered to the patient is the same across the treatment field, the profile of the beam should be flat in the plane which is parallel to the incident plane of the treatment field (Fig. 7.5). The flatness of the beam is measured at right angles to the central axis, across the width and length of the field and across the diagonals, for a 10 cm × 10 cm field, a 30 cm × 30 cm field and at maximum field size. Symmetry is the overall balance between two halves of a radiation beam and during radiotherapy treatment delivery is constantly monitored by the treatment machine which uses a segmented ionisation chamber (Greene 1986).

In practice it is not possible to achieve a perfectly flat beam under all conditions, but the flatness and symmetry must meet the specified standard. Typically the difference between measured outputs across the major axes of the field, including diagonals must not exceed 3%.

Output calibration

During this process the amount of radiation emitted from the linac is measured under specified conditions (ICRU 1969). This entails calibration of the linac's own radiation monitor for field size, distance, modality and wedge, against an external standard dosemeter. Thus, the machine's output is measured in monitor units (MU) per gray. For a linac this output measurement is standardised for the field size 10 cm × 10 cm, where 100 monitor units delivers a dose of 1 Gy at the dose maximum point. As the field size decreases, the aperture of the radiation beam is smaller, there is less scatter in the irradiated body and therefore it is necessary to give more monitor units to deliver 1 Gy. The reverse applies when the field size is increased. Also the output will decrease with increasing treatment distance. The practical consequences of this for dose calculation will be dealt with later in this chapter.

In practice it is important to know that the treatment machine delivers the same dose per monitor unit regardless of the number of MU set; this is known as linearity.

Initial output calibration is carried out in a water phantom, but as this is not used for daily output measurements, it is cross-checked with the phantom and measuring device to be used for daily checks.

Completing the collection of dosimetry data

The procedures described below are necessary to ensure that the outcome of any treatment process may be accurately predicted, in terms of the area covered by the radiation beam, the amount of radiation received at any point within the patient and the effect of any beam modifiers. The actual measurements and equipment used do not differ in practice from those described above, but for clarity are described separately.

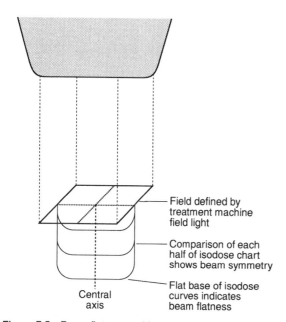

Field defined by treatment machine field light

Comparison of each half of isodose chart shows beam symmetry

Flat base of isodose curves indicates beam flatness

Central axis

Figure 7.5   Beam flatness and beam symmetry.

Measurement of isodose curves

The measurement of isodose curves for all treatment conditions is no longer necessary, as computerised treatment planning systems are able to generate these. However, it is prudent to collect sufficient isodose curves for data comparison with the planning system. Typically isodoses generated will include isodoses at various f.s.d.s., with and without beam-modifying wedges, and away from the central axis. Figure 7.6 shows some examples of isodose curves measured under these conditions.

Central axis depth–dose data

Central axis depth–dose data is collected for many combinations of field size, wedge and f.s.d., and is used in combination with the beam profiles, described below, as the raw data for many planning computers.

Beam profiles

Detailed measurements in the penumbra region of the radiation beam are taken at many depths. This is carried out for all wedges and f.s.d.s. The data acquired gives accurate information about the fall-off of the radiation beam at the edges of the field. This percentage depth dose data gives detailed information about the dose delivered at depth. If all this information is combined it is possible to generate isodose curves. This is the basis of operation of modern planning computers.

Output

The output variations with f.s.d. and field size must be checked across the range of intended treatment parameters, because although it is possible to calculate output variations, in practice these vary with the target and collimators. Thus each set of linac outputs is unique.

It is necessary to modify the shape of some treatment fields with lead blocks. These are suspended between the linac head and the patient. The introduction of this support mechanism, the lead platform, causes some of the

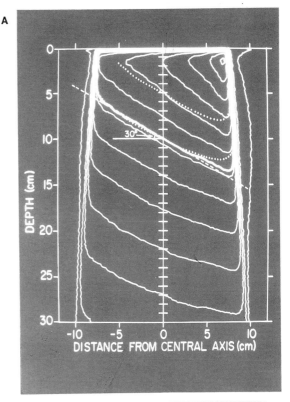

A

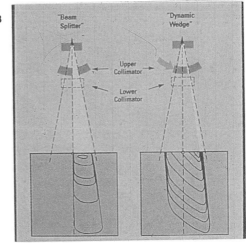

Figure 7.6. **A** Wedged isodose chart. (Courtesy of Varian Oncology Systems.) **B** Off-axis isodose chart. (Courtesy of Varian Oncology Systems.)

radiation to be absorbed. The radiation absorbed by a lead platform is constant for any beam energy. Therefore the amount of radiation absorbed by the platform is measured and a factor produced which is incorporated into the output calculation to correct for the loss of radiation. This is known as a transmission factor. Transmission factors may also be used for wedge fields where the reduction in radiation is not incorporated into the isodose curves (Mould 1982).

PRESENTATION OF DOSIMETRY DATA FOR DAILY PRACTICE

The data collected during commissioning is processed and documented in a format agreed by the radiotherapy department. The content of the data is essentially the same in every department, but the way in which it is presented varies considerably.

For ease of presentation and dose calculation the variation of machine data with changing field size is presented using equivalent squares. The equivalent square of any treatment field is the equivalent irradiated area to that if the treatment field were square, i.e. equivalent scatter conditions. Therefore before dose calculation is possible it is necessary to find the equivalent square of the prescribed treatment field. Typically tables are provided (Table 7.1) where the length of each axis of the treatment field is displayed and the equivalent square is shown where both the axis lengths intersect.

To calculate radiotherapy doses for patients whose treatment does not require a computerised treatment plan, some or all of the information subsequently described is necessary and will be found in the treatment calculation folder on all treatment machines.

Central axis depth–dose data

Central axis depth–dose data is necessary to find the percentage depth dose delivered to the area of interest under prescribed treatment conditions. This data may be documented in graph form or in table form (Table 7.2). In table form it is possible to demonstrate the changes in central axis depth dose with changing equivalent square and depth

for each f.s.d. in common clinical use. This presentation is simple and easy to interpret.

Typically this data is used to calculate the midplane dose for parallel opposed pairs and may be further processed to produce a table of midplane doses for a given f.s.d. (Table 7.3). This table can prove useful in practice if parallel opposed pairs are routinely treated at normal f.s.d.

Machine output data

Machine output data is necessary to calculate the time or monitor units needed to give the required dose under the treatment conditions. Machine output varies with the equivalent square of the treatment field to be irradiated and the f.s.d. at which the treatment is to be given.

Output can be described in one of two ways, either monitor units per gray or gray per monitor unit. Both are acceptable but must be applied to the dose calculation in different ways.

For monitor units per gray:

$$\text{Given dose} \times \text{monitor units/gray} = \text{monitor units}$$

For gray per monitor unit:

$$\text{Given dose} \div \text{gray/monitor units} = \text{monitor units}$$

Output data for fixed f.s.d. treatments

Presentation of machine output data may be in table or graph form (Table 7.4). Where a table format is used, an output over a range of equivalent squares is given. This is not inaccurate as there is little change in the output across the range.

Outputs for extended f.s.d. or reduced f.s.d. are not strictly necessary as they can easily be calculated from the output table for the standard f.s.d. Where the standard f.s.d. is 100 cm, the following equation can be used to calculate the output at any f.s.d. in MU/Gy:

$$\begin{array}{l}\text{Output at} \\ \text{required f.s.d.}\end{array} = \frac{\text{f.s.d.}}{100} \times \frac{\text{f.s.d.}}{100} \times \begin{array}{l}\text{output at} \\ 100 \text{ cm f.s.d.}\end{array}$$

Table 7.1 Equivalent square of rectangular fields

Long axis, cm	Short axis, cm																				
	0.5	1	2	3	4	5	6	7	8	9	10	11	12	13	14	15	16	17	18	19	20
0.5	0.5																				
1	0.7	1.0																			
2	0.9	1.4	2.0																		
3	1.0	1.6	2.4	3.0																	
4	1.1	1.7	2.7	3.4	4.0																
5	1.1	1.8	2.9	3.8	4.5	5.0															
6	1.2	1.9	3.1	4.1	4.8	5.5	6.0														
7	1.2	2.0	3.3	4.3	5.1	5.8	6.5	7.0													
8	1.2	2.1	3.4	4.5	5.4	6.2	6.9	7.5	8.0												
9	1.2	2.1	3.5	4.6	5.6	6.5	7.2	7.9	8.5	9.0											
10	1.3	2.2	3.6	4.8	5.8	6.7	7.5	8.2	8.9	9.5	10.0										
11	1.3	2.2	3.7	4.9	6.0	6.9	7.8	8.5	9.3	9.9	10.5	11.0									
12	1.3	2.2	3.7	5.0	6.1	7.1	8.0	8.8	9.6	10.3	10.9	11.5	12.0								
13	1.3	2.2	3.8	5.1	6.2	7.2	8.2	9.1	9.9	10.6	11.3	11.9	12.5	13.0							
14	1.3	2.3	3.8	5.1	6.3	7.4	8.4	9.3	10.1	10.9	11.6	12.3	12.9	13.5	14.0						
15	1.3	2.3	3.9	5.2	6.4	7.5	8.5	9.5	10.3	11.2	11.9	12.6	13.3	13.9	14.5	15.0					
16	1.3	2.3	3.9	5.3	6.5	7.6	8.6	9.6	10.5	11.4	12.2	12.9	13.7	14.3	14.9	15.5	16.0				
17	1.3	2.3	3.9	5.3	6.5	7.7	8.8	9.8	10.7	11.6	12.4	13.2	14.0	14.7	15.3	15.9	16.5	17.0			
18	1.3	2.3	3.9	5.3	6.6	7.8	8.9	9.9	10.9	11.8	12.6	13.5	14.3	15.0	15.7	16.3	16.9	17.5	18.0		
19	1.4	2.3	4.0	5.4	6.6	7.8	8.9	10.0	11.0	11.9	12.8	13.7	14.5	15.3	16.0	16.7	17.3	17.9	18.5	19.0	
20	1.4	2.3	4.0	5.4	6.7	7.9	9.0	10.1	11.1	12.1	13.0	13.9	14.7	15.5	16.3	17.0	17.7	18.3	18.9	19.5	20.0
22	1.4	2.4	4.0	5.5	6.8	8.0	9.1	10.2	11.3	12.3	13.3	14.2	15.1	16.0	16.8	17.6	18.3	19.0	19.7	20.3	20.9
24	1.4	2.4	4.0	5.5	6.8	8.1	9.2	10.4	11.4	12.5	13.5	14.5	15.4	16.3	17.2	18.0	18.8	19.6	20.3	21.0	21.7
26	1.4	2.4	4.1	5.5	6.9	8.1	9.3	10.5	11.6	12.6	13.7	14.7	15.7	16.6	17.5	18.4	19.3	20.1	20.9	21.6	22.4
28	1.4	2.4	4.1	5.5	6.9	8.2	9.4	10.5	11.7	12.7	13.8	14.8	15.8	16.8	17.8	18.7	19.6	20.5	21.3	22.1	22.9
30	1.4	2.4	4.1	5.6	6.9	8.2	9.4	10.6	11.7	12.8	13.9	15.0	16.0	17.0	18.0	18.9	19.9	20.8	21.6	22.5	23.3
32	1.4	2.4	4.1	5.6	6.9	8.2	9.4	10.6	11.8	12.9	14.0	15.0	16.1	17.1	18.1	19.1	20.1	21.0	21.9	22.8	23.7
34	1.4	2.4	4.1	5.6	6.9	8.2	9.5	10.7	11.8	12.9	14.0	15.1	16.2	17.2	18.2	19.2	20.2	21.2	22.1	23.1	24.0
36	1.4	2.4	4.1	5.6	7.0	8.2	9.5	10.7	11.8	13.0	14.1	15.2	16.2	17.3	18.3	19.3	20.4	21.3	22.3	23.3	24.2
38	1.4	2.4	4.1	5.6	7.0	8.3	9.5	10.7	11.9	13.0	14.1	15.2	16.3	17.4	18.4	19.4	20.5	21.5	22.4	23.4	24.4
40	1.4	2.4	4.1	5.6	7.0	8.3	9.5	10.7	11.9	13.0	14.1	15.2	16.3	17.4	18.5	19.5	20.5	21.5	22.6	23.5	24.5
45	1.4	2.4	4.1	5.6	7.0	8.3	9.5	10.7	11.9	13.1	14.2	15.3	16.4	17.5	18.5	19.6	20.7	21.7	22.7	23.7	24.8
50	1.4	2.4	4.1	5.6	7.0	8.3	9.5	10.7	11.9	13.1	14.2	15.3	16.4	17.5	18.6	19.7	20.7	21.8	22.8	23.8	24.9
55	1.4	2.4	4.1	5.6	7.0	8.3	9.5	10.8	11.9	13.1	14.2	15.3	16.4	17.5	18.6	19.7	20.8	21.8	22.9	23.9	24.9
60	1.4	2.4	4.1	5.6	7.0	8.3	9.5	10.8	11.9	13.1	14.2	15.4	16.5	17.6	18.6	19.7	20.8	21.8	22.9	23.9	25.0
Inf.	1.4	2.4	4.1	5.6	7.0	8.3	9.5	10.8	11.9	13.1	14.2	15.4	16.5	17.6	18.6	19.7	20.8	21.9	22.9	24.0	25.0

All dimensions in cm

Table 7.2 Central axis depth–dose data. Percentage depth doses for the SL75–14 8 MV, at 100 cm f.s.d.

Depth, cm	Equivalent square, cm															Depth, cm
	4.0	5.0	6.0	7.0	8.0	9.0	10.0	12.0	15.0	17.0	20.0	25.0	30.0	35.0	40.0	
0	10.5	11.5	12.5	13.5	14.5	15.5	16.5	18.5	21.4	23.2	26.0	29.6	30.8	31.1	31.4	0
1	94.0	94.3	94.4	94.5	94.6	94.7	95.0	95.6	96.4	96.9	97.4	97.9	98.1	98.2	98.3	1
2	100.0	100.0	100.0	100.0	100.0	100.0	100.0	100.0	100.0	100.0	100.0	100.0	100.0	100.0	100.0	2
3	97.3	97.3	97.4	97.4	97.4	97.4	97.5	97.5	97.6	97.7	97.9	97.8	97.8	97.8	97.8	3
4	93.0	93.2	93.5	93.5	93.6	93.6	93.7	93.8	93.8	93.9	94.0	94.0	94.0	94.0	94.0	4
5	88.3	88.9	89.2	89.2	89.4	89.4	89.8	89.9	90.0	90.0	90.2	90.3	90.4	90.6	90.8	5
6	84.0	84.4	85.1	85.1	85.3	85.6	85.8	85.9	86.1	86.5	86.8	86.9	87.0	87.1	87.3	6
7	79.9	80.3	80.7	81.4	81.4	81.9	81.9	82.1	82.6	82.8	83.0	83.1	83.7	83.9	84.2	7
8	75.5	76.2	76.9	77.3	77.4	78.0	78.3	78.8	79.2	79.6	79.8	80.0	80.5	80.8	80.9	8
9	71.4	72.4	73.1	73.6	73.8	74.2	74.7	75.3	75.8	76.2	76.8	76.9	77.2	77.6	77.8	9
10	67.8	68.7	69.3	70.0	70.3	70.9	71.2	71.8	72.5	73.1	73.4	73.6	74.3	74.6	74.7	10
11	64.0	65.2	65.8	66.5	67.1	67.6	68.0	68.6	69.4	69.9	70.5	70.7	71.3	71.8	72.2	11
12	60.6	61.7	62.5	63.2	63.7	64.4	64.8	65.4	66.2	66.8	67.5	67.9	68.3	68.9	69.1	12
13	57.4	58.4	59.3	59.9	60.5	61.2	61.5	62.4	63.4	63.9	64.7	65.2	65.5	65.9	66.5	13
14	54.4	55.4	56.3	57.2	57.5	58.4	58.8	59.5	60.4	61.2	62.1	62.4	62.9	63.6	63.8	14
15	51.5	52.4	53.4	54.1	54.6	55.4	55.8	56.7	57.8	58.3	59.2	60.0	60.4	60.9	61.3	15
16	48.7	49.7	50.7	51.4	52.0	52.6	53.2	54.3	55.2	55.8	56.6	57.4	57.8	58.3	58.7	16
17	46.3	47.1	48.0	48.7	49.3	49.4	50.6	51.5	52.4	53.5	54.3	54.8	55.3	55.9	56.5	17
18	43.8	44.6	45.5	46.3	46.9	47.6	48.1	49.1	50.2	50.9	51.9	52.4	52.9	53.5	54.1	18
19	41.4	42.3	43.3	44.1	44.6	45.2	45.7	46.8	47.9	48.5	49.5	50.5	50.8	51.7	51.8	19
20	39.3	40.2	41.0	41.9	42.3	43.0	43.7	44.6	45.8	46.3	47.1	48.0	48.6	49.1	49.6	20
21	37.4	38.1	38.9	39.8	40.3	40.9	41.4	42.3	43.6	44.2	45.2	45.9	46.6	47.4	47.6	21
22	35.5	36.1	36.9	37.7	38.3	39.0	39.4	40.4	41.7	42.1	43.1	43.9	44.7	45.5	45.7	22
23	33.5	34.4	35.3	35.7	36.3	37.0	37.6	38.5	39.7	40.3	41.2	42.1	42.8	43.6	43.8	23
24	31.8	32.5	33.3	33.9	34.5	35.2	35.8	36.7	37.8	38.5	39.4	40.2	40.9	41.7	42.0	24
25	30.2	30.9	31.5	32.3	32.8	33.6	34.1	35.0	36.2	36.8	37.7	38.5	39.2	39.9	40.3	25
26	28.5	29.3	30.0	30.7	31.2	31.9	33.3	33.1	34.4	35.1	35.8	36.8	37.5	38.3	38.6	26
27	27.1	27.7	28.5	29.1	29.6	30.3	30.8	31.6	32.8	33.5	34.3	35.3	35.9	36.4	36.9	27
28	25.7	26.3	27.2	27.6	28.2	28.8	29.2	30.2	31.3	31.9	32.5	33.6	34.4	35.0	35.4	28
29	24.5	25.0	25.7	26.5	26.8	27.4	27.9	28.8	29.8	30.4	31.4	32.1	32.9	33.6	33.9	29
30	23.2	23.8	24.5	25.1	25.6	26.2	26.6	27.3	28.4	29.0	29.9	30.8	31.6	32.1	32.6	30
Tissue–air ratio (TAR) at 2.0 cm	1.014	1.018	1.021	1.023	1.026	1.028	1.031	1.036	1.042	1.046	1.051	1.056	1.058	1.059	1.060	

Table 7.3 Midplane doses for parallel opposed pair for fixed f.s.d. treatments (SL75–14 8 MV, at 100 cm f.s.d.). Tissue max is the maximum dose delivered to the tissue

Separation, cm		Equivalent square, cm												
		4.0	5.0	6.0	8.0	10.0	12.0	15.0	17.0	20.0	25.0	30.0	35.0	40.0
10	Centre	177	178	178	179	180	180	180	180	180	181	181	181	182
	Tissue max	175	176	176	177	178	178	179	179	179	180	180	180	180
11	Centre	172	173	174	175	176	176	176	177	177	177	177	178	178
	Tissue max	171	172	173	173	174	175	175	176	176	176	177	177	177
12	Centre	168	169	170	171	172	172	172	173	173	173	173	174	174
	Tissue max	167	168	169	170	171	171	172	173	173	173	174	174	174
13	Centre	164	165	166	167	168	168	169	169	170	170	171	171	172
	Tissue max	164	165	165	167	168	168	169	169	170	170	171	171	172
14	Centre	160	161	161	163	164	164	165	166	166	166	167	168	168
	Tissue max	160	161	162	163	164	165	166	166	167	167	168	168	169
15	Centre	155	157	158	159	160	161	162	162	163	163	164	165	165
	Tissue max	157	158	159	160	161	162	163	163	164	165	165	165	166
16	Centre	151	152	154	155	157	158	158	159	160	160	161	162	162
	Tissue max	154	155	156	157	158	159	160	161	162	162	162	163	163
17	Centre	147	149	150	151	153	154	155	156	157	157	158	158	159
	Tissue max	151	152	153	154	155	156	157	158	159	160	160	160	161
18	Centre	143	145	146	148	149	151	152	152	154	154	154	155	156
	Tissue max	148	149	150	152	153	154	155	155	156	157	157	158	158
19	Centre	139	141	142	144	146	147	148	149	150	151	152	152	153
	Tissue max	146	147	148	149	150	151	152	153	154	154	155	155	156
20	Centre	136	137	139	141	142	144	145	146	147	147	149	149	149
	Tissue max	143	144	145	146	148	149	150	150	151	152	152	153	154
21	Centre	132	134	135	137	139	140	142	143	144	144	146	146	147
	Tissue max	141	142	143	144	145	146	147	148	149	150	150	151	151
22	Centre	128	130	132	134	136	137	139	140	141	141	143	144	144
	Tissue max	139	140	141	142	143	144	145	146	147	148	148	149	149
23	Centre	125	127	128	131	133	134	136	137	138	139	140	141	141
	Tissue max	137	138	138	140	141	142	143	144	145	145	146	147	147
24	Centre	121	123	125	127	130	131	132	134	135	136	137	138	138
	Tissue max	135	136	136	138	139	140	141	142	143	143	144	145	145
25	Centre	118	120	122	124	126	128	130	131	132	133	134	135	136
	Tissue max	133	134	135	136	137	138	139	140	141	142	142	143	143
26	Centre	115	117	119	121	123	125	127	128	129	130	131	132	133
	Tissue max	131	132	133	134	135	136	137	138	139	140	140	141	142
27	Centre	112	114	116	118	120	122	124	125	127	128	128	130	130
	Tissue max	130	130	131	132	134	135	136	136	137	138	139	139	140
28	Centre	109	111	113	115	118	119	121	122	124	125	126	127	128
	Tissue max	128	129	130	131	133	133	134	135	135	136	137	138	138
29	Centre	106	108	110	112	115	116	118	120	121	122	123	125	125
	Tissue max	127	127	128	129	130	131	132	133	134	135	135	136	136

Table 7.4 Output chart for the SL75–14 8 MV. Data are given in monitor units/Gy

Equivalent square of diaphragm setting	f.s.d., cm				
	100	120	130	150	180
4.0–4.1	107.5	154.8	181.7	241.9	348.3
4.2–4.4	107.0	154.1	180.8	240.8	346.7
4.5–4.7	106.5	153.4	180.0	239.6	345.1
4.8–5.0	106.0	152.6	179.1	238.5	343.4
5.1–5.3	105.5	151.9	178.3	237.4	341.8
5.4–5.6	105.0	151.2	177.4	236.3	340.2
5.7–5.9	104.5	150.5	176.6	235.1	338.6
6.0–6.3	104.0	149.8	175.8	234.0	337.0
6.4–6.7	103.5	149.0	174.9	232.9	335.3
6.8–7.2	103.0	148.3	174.1	231.8	333.7
7.3–7.7	102.5	147.6	173.2	230.6	332.1
7.8–8.2	102.0	146.9	172.4	229.5	330.5
8.3–8.7	101.5	146.2	171.5	228.4	328.9
8.8–9.2	101.0	145.4	170.7	227.3	327.2
9.3–9.7	100.5	144.7	169.8	226.1	325.6
9.8–10.4	100.0	144.0	169.0	225.0	324.0
10.5–11.1	99.5	143.3	168.2	223.9	322.4
11.2–11.9	99.0	142.6	167.3	222.8	320.8
12.0–12.9	98.5	141.8	166.5	221.6	319.1
13.0–13.9	98.0	141.1	165.6	220.5	317.5
14.0–15.1	97.5	140.4	164.8	219.4	315.9
15.2–16.5	97.0	139.7	163.9	218.2	314.3
16.6–18.2	96.5	139.0	163.1	217.1	312.7
18.3–20.8	96.0	138.2	162.2	216.0	311.0
20.9–24.0	95.5	137.5	161.4	214.9	309.4
24.1–27.7	95.0	136.8	160.6	213.8	307.8
28.8–31.7	94.5	136.1	159.7	212.6	306.2
31.8–35.6	94.0	135.4	158.9	211.5	304.6
35.7–40.0	93.5	134.6	158.0	210.4	302.9

Output calculations for isocentric treatments

All the output calculations described above assume that the patient is positioned at a set f.s.d. away from the treatment machine. However, when isocentric treatment techniques are employed, the radiation beam does not hit the surface of the patient at the normal treatment f.s.d. (see Fig. 9.14). Therefore it is necessary to take this into consideration when calculating outputs for isocentric treatment.

There are two main systems in use for the calculation of output for isocentric treatments. The method of calculation of the output depends on the planning method employed by the planning computer. If the planning computer produces plans by the combination of isodose curves at different f.s.d.s, then the output is calculated using the same equation described above as it is assumed that the radiation beams of the isocentric plan are a series of beams delivered at different f.s.d.s.

Alternatively the output is calculated by measuring how much air and tissue the radiation beam must travel through to reach the isocentre (tissue air ratio) (Mould 1982), which is by definition at a standard distance. More of the radiation is absorbed in tissue than in air, therefore the more tissue the radiation beam travels through to reach the isocentre, the greater the output in MU/Gy needed to give the required dose. This amount of tissue can be calculated during the computer planning process and the resultant output in MU/Gy required given on the treatment plan. This output is only correct if the radiation beam travels through the correct amount of tissue before reaching the isocentre. The amount of tissue is easily measured in practice when the patient is in the treatment position. A rangefinder reading is taken with the treatment head in the treatment field position. This reading is taken away from the normal treatment f.s.d. This reading is sometimes known as tumour centre–skin distance or t.s.d. (see Fig. 15.11). To allow alterations to the output to be made, tables can be provided which give the outputs for all normal t.s.d. and equivalent square combinations.

Transmission factors

The transmission factors can be documented in two ways, either as the percentage of the radiation beam absorbed, or the percentage of the beam transmitted. The final output applied to the treatment dose must include correction for any absorber used.

Wedged fields

When wedges (see Ch. 8) are used in treatment delivery they act as an absorber in the same way as a lead tray. The reduction in dose received by the tumour may be corrected in one of two ways:

• The application of a transmission factor to the output calculations.
• The isodoses used to generate the treatment plan take into account the reduced dose delivered at depth. It is not necessary to include a transmission factor in the output calculation using this method, i.e. the peak isodose level is less than 100% (Mould 1981).

DOSE CALCULATION

Dose calculation can be divided into two distinct parts:

• Determination of the percentage depth dose delivered to the area of interest.
• Calculation to determine the monitor units required to deliver the specified dose under the treatment conditions.

More complex dose calculations required for multifield isocentric set-ups are carried out during the computer planning process. Manual dose calculations are usually only carried out for simple single- or two-field treatments, the most common of these being the parallel opposed pair.

The treatment prescription

The dose of radiation to be received by the patient and the number of treatments to be used are documented by a radiotherapist on the treatment prescription. Details of the field size, energy and patient position will also be part of this document. Ideally the treatment card should be a complete description of the treatment procedure.

Treatment calculation for a parallel opposed pair at fixed f.s.d.

Calculation of the percentage depth dose delivered to the tumour

The depth of the tumour in relation to the skin surface could be measured on a lateral X-ray film, but commonly is assumed to be in the middle of the patient. This assumption is not as inaccurate as it sounds, as the isodose distribution for a parallel opposed pair (Fig. 7.7) shows a large area of equal dose. When the field position is planned, a measurement of the thickness of the patient is taken at the central axis (patient separation) of the beam (Fig. 7.8). This may be supplemented with other separations at the top and bottom of the field, if the surface of the patient is so uneven that the result of the calculation to find the percentage depth dose in the centre of the treatment field would be very different from the same calculation at the field edges.

As percentage depth dose is affected by depth in tissue, beam energy and field size of the radiation beam, it is necessary to determine the percentage depth dose delivered to the tumour under the treatment conditions.

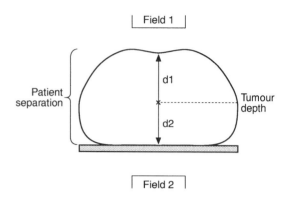

Figure 7.8 Patient separation and depth of the tumour. With a central tumour, d1 is the depth of tissue traversed by field 1, d2 the depth traversed by field 2, to reach the tumour; d1 + d2 = patient separation.

1. Using the equivalent square charts, such as Table 7.1, the equivalent square of the field size to be treated is found. The depth of the tumour in the patients, usually assumed to be in the middle of the patient and therefore at a depth equal to half the patient separation, is found.

2. Using the depth–dose data provided for the energy of radiation beam to be used, the percentage depth dose delivered at the depth of the tumour is found, as in Table 7.2.

This is the percentage depth dose delivered by one of the radiation fields to the tumour. Assuming that the field size, depth of the tumour in the patient, and energy of the beam are the same for the second field, the total percentage depth dose received by the tumour is found by doubling the percentage depth dose found for the first field.

Calculation of MU required

The tumour dose will be documented on the treatment prescription. This dose, expressed in grays, is equaled to the percentage depth dose found using the method described above.

Each of the fields contributing to the percentage depth dose delivers a given dose, which is defined as 100%. Therefore the calculation to ascertain the given dose required is:

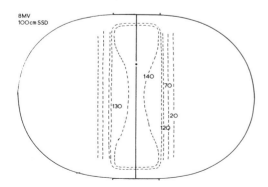

Figure 7.7 Isodose chart for parallel opposed pair. (Reproduced from Walter et al 1982.)

$$\text{Given dose (in grays)} = \frac{\text{Tumour dose (in grays)}}{\text{Percentage depth dose}} \times 100$$
$$\text{(summation from both fields)}$$

The doses calculated are the total dose for the whole treatment and must be divided by the number of treatments to give the daily doses.

Using the equivalent square, find the output for the treatment fields from the output charts. If this output is not for the required f.s.d. then apply the equation described above.

Combine the output and the daily given dose in the correct manner, e.g. if monitor units/gray are used then the daily given dose should be multiplied by the output.

The use of any radiation absorbers must be compensated for using the appropriate transmission factor.

The resultant monitor units are applied daily from each treatment field to deliver the required tumour dose.

Calculation of dose from a treatment plan

The format of the treatment plan will vary from department to department but all the information necessary to calculate the given doses and the monitor units will be present.

The process for dose calculation is identical to that described for parallel opposed pairs, except that the percentage depth doses are replaced by the isodoses on the treatment plan. Therefore a dose will be prescribed for the tumour, from which the given doses for all fields are calculated.

Often the given doses for each field are not identical; this is known as field weighting. Instead of the given doses being annotated as 100% the summation of the percentage depth doses to tumour volume is called 100% and the given doses are a percentage of the tumour dose (see Ch. 14). This is known as normalisation of the tumour dose. Thus to calculate given dose from the tumour dose the following equation is used:

$$\text{Given dose} = \frac{\text{Tumour dose}}{100} \times \frac{\text{Weight}}{\text{percentage for the field}}$$

Calculation of the monitor units for each field

To calculate the monitor units required for each treatment field an output factor must be applied to the given dose. The method of determining this output is described earlier in this chapter. However, it is important to point out that if the plan is for an isocentric set-up, then the output must take into consideration the amount of tissue through which the radiation beam has travelled and include transmission factors for wedged fields where appropriate.

In some centres the treatment plan will include the output for each treatment field taking into consideration all the treatment conditions. For fixed f.s.d. treatments the output charts provided can be used.

Standardisation of dose prescription from a treatment plan

Sometimes the 100% isodose curve does not adequately cover the tumour on the treatment plan. Under these circumstances the plan may be prescribed by the radiotherapist using the percentage depth dose which best fits the tumour to be treated.

The main problem, where the radiotherapist chooses an isodose curve on which to base the treatment calculations, is that it is difficult to compare the dose delivered if there is no standard method for prescribing from a treatment plan. A standard format for dose specification is currently available (ICRU 1992) which, if used internationally, would permit direct comparison of treatment prescriptions from centre to centre.

PRACTICAL TREATMENT DELIVERY

It is important to realise that dose distribution and calculation for radiotherapy is imperfect. The responsibility for dose calculation and delivery rests with the radiographer. It is therefore of value to examine some of the factors which are relevant when deciding whether a dose calculation or distribution is acceptable or not.

Firstly the output from a linac is clinically acceptable at plus or minus 3%; at the threshold of these limits the patient would be over- or underdosed by this amount. Planning computers are expected to generate plans which describe the dose distribution to within 5%, but the method of patient outline generation may not be perfect (see Ch. 14) which will affect the dosimetry of the treatment plan.

Decision-making during treatment delivery

Making the decision not to alter a treatment calculation, for the sake of one monitor unit per fraction, is often harder for some than deciding that a treatment plan does not fit the patient. The risks of error associated with calculating and delivering an extra monitor unit must be offset against the potential gain (see Ch. 10). Modern linacs with computer verification will require overriding and updating which have risk factors of their own. Above all else the patient must be in the right position underneath the treatment machine (see Chs 12, 13) and any decisions to adjust the prescription must not jeopardise this.

QUALITY ASSURANCE OF DOSE DELIVERED
External dosemeters

The quality of treatment delivery can be mea-sured in terms of the accuracy of position of the fields and of the dose delivered to the patient. The latter can be measured using external dosemeters.

Thermoluminescent crystals

These are provided in the form of capsules of lithium fluoride. They absorb energy from the beam, which can be measured in the form of light emitted when the capsules are heated. They have the advantage that very small capsules can be constructed which can be fitted under a beam direction shell (see Ch. 17).

Semiconductors

These provide a method of real-time in vivo dosimetry. The equipment involved requires regular calibration to ensure the accuracy of the readings. Furthermore, correction factors may have to be applied depending upon the energy of the treatment beam used.

Practical considerations

The siting of the dosemeters in the treatment beam is often a limitation in verifying tumour doses. As the dosemeters can only be sited on the skin surface or, more unusually, in a body orifice, it may be necessary to relate the measurement obtained to the point of interest (Leunens et al 1990). When the measurement is taken on a body surface it may or may not be relevant to add build-up, depending on the point of interest.

REFERENCES AND FURTHER READING

British Institute of Radiology 1983 Central axis depth dose data for use in radiotherapy. British Journal of Radiology, (Suppl 17)

Greene D 1986 Linear accelerators for radiation therapy. Adam Hilger, Bristol

Institute of Physical Sciences in Medicine 1988 Commissioning and quality assurance of linear accelerators. Institute of Physical Sciences in Medicine, York

International Commission on Radiation Units and Measurements 1969 Radiation dosimetry: X-rays and gamma rays with maximum photon energies between 0.6 and 50 MeV. ICRU, Washington

International Commission on Radiation Units and Measurements 1992 Prescribing recording and reporting photon beam therapy. Report No 50. ICRU, Washington

Kron T, Schneider M, Murray A, Hameghan H 1993 Clinical thermoluminescence dosimetry: how do expectations and results compare? Radiotherapy and Oncology 26: 151–161

Leunens G, Van Dam J, Dutreix A, Van der Schueren E 1990 Quality assurance in radiotherapy by in vivo dosimetry. 2: Determination of target absorbed dose. Radiotherapy and Oncology 19: 73–87

Mould R F 1981 Radiotherapy treatment planning. Adam Hilger, Bristol

Walter J, Miller H, Bomford C K 1982 A short textbook of radiotherapy, 4th edn. Churchill Livingstone, Edinburgh

8

Beam modification

The rectangular and square radiation fields with flat-base isodose curves are suitable, as they stand, for the treatment of many body sites. However, it is possible to modify both the field shape and the shape of the isodose curves to achieve treatment beams tailored to the individual tumour shape and site.

MODIFYING THE SHAPE OF THE RADIATION FIELD

A rectangular treatment field is commonly shaped by placing shielding blocks in the beam. The thickness of the block depends upon the energy of radiation and the material of the block. Typically a block of lead 9 cm thick will absorb 98% of an 8 MV X-ray beam (Marrs et al 1993).

For high energy treatment machines the blocks are placed in a lead tray which is attached to the treatment head. This is because:

- the blocks are too heavy to rest on the skin
- the number of secondary electrons, produced by interactions of the radiation beam with the lead and tray, which reach the patient is minimised (Morgan 1987, unpublished).

Shaping the beam using straight-sided blocks

A dose gradient known as the penumbra occurs at the edge of treatment beams (see Ch. 3) and around the edge of lead blocks. This is a result of the divergent nature of the radiation beam.

Because only the central ray of the beam is normal to a plane across the beam, the shadow cast by a straight-sided block depends upon its position in the field. The further the block is placed from the central axis, the larger the penumbra produced by the block (Meredith & Massey 1968). The shadow cast will have a portion of full shielding surrounded by a penumbra of unknown width.

Difficulties in defining the fully shielded area

Defining the area of full shielding within the shadow cast by the block is not routinely possible. A portal film will show the whole shadow cast but defining the area of full shielding requires complex photodensitometry.

Simulation (see Ch. 11) of leaded treatment fields using straight-sided blocks of the correct thickness gives a better indication of the area shielded by the straight-sided blocks than outlining the leaded area with solder wire. However this is not possible on all simulators as suitably designed lead trays are not always provided.

Therefore the shadow is normally accepted as being the shielded area, since only areas outside the shadow will presumably be expected to receive the full dose.

Construction of blocks

Straight-sided blocks are usually machined out of lead and they should be coated with a nontoxic material for safe handling.

To enable the blocks to be located in the lead tray when the treatment machine is used away from the vertical position, a screw may be attached to one side, which will locate in a slotted tray. Alternatively a compression lead tray may be used, in which the blocks are clamped between two perspex sheets, and the ends of the lead must be covered in a soft fabric such as felt to prevent the tray from being scratched.

Shielding using beam-shaped blocks

For more precise or complex beam shaping, where critical organs are in close proximity to areas requiring full treatment doses, for example mantles or craniospinal irradiation, the extra shadowing effect described for straight-sided blocks must be avoided by using beam-shaped blocks (Fig. 8.1).

The beam-shaped shielding blocks are constructed so that their sides are coincident with the rays in the part of the treatment field in which they are located. The shadow then thrown replicates the exact block shape and represents full shielding.

Orientation and positioning of the blocks

Accurate orientation and positioning of these shaped blocks in the radiation beam is vital to ensure that the shadow cast represents full shielding. This is best achieved if the blocks are attached to a rigid plate which is slotted into the treatment head (Fig. 8.2). Many lead trays provide a system for coding the rigid plates, so that when used with a verification system, only the correct plate in the correct orientation can be used.

Construction of the blocks

The method of construction of these blocks using low melting point alloy is widely documented (Walter et al 1982).

Care of shielding blocks

All shielding blocks are made from soft metals and are easily damaged. Damaged blocks may cast inaccurate shadows giving rise to under- or overshielded fields. Therefore it is essential that the library of straight-sided blocks routinely kept

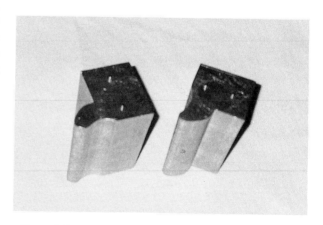

Figure 8.1 Divergent blocks with pegs to accurately locate them in a perspex plate.

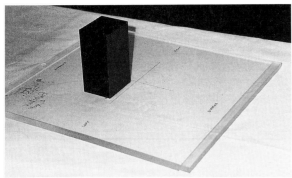

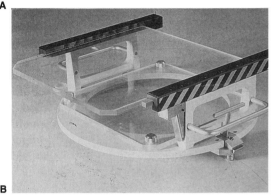

Figure 8.2 **A, B** Fixed block with coded base plate. The small drilled dip on the left of the perspex plate can only be aligned with the coding device located in the runners of the lead tray, thus preventing orientation errors. (Courtesy of Philips Medical Systems.)

on the treatment machine is regularly checked for misshapen edges, cracks or any other damage which may affect adequacy. The protective covering must remain intact to protect the radiographers handling it.

Positioning the blocks in the radiation beam

Accurate shielding is an important part of quality treatment delivery. Small discrepancies in the position of the blocks at tray level is magnified by the tray–skin distance, thus minute changes in the block position at the tray can lead to large errors particularly at extended f.s.d.s.

Manually placed blocks

If unmounted blocks are used without a fixation

system, shielding will not be accurately repeated at each treatment.

Placing blocks to a line by eye is a subjective procedure, the tendency being to position the block so that its shadow obscures the line, leading to overshielding. In addition, manual positioning of blocks is time-consuming for the radiographer particularly as many pieces of lead are used for one field. This problem can be overcome by fixed lead systems.

Fixed lead systems

Mounted blocks overcome the problem of daily variation in block position, as the blocks are mounted on a plate which is fixed in relation to the radiation beam (Fig. 8.3). There should be no play in the lead tray (Fig. 8.4) or its locating system.

The blocks can be fixed permanently to the mounting sheet. This is essential for shielding with the machine in the lateral position, but the sheet and the blocks are likely to be very heavy.

Alternatively the blocks can be individually located in the mounting sheet by a peg-and-socket system. This is only possible for set-ups where the gantry is set at zero.

Differences between machines

Where a tray with fixed blocks is interchanged between the simulator and the treatment machine, problems may occur with field symmetry about the blocks if there is any variation in tray

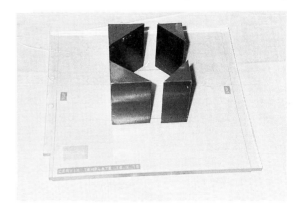

Figure 8.3 Fixed straight-sided lead for standard field shaping.

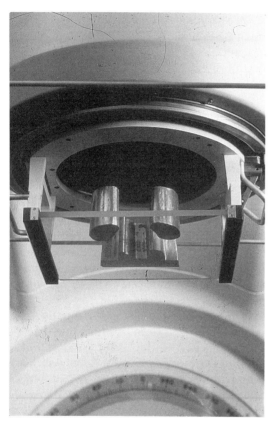

Figure 8.4 Divergent blocks fixed to perspex sheet and located in the lead tray, which in turn is located in the treatment machine head. (Courtesy of Philips Medical Systems.)

location between the two, e.g. blocks may be nearer to one edge of the field than expected. This effect may also be seen if the light/radiation beam/central axis relationships differ between the simulator and the treatment machine (see Fig. 18.8).

Similarly, because the relationships are imperfect and variable, variations in the blocked field symmetry may occur if a different collimator angle is used on the same machine, for example 0°, 180°. Variations will also occur if the patient is transferred to another machine.

Effect of shielding blocks on dosimetry

The use of a shielding block has various effects on dosimetry. The scatter conditions and ultimately the dose delivered to the patient change with the shape and size of the treatment field, so

that an output factor compensating for the reduced effective equivalent square may be required. Normal practice is that output factors are only necessary when more than one-third of the field is leaded, as smaller shielded areas make little difference to the final output.

The dosimetric effect of shielding the field down to small, and particularly to narrow, shapes is that full scatter conditions are not reached. This results in a lower dose being received near the shielding than would be expected for the overall field size. This is particularly important for the calculation of equivalent squares for irregular, long narrow fields, e.g. mantles and doglegs (Ch. 18); often this calculation is carried out using the planning computer, so that the dosimetry around the blocks can be visualised and an accurate equivalent square calculated.

Finally it is important to note that scatter and penumbra effects around the blocks result in up to 20% of the prescribed dose (for parallel opposed pairs) being received by tissue in the shielded area, even with beam-shaped blocks. This is particularly significant when cord shielding is applied (see Fig. 18.6).

Multileaf collimators

Multileaf collimators facilitate customised beam shaping without the use of lead blocks. The detail of the design of this collimating system varies between manufacturers. The multileaf collimators described are manufactured by Philips Medical Systems (Fig. 8.5) and are contained within a normal-sized treatment machine head.

One of the pairs of collimators is split into two, the lower half of each collimator is then sliced, creating 40 pairs of leaves. The leaves are mounted directly opposite each other in the treatment head, and can move to any position across the radiation beam.

Each leaf casts a shadow 1 cm wide at the isocentre, and thus a field size of up to 40 cm at 100 cm f.s.d. can be treated. The position of the leaf is controlled and monitored by a dedicated computer.

Complex tumour-shaped beams can be created (see Ch. 23) around the tumour (Fig. 8.6). This method of beam shaping can potentially speed

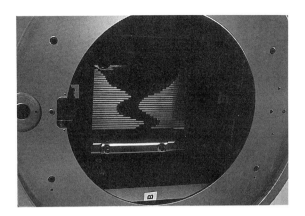

Figure 8.5 The multileaf collimators within the treatment head. (Courtesy of Philips Medical Systems.)

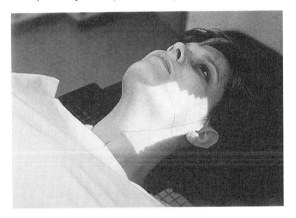

Figure 8.6 A shaped field using multileaf collimators. (Courtesy of Varian Oncology Systems.)

up the process of treatment delivery as few fields will then require the manual positioning of shielding blocks.

Shaping the beam using multileaf collimators

There are two ways in which the required field shape can be defined.

The shape library. A set of predefined field shapes is provided by the manufacturer. The predefined shapes can be manipulated to produce the desired field shape. This system restricts the potential of the system slightly but many shapes in routine use can be created.

Customised beam shaping. Customised beam shaping requires complicated planning of the leaf positions to fit the treatment volume drawn on the planning film. This method permits an almost infinite number of beam shapes from which a shape can be found to fit the shape of the tumour to be treated (Hounsell et al 1992).

MODIFYING THE SHAPE OF THE ISODOSE CURVES

The shape of the isodose curves of a radiation beam can be modified by the introduction of an absorber into part or all of the beam. The purpose of this is to modify the isodose curves to obtain a distribution more suitable for certain applications. Examples include the use of the linac beam flattening filter, customised cervix filters used in conjunction with brachytherapy (see Ch. 23) and wedge filters.

Use of wedge filters

The dosimetry across the beam may be graduated so that a higher dose is delivered at one edge of the beam than at the other, by insertion of a wedge-shaped absorber into the beam. The resultant wedge-shaped isodose (see Fig. 7.6A) can be used in a number of ways, for example:

- to compensate for the missing tissue of an oblique skin surface
- to ensure an even dose distribution where multiple beams converge, e.g. multifield isocentric plans (see Fig. 15.8).

Definition of the wedge angle

The wedge angle is defined as the slope of the 50% isodose curve relative to the original plane (Fig. 8.7). A linac can be provided with a range of wedge-shaped beam absorbers which will provide a number of standard wedge angles; these are usually 15°, 30°, 45° and 60°. Other wedge angles can be achieved by manufacturing custom wedges on site. These could include half wedges which only wedge half the field, and are sometimes useful for tissue compensation in head and neck treatments (see Ch. 17).

Fixed angle wedges

There are two basic types of fixed wedges in use, either located within the treatment head (internal

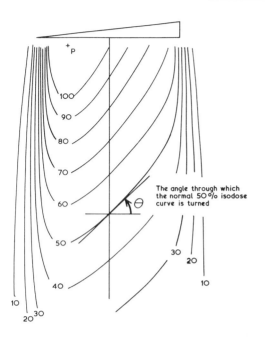

Figure 8.7 A wedged isodose curve demonstrating the measurement of wedge angle. (Reproduced from Walter et al 1982.)

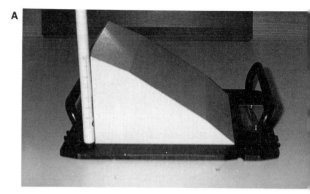

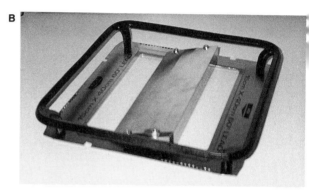

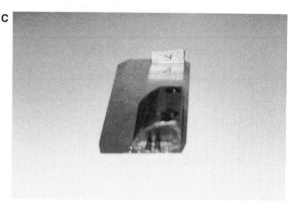

Figure 8.8 A comparison of **A, B** the external wedges, with **C** the internal wedge, demonstrates the advantages of the latter in terms of size and weight.

wedges), or fixed to the outside (external wedges). As a result of the divergent nature of the beam, internal wedges have the advantage of being much smaller and lighter than the equivalent external wedge (Fig. 8.8).

Care of fixed wedges

The shape of the wedges and their position in the treatment head is critical for correct dosimetry. Wedges in regular use are prone to wear and tear and accidental damage. It is important that they are inspected daily for damage to the wedge shape or insecure coupling to the wedge plate. Any alterations or repairs should be followed by calibration to ensure the wedge is in the correct position in the beam.

Motorised wedges

Manually loaded fixed angle wedges are now being superseded by a single wedge mounted permanently in the treatment head, on a motorised plate (Fig. 8.9). The wedge is auto-

matically inserted into the radiation beam for a number of monitor units, programmed by the radiographers.

The motorised wedge has a wedge angle of approximately 60° when inserted in the beam for the whole of the treatment field time. All other wedge angles are achieved by the wedge

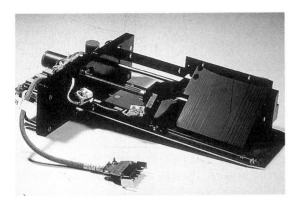

Figure 8.9 A motorised wedge with associated drive mechanism. (Courtesy of Philips Medical Systems.)

being in the beam for part of the treatment field time (Fig. 8.10),'then being automatically withdrawn for the remaining time. Variation of the proportion of the wedged to unwedged treatment field time results in different effective wedge angles. Calculation of the effective wedge angle is well documented (Tatcher 1970; Mansfield et al 1974).

Advantages of motorised wedges

- They are not handled by the radiographers and therefore less likely to be damaged.
- There is a health and safety gain for patients and staff, since the wedges are not handled.
- Treatment set-up times are reduced.
- Greater flexibility of wedge angle.
- The field-defining light is not obscured when the wedge is in position.

Calculation of the wedged treatment time

When a motorised wedge is used it is no longer meaningful to annotate a wedge angle. Instead the percentage of treatment field time to be wedged may be given in the form of a factor, e.g. 0.765. The overall number of monitor units for the field are multiplied by this factor to calculate the number of wedged monitor units.

This information is then entered into the microprocessor of the treatment machine in one of two ways:

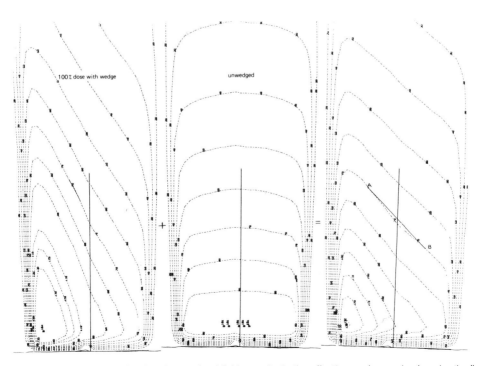

Figure 8.10 The summation of the wedged and unwedged fields results in the effective wedge angle given by the line AB. (Courtesy of Philips Medical Systems.)

1. The total number of monitor units for the whole field is entered plus the number of these to be wedged.

2. The field is split into two distinct segments, the number of monitor units for the unwedged and wedged segment being entered separately. The total number of monitor units for the field is a summation of the two.

The treatment field is delivered in two portions with a pause while the wedge is automatically withdrawn.

Creating wedged fields using the collimators

This is an alternative method of providing an infinitely variable wedge angle by programming one diaphragm to travel across the beam during the exposure (Leavitt et al 1988). The collimator is open for longest at the field edge which corresponds to the thin end of the wedge (Fig. 8.11), thus creating a dose gradient across the beam similar to that produced by a wedge.

This system has the potential advantage of being able to produce wedged fields of different profiles permitting optimisation of the treatment plan to an individual patient.

The speed of treatment delivery will depend upon the diaphragm travelling across the beam during the exposure. At present the radiation beam switches off whilst the diaphragm is in transit, prolonging the treatment times.

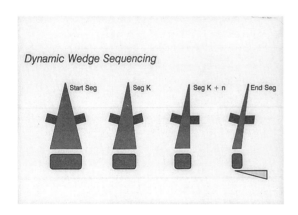

Figure 8.11 The dynamic collimator movement required to produce a wedged field. (Courtesy of Varian Oncology Systems.)

Using the system for different types of isodose shaping

More complex isodose shaping is potentially possible using the moving diaphragms, e.g. correction of dose inhomogeneity. However, this will require complex planning and treatment machine control.

Modifying the relationship of isodose curves with tissue shape using bolus

Bolus is material which has properties equivalent to tissue when irradiated. It is used widely in practice but its functions fall into one of the following two categories.

Compensating for missing tissue or irregular tissue shape. For this purpose it must be possible to mould the bolus and fill the tissue space. Lincolnshire and Spier's bolus, loosely packed in polythene bags, is suitable as the bolus bags take the shape of the skin surface and are easily smoothed to achieve a flat surface incident to the radiation beam.

Modifying doses at the skin surface and at depth. A specified thickness of bolus can be applied to the skin to alter the dose received at depth in the tissue and on the skin surface. A typical example of this is the application of a defined thickness of bolus to a chest wall for breast treatment, to increase the skin dose. The thickness of bolus applied is dependent on the skin dose required and the angle of incidence of the treatment beams. For example if oblique 6 MV beams are used for a tangential pair, 1 cm of bolus effectively becomes 1.5 cm, i.e. 'full bolus' (Fig. 8.12).

When full bolus is applied, bolus thickness equal to the depth of the build-up region removes the skin-sparing effect of a megavoltage X-ray beam.

Pliable bolus

Suitable materials must be pliable and easily moulded to the skin surface, but retain a constant thickness. Examples include paraffin gauze and 'Superflab' – a pliable non-sticky plastic gel (expensive).

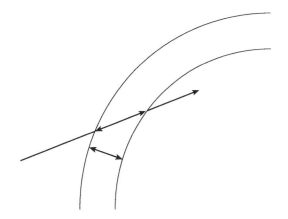

Figure 8.12 The effect of beam obliquity on effective bolus thickness.

Modifying the isodose curves using a remote tissue compensator

Tissue compensators are used to correct the isodoses for tissue shape and/or correct for dose inhomogeneity (Fig. 8.13). They can replace a wedge or bolus and have the advantage of being custom-made for the patient's shape (Fig. 8.14).

Constructed of aluminium blocks (Walter et al 1982) mounted on a base plate, tissue compensators are sited in the treatment head and thus the skin-sparing effect of megavoltage is retained.

Rigid bolus

For smaller areas which do not required the bolus to be moulded over the skin, perspex can be used. The use of perspex bolus is advantageous for electron set-ups because it is transparent. Since the f.s.d. for most electron fields (see Ch. 21) is 95 cm, so that the movements of the couch are not isocentric (see Ch. 9), inaccuracies may arise for aligning angled fields when opaque bolus is inserted.

Positioning bolus in the treatment beam

To ensure that the required dose is received by the patient, bolus of the right thickness must be placed correctly. Therefore bolus requirements must be clearly documented in the setting-up instructions of the treatment card. When using bolus to compensate for missing tissue, the whole of the bolussed area must be level with the point on the patient where the f.s.d. is set, to ensure dose homogeneity.

Where bolus is used to reduce the skin-sparing effect, the bolus does not necessarily need to touch the skin all over the bolussed area as the scatter is of sufficiently high energy to be unaffected by an air gap. However, it is important that the bolus is of uniform thickness. Some bolus materials are easily squashed and must be carefully stored and measured at regular intervals.

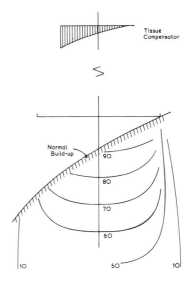

Figure 8.13 Tissue compensation using a remote tissue compensator to maintain the skin-sparing effect of a megavoltage X-ray beam. (Reproduced from Walter et al 1982.)

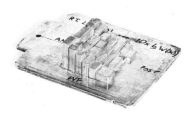

Figure 8.14 A tissue compensator with clear labelling indicating required positioning and orientation. (Reproduced from Walter et al 1982.)

Orientation of tissue compensators

The correct orientation of compensators requires a good communication system between planning and the mould room. Ideally it should only be possible to position the compensator in one orientation in the treatment head. Where this is not possible the compensator should be clearly labelled.

Further uses for tissue compensators

More recently tissue compensators have been used to change the intensity of the beam across the treatment field. The aim is to deliver a higher daily dose to the tumour than to the surrounding tissue, thus delivering the boost dose to the tumour at the same time. This treatment technique is known as the 'concomitant boost' (see Ch. 23).

REFERENCES AND FURTHER READING

Hounsell A R, Sharrock P J, Moore C J, Shaw A J, Wilkinson J M, Williams P C 1992 Computer-assisted generation of multi-leaf collimator settings for conformal therapy. British Journal of Radiology 65: 321–326

Leavitt D D, Martin M, Moeller J H, Lee W L 1990 Dynamic wedge field techniques through computer controlled collimator motion and dose delivery. Medical Physics 17: 87–91

Mansfield et al 1974 Experimental verification of a method for varying the effective angle of wedge filters. American Journal of Radiology 120: 699–702

Marrs J E, Hounsell A R, Wilkinson J M 1993 The efficacy of lead shielding in megavoltage radiotherapy. The British Journal of Radiology 66: 140–144

Meredith W J, Massey J B 1968 Fundamental physics of radiology. Wright, Bristol

Tatcher J 1970 A method for varying the effective wedge angle of wedge filters. Radiology 97: 132

Walter J, Miller H, Bomford C K 1982 A short textbook of radiotherapy, 4th edn. Churchill Livingstone, Edinburgh

9

Ancillary equipment

In order to treat the patient by using the radiation beam, he or she needs to be supported in a specific way at a particular point relative to the isocentre of the machine. This is achieved by the use of a variety of ancillary equipment, including a specially designed treatment 'couch' supplied and installed with the machine. The principles applied in positioning the patient on the couch, and treatment techniques and methods, will be covered in later chapters; here we are concerned with the use and function of ancillary equipment. It is an important subject as the effectiveness of patient set-up, and therefore treatment, depends on the methods and thought employed in the use of these devices.

The equipment cannot be perfectly accurate and accepted tolerances are defined for each parameter. Checks ensure that all equipment is operating within these limits, at commissioning and during routine quality assurance programmes. However, accuracy of operation is specified under certain conditions of use but any inaccuracy may be greatly increased when other conditions pertain. Potential sources of inaccuracy and their avoidance will become clear on applying the content of this chapter to the treatment principles which follow later.

TREATMENT MACHINE AND COUCH FEATURES

The nature of machine movements and the isocentre

Isocentrically mounted treatment machines rotate around an axis on which lies the isocentre. The isocentre is an important point, not only in relation to the specification of dose (see Chs 2 and 7), but also for 'setting up' the patient at the correct point in the treatment beam. For routine treatment techniques the isocentre is required to be at a specified point in the patient or on the surface of the patient. The design of the treatment couch and various ancillary devices influences the processes required to achieve the desired set-up. The light beam representing the radiation beam, and the cross representing the beam central axis (see Ch. 2) or beam applicators are also used in the setting-up process.

The treatment couch and its movements

Couch support systems, vertical and rotational movements

The couch is supported by a structure which allows both vertical and rotational movement. This may be a cylindrical ram (Fig. 9.1) which requires some depth of pit so that it can extend below floor level. Alternatively the support may be a pedestal structure (Fig. 9.2), attached to a rotatable floor section. For flexibility in use, a couch rotation range well in excess of 180° is required. Some models are limited to ±90° which restricts the usefulness of the treatment machine, being impractical for some types of set-up.

The range of vertical movements of the couch should be large, so that a low height is available to facilitate patient access, and for extended f.s.d. treatments. The ram type allows a lower minimum height and is less bulky, allowing more freedom for under-couch set-ups as well as complete tabletop removal and ram retraction to leave a clear floor area for special applications. Extra height should be available where long f.s.d. under-couch fields, e.g. whole trunk, are to be used. Both systems may provide this if an appropriate model is chosen; however, the ram type, although allowing more height extension, requires a deep pit which is an expensive installation feature. The specified accuracy allows that a point on the treatment couch may move up to 1 mm in any direction during a 10 cm vertical couch movement.

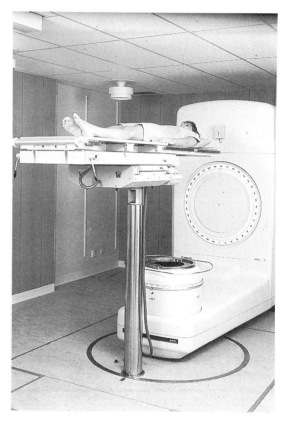

Figure 9.1 Ram-mounted treatment couch, at extended height. (Courtesy of Philips Medical Systems.)

Isocentric couch mounting and couch rotation. On linacs and cobalt units the couch is installed so that it rotates around a vertical axis which crosses the isocentre. This is termed isocentric couch mounting (Fig. 9.1), and gives simplified use of couch movements during set-up. Again, the accuracy of isocentric couch rotation is not absolute, and a movement of 2 mm in any direction may occur during a rotation of 90°.

In addition to isocentric couch rotation, some couches allow a nonisocentric rotation of the couch top about its support structure. This is occasionally useful to gain extra clearance laterally, for example to treat a limb extending out over the side of the couch. If the couch rotation (vertical) axis is not coincident with the isocentric axis, a rotational movement of the couch results in lateral/longitudinal movement of the couch with relation to the isocentre, rather than a

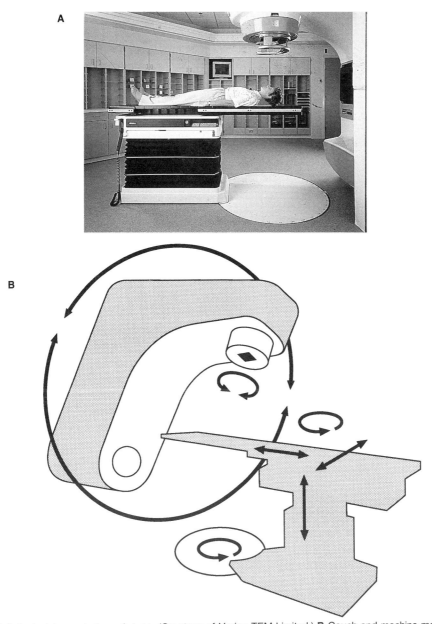

Figure 9.2 **A** A Pedestal-mounted couch type. (Courtesy of Varian-TEM Limited.) **B** Couch and machine movements.

rotation around the isocentre (Fig. 9.3). Such additional movements require constant correction in both directions during couch rotations, so that the setting-up process is unacceptably tedious for both staff and patient. This problem also occurs for some types of set-up carried out at an f.s.d. which differs from the isocentric distance, as for electron set-ups (see Ch. 21).

Couch top dimensions, lateral and longitudinal movements

The treatment couch should have motorised-movements in the vertical, longitudinal, lateral and rotational directions. A 'free float' facility for the couch top, allowing longitudinal and lateral movements, speeds the setting-up process as

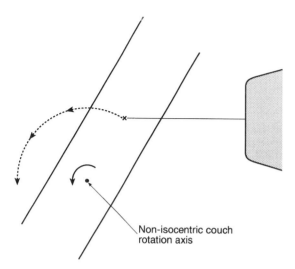

Figure 9.3   The path of movement of a point, relative to the isocentre, when nonisocentric couch rotation occurs. Lateral and longitudinal movement of the couch is required to bring the point back to the isocentre or its original position.

there is less use of relatively slow motorised movements.

The treatment couch should be versatile. It should be wide enough for a large patient, and for allowing rulers or other devices to stand adjacent to the patient. It should be narrow enough to allow a suitable clearance between it and the machine, if laterally positioned, when shielding trays or compensators are attached to the accessory mount. Good clearance is necessary to allow isocentric lateral treatment without moving the patient across the couch between fields.

The top should be long enough to accommodate tall patients for a wide range of treated sites, with a removable end section to increase the range of uses. A detachable headrest at the end of the couch is useful for treating posterior oblique fields on a patient lying supine. However, to use this to full advantage, for set-ups such as a superior head field with the gantry lateral and the couch turned through 90°, the extent of the couch travel in the longitudinal direction becomes critical for achieving the required treatment distance setting (Fig. 9.4).

The couch should not be free to move in any direction once locked. However, since this is rarely the case, radiographers should avoid leaning or knocking against it after set-up.

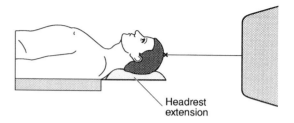

Figure 9.4   The longitudinal movement range of the couch should allow an f.s.d. treatment to be set on a patient positioned on the extremity of the couch, or on a headrest extension.

The effect of couch top sag, tilt or flex

The couch top should be rigid and flat, and have minimal sag or flexing when various weights are placed on it, remaining horizontal in both directions.

Lateral tilt. A couch top with a tilt in the lateral direction leads to various treatment discrepancies, for example in techniques using lateral beams which are expected to travel horizontally through the patient, i.e. parallel with the surface plane of the couch (Fig. 9.5).

Longitudinal tilt or flex. A longitudinal tilt results in different types of discrepancy, some of which can be overcome with knowledge and cunning. There are two effects, firstly that the patient may not be exactly horizontal in the beam in the longitudinal direction (Fig. 9.6). However, the degree of tilt is small compared with the average

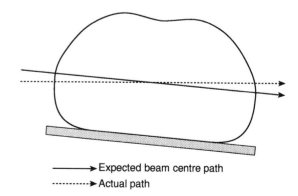

Figure 9.5   Where the couch has a lateral tilt, the beams will not follow the planned path through the patient unless the patient is rotated.

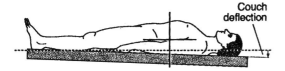

Figure 9.6 If the couch top flexes with patient weight, the patient is not horizontal and the height of the couch registered on the readout may not be the height of the patient at the point of interest.

length of a body site requiring treatment, and the general trend of the tilt will be similar on a diagnostic or simulation unit used in planning (the significance of this will become clear in later chapters), so that the effect is likely to be negligible for many treatments.

The main problem then is that of establishing the exact height of the patient/couch surface, since most couch height scales or display readings do not take account of couch sag or flexing. This problem will be further discussed in Chapter 13.

Couch sections, construction and sag effects. Special, less dense, top sections, which allow treatment through the couch should be available. These are often provided as window sections with a 'tennis racquet' type of webbing, overlaid with a thin layer of plastic material (mylar). These sections may be 60 cm long, the full width of the couch (Fig. 9.7) and with an all-round supporting frame. There are also substantial fixed lateral couch support bars, or supporting arms, which can be swung from the lateral to the central

couch position. These are called C-arm sections (Fig. 9.8) and give more flexibility since a fixed supporting frame can obstruct some types of set-up. The C-arm can be moved as required out of the beam path.

Some window sections are half the couch width and 25–30 cm long. These may be of the same 'tennis racquet' construction but with a central couch bar to support the patient, and they allow unobstructed treatment of oblique fields well below 90° (Fig. 9.7), but the section frame itself obstructs fields at or near 90°.

Other types of couch have various sections, any one or more of which can be removed, leaving a thin mylar covering to support the patient. This, like the tennis racquet, allows unobstructed treatment of some types of large field through a large window area (Fig. 9.9A), although it is not suitable for complex fields where precision is required (see Ch. 18). An advantage

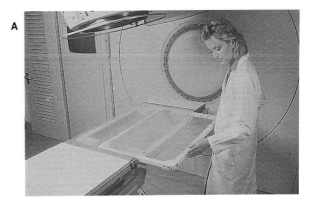

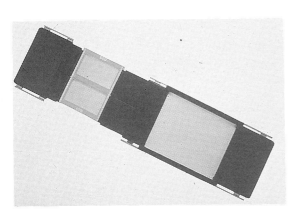

Figure 9.7 Couch top with removable 'tennis racquet' sections. (Courtesy of Varian-TEM Limited.)

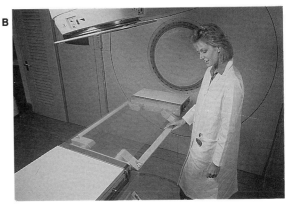

Figure 9.8 A, B Couch top with C-arm section. (Courtesy of Philips Medical Systems.)

is that sections can be removed or exchanged while the patient remains on the couch, if this should be necessary.

Tennis racquet sections or mylar windows are not rigid enough to support the patient (Fig. 9.9B) without a considerable sag (up to 16 mm for tennis racquet, 20 mm for mylar). The sag is not consistent from day to day for the same patient lying at the same point on the couch (Quinn 1992), and differs with patient position, being greatest for chest patients lying supine (Fig. 9.9C). Thus an extra support is required to improved rigidity. A large rigid area should be available on any couch top, and some of the window sections should be made rigid, so that an accurate couch height can be set when required, for isocentric treatments using under-couch oblique or vertical fields. Carbon fibre sections of reasonably uniform thickness may provide the answer.

Most couches do not have all these features, and techniques used on a particular piece of equipment must be designed according to the features available.

Equipment controls, readouts and scales

Equipment settings are carried out either by manual or manual plus computer control. Manual controls for gantry and couch movements are usually combined on one handset or stand-alone unit, and additional couch controls are often available sited on the couch itself. Controls which allow variable-speed movements, ranging from smooth fine adjustment to fast movement, are required for speedy, accurate set-ups and 'patient-friendliness'. A jerky couch is unsatisfactory (for both staff and patients!).

Well-designed mechanical scales are much easier to use than digital readouts, as they allow visualisation of the movement required. It is often necessary to reverse collimator angles between fields. For example a collimator angle several degrees from a quarter-circle angle (0°, 90°, 180°, 270°) may require reversal. With a digital readout the only information available is a number, e.g. 257, but if the scale is displayed

round the collimator covers (see Fig. 2.5), no mental addition or subtraction is required: the move can be visualised on the scale and degrees easily counted as the collimators are turned.

Movement controls

Design. The design of the controls is important for their effective use. Handsets hanging from overhead supports, or attached to the gantry (Fig. 9.10) are preferable to those attached to the foot of the couch, which are too distant from where they are used, i.e. the vicinity of the isocentre. With remote attachments, staff trip over trailing wires and must walk the length of the couch to return the handset when they need both hands free.

There must be clear and simple indications of which movements (and in which direction) are controlled by each button. Each button may be used for multiple functions by switching modes (Fig. 9.11A), or each button may have a single function (Fig. 9.11B). If the buttons are too close together or the layout is confusing, inadvertent changes of other parameters occur. The movements available should be smooth and of variable speed from slow, for fine adjustment, to fast, and should allow a precise stop at the required setting. Some movements, such as collimator setting, are more difficult to set manually if the machine is computer controlled. Two sets of controls or two handsets allow more efficient use of the equipment.

Scales and readouts

Parameter and machine settings are monitored via mechanical scales and/or digital readouts, the design and location of which vary with the machine model.

Accuracy and reliability. All equipment scales, whether analogue or digital, can be unreliable (Hoornaert et al 1993), and need to be regularly checked under exactly the same conditions in which they will be used. It is essential to have a backup scale and/or visual check using lasers and rulers where settings are critical, particularly lateral, longitudinal and vertical settings or movements of the couch.

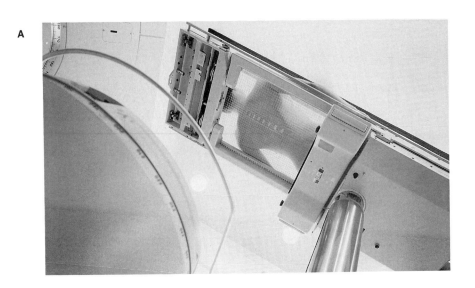

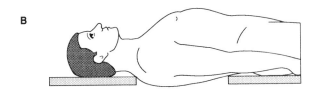

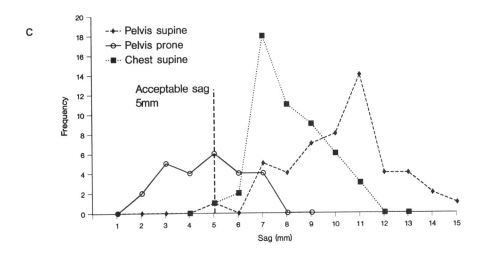

Figure 9.9   **A** Unobstructed treatment of a large field through a mylar window. (Courtesy of Philips Medical Systems.) **B** Supine patient on a tennis racquet or mylar couch panel, showing sag effect. **C** Frequency and amount of couch top sag (tennis racquet panel) with different patient positions (Quinn 1993).

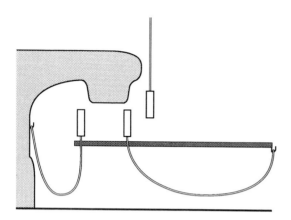

Figure 9.10   Common handset mounting points.

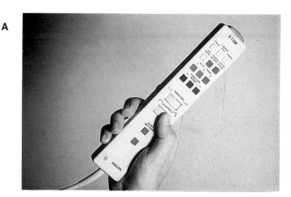

A

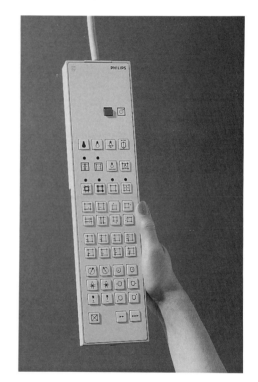

B

Angulation scales must be accurate to within ±0.5°. Any alignment inaccuracy at the isocentre which results from either a gantry or collimator angle discrepancy is magnified at increased f.s.d.s and can become significantly large (see Ch. 18).

Design issues. The controls and their readouts should be designed so that they are visible during set-up, i.e. they are not obscured by the patient in the vicinity of the required treatment position. Labels and readouts should be illuminated or fluorescent. Setting-up takes place under conditions of dimmed lighting so that field illumination can be seen on the patient surface (see Fig. 2.13).

ADDITIONAL ACCESSORY DEVICES

Lasers

Lasers are used extensively in patient positioning, and for setting the patient at the correct point in the treatment beam. They are used as a supplement to the light field and rangefinder. The parameters which are accurately defined by the lasers must be understood as a basic equipment principle. Common usage will be discussed in Chapter 13 and other specific uses throughout Section 2.

Laser crosses

The sagittal laser coincides with the overhead and lateral crosses at the isocentre only, since the

Figure 9.11   A Handset showing multifunction control button layout. **B** Handset showing single function button layout. (Courtesy of Philips Medical Systems.)

crosses are accurate only in the region of the isocentre. At 15 cm from the isocentre there may be a 2 mm discrepancy in the laser cross position, with a tendency for this to increase further from the isocentre (Fig. 9.12).

The isocentre is accurately defined by the laser crosses, which may therefore be used for setting-up purposes and as a check on the rangefinder setting. Where the rangefinder is not visible,

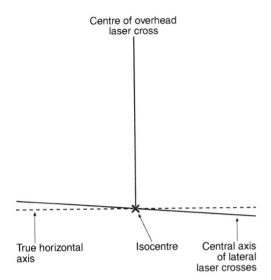

Figure 9.12 Laser crosses defining the isocentre position. The lateral crosses may not be perfectly horizontal and are therefore less accurate further from the isocentre.

lasers may be used for setting 100 cm f.s.d., i.e. the isocentre is where two orthogonal lasers meet. Laser alignment should be checked at least daily, as should other devices such as the range-finder.

Sagittal lasers

A sagittal laser is set up so that it runs straight and centrally along the longitudinal axis of the radiation beam at all couch heights. It can be used as a check on the alignment of the light field and of the centre cross which defines the centre of the light/radiation beam. The arms of this centre cross do not always run parallel to the edges of the light field (Fig. 9.13), and are not, at present, specifically required to do so. The laser is used in place of the machine centre cross in some situations. Sagittal, lateral and overhead cross lasers should be available on the CT scanner, the simulator, and the mould room and treatment units. They are used in correctly positioning the patient along a particular axis.

Immobilisation devices

For many sites the patient can be positioned well enough to ensure that treatment is given to within an accuracy of a few millimetres by using skin tattoos. For treatment of the head and neck region (where tattoos are illegal in the UK), or mobile parts such as the forearm, immobilisation equipment may be required.

The device may simply be a headrest system, with the means to hold the chin and forehead in position relative to the neck. Headrest design will be discussed in Chapter 17. There are a number of products on the market which can be moulded to the patient's shape during planning, so that an individually moulded support is produced for each patient to lie on during treatment in order to reproduce their position at each treatment. Some of these systems have products which are re-mouldable for cost-effective use, such as evacuated polystyrene bead bags. The usefulness of such devices is limited if they may obscure visibility of the treated area from some machine angles. They also tend to lose their shape early in the treatment course.

Some immobilisation devices are provided as accessory equipment, such as adjustable hand-grips, armpoles, footrests and variable angle tilting chestboards. Each can be valuable if used appropriately.

Beam direction shells

The most commonly used immobilisation device is a plastic shell made individually for each patient, fitting the treated region (Chandler 1988). Beam direction shells are used for the majority of head and neck treatments, and carry field, shielding and beam direction marks. If well constructed and well fitting, these may allow accurate treatment and spare the patient the necessity of skin marks on the head or neck. The design of the shell and its method of attachment to the headrest system influences its effectiveness (see Ch. 17). However, there is some research evidence that the use of a shell does not in itself lead to the millimetre accuracy expected. A study by Huizenga et al (1988) showed that patient movement within a head and neck cast was clearly an error source with errors of average 5 mm and 5.6 mm standard deviation (see Ch. 12).

In some centres, whole body shells are used to direct treatment to areas of the trunk, on the basis

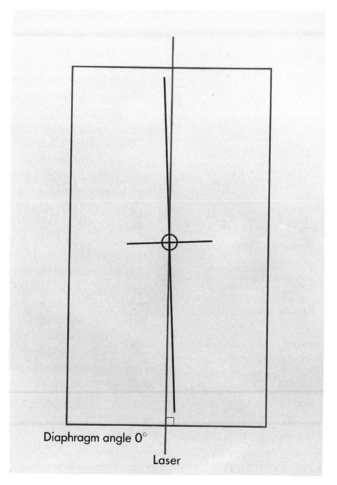

Diaphragm angle 0°

Laser

Figure 9.13 The field centre cross may not always run parallel with the field edges and is therefore not coincident with the sagittal laser except at the central axis.

that they must give greater accuracy. The authors know of little evidence to support this concept, and have established techniques to treat areas of the trunk with a high degree of accuracy without such devices. A study conducted in Belgium (Hulshof et al 1989) showed that large shells used for immobilising the trunk were unsuited to the purpose owing to distortion.

Distance setting devices

Rangefinder. The rangefinder is used to check the distance between a point on the patient's surface and the isocentre. A set-up at standard f.s.d. is achieved by moving the couch and thus the patient until the required reading of the rangefinder shows at the field centre on the skin surface (see Fig. 2.13). Where an f.s.d. treatment is given using opposed vertical fields (see Ch. 15), the couch height is adjusted to the correct rangefinder reading at the patient surface, both for overhead and under-couch fields. Where an extended f.s.d. is required the appropriate rangefinder reading is set (Fig. 9.14).

Lasers. Distance setting can also be achieved in some circumstances by using one or more lasers, since these define the isocentre position (Fig. 9.12).

Measurement. For extremely long f.s.d. techniques, such as for whole body treatments at 400

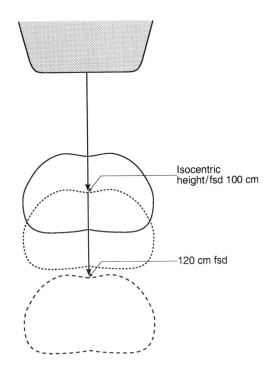

the obliquity of the scale. The rangefinder should not be projected in such a way that it traverses the lead tray, as this leads to distortion of the scale (with a perspex tray base) and necessitates removal of the tray base to set the distance accurately. This is tedious but is especially important on oblique fields or irregular surfaces where a 'standard' correction cannot be applied.

Beam direction aids

Some treatments require use of a system to help set the gantry and floor angles appropriately, so that the beam passes through the patient in the required direction and thus will exit the body at a predictable point (assuming that the patient's position is correct, see Ch. 13). One system is to mark a point on the patient's surface where the centre of a particular field should exit from the patient. This is called an exit point and may be used on beam direction shells for f.s.d. treatments. (It is not required for isocentric treatments which are directed by using a specified gantry and table angle.)

Figure 9.14 The principle of isocentric, normal f.s.d. and extended f.s.d. overhead set-ups.

cm f.s.d. with the gantry lateral, the distance beyond the isocentre can be measured along the floor of the room. A vertical rule at that distance may then be used to align the patient at the correct f.s.d., accurately enough for the purpose. The effect of a 1 cm discrepancy at 400 cm f.s.d. is much less than at 100 cm f.s.d.. Also the patient surface is irregularly shaped and an f.s.d. setting point is not specified.

Rangefinder design

The design of the rangefinder, in particular its angle of incidence or obliquity, which affects the spacing of points and numbers on the scale, is important for its accuracy in routine use. Scale points should be spaced so that 1 cm difference in f.s.d. is equivalent to a similar distance on the scale. With smaller ratios, it is difficult to set or read to the nearest millimetre. Readings also become subjective and can appear different from either side of the couch, which may be related to

Backpointers

Backpointing devices, which indicate the centre of the beam on the distal surface of the patient, are available as equipment accessories (Fig. 9.15).

Mechanical backpointers. Mechanical backpointers are cumbersome to use, and are prone to inaccuracy due to damage to the pointer, which easily becomes bent during frequent demounting. (They are mounted on to the gantry only for setting-up, and are then removed.) Where only a mechanical backpointer is available, this should

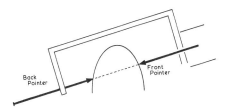

Figure 9.15 Front and backpointers as beam direction indicators. Both pointers follow the line of the beam central axis. (Reproduced from Walter et al 1982.)

be checked regularly for straightness and accuracy. This can be achieved by attaching the pointer and checking that its point aligns with the field central axis indicator, from the isocentre outwards throughout the range of movement of the pointer. If the tip of the pointer describes a circle when rotated in the holder, this indicates that the pointer is bent.

Laser backpointers. Most linacs now have integral laser backpointers which are easy and accurate to use. A single laser line intersects the lateral arm of the lateral or overhead laser cross to indicate the point of beam exit. When the field is correctly aligned on the entry side, then a backpointer is used while adjusting gantry and floor angles so that the beam exits at the specified point. In some cases, for true lateral fields, the room laser crosses can be used to check the beam exit point.

Front pointers and applicators. As an alternative to the backpointer, other devices may be used at the proximal side of the patient to indicate the field entry point (Fig. 9.15). Mechanical front pointers indicate the direction of entry of the beam, via the alignment of the pointer itself. However, a backpointer is usually needed in conjunction with a front pointer to check beam direction. Alternatively for 'direct' single fields (see Ch. 15), a flat plate normal to the central ray may be attached to the pointer for alignment with a surface on the patient. This approximates to the use of an applicator (see Ch. 4) as it also indicates the f.s.d.

A retractable graduated front pointer can be useful for checking the distance between the patient surface and the isocentre, in set-ups where the rangefinder is obstructed by the couch or accessories.

Optical front pointer. This type of front pointer may be used under certain conditions to set the gantry and floor angle. The device consists of a convex lens mounted in a plate attaching directly to the treatment head (Fig. 9.16). It is inserted into the light beam and converges it to form a light spot at a distance from the lens. (When used with f.s.d.s other than 100 cm, the spot becomes less well focused.)

A rigid reflecting surface which is normal to the

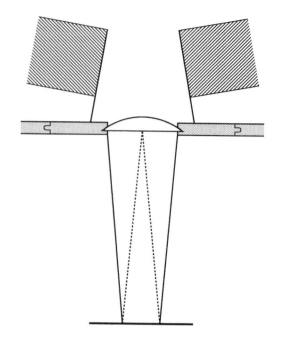

Figure 9.16 The principle of the optical front pointer device. The field light beam is converged by a lens, and reflected back to the lens from a beam direction device which is normal to the central ray.

required beam entry axis, i.e. a beam directing device attached to the patient, is positioned in the converging light beam, and the light is reflected back towards the lens. When the reflecting surface is exactly normal in both planes to the central ray, the light beam hits an opaque spot in the centre of the lens. The system can be very accurate since any small deviation in angle is doubled on reflection and the light spot moves considerably. However, any flexibility in the position of the reflecting surface during use leads to inaccuracy, as does any variation in the attachment of the device to the patient. This can be a difficult problem to overcome. The reflecting surface must also be accurately constructed and checked during the planning procedure, and damage to it during treatment necessitates reconstruction and rechecking. If used with a suitably rigid reflecting surface, this device gives an accurate indication of gantry angle and floor or couch angle setting, after the f.s.d. is set. Subsequent longitudinal or lateral movement of the couch in finally adjusting the field does not necessitate reusing the device, as would be the case with a backpointer. This is because the optical plate is effectively used at the isocentre, whereas a back- pointer is used at a distance from the isocentre and its use is therefore affected by couch movement (see Fig. 9.3).

REFERENCES AND FURTHER READING

Chandler M 1988 Behind the mask (A radiotherapy mould room guide). Change, Stoke-on-Trent

Hoornaert M Th, Van Dam J, Vynckier S, Bouiller A 1993 A dosimetric quality audit of photon beams by the Hospital Physicist Association. Radiotherapy and Oncology 28: 37–43

Huizenga H, Levendag P C, De Porre P M Z R, Visser A G 1988 Accuracy in radiation field alignment in head and neck cancer: a prospective study. Radiotherapy and Oncology 11: 181–187

Hulshof M, Vanuytsel L, Van den Bogaert W, Van derSchueren E 1989 Localization errors in mantle-field irradiation for Hodgkin's disease. International Journal of Radiation Oncology, Biology and Physics 17: 679–683

Quinn G 1993 An investigation into radiotherapy treatment couch sag. Radiography Today 59: 9–12

Walter J, Miller H, Bomford C K 1982. A short textbook of radiotherapy, 4th edn. Churchill Livingstone, Edinburgh

10

Computers in radiotherapy

Computers have had a significant impact on the processes involved in the planning and delivery of radiotherapy treatment in the last decade. Tumour definition and imaging, tumour localisation (see Ch. 11), treatment planning (see Ch. 14) and treatment delivery have benefited from computer-aided advances.

Radiographers are now required to have some computer or keyboard skills to operate most of the equipment in modern radiotherapy departments, as the radiographer–machine interface is commonly a keyboard with a few additional specialised function keys (Fig. 10.1).

These technological advances have necessitated a change ·in the patterns of work for all radiographers. The need for specialist staff to advance technical practice (see Ch. 26) is vital if radiotherapy is to provide the maximum benefit from the technology afforded by the current generation of equipment.

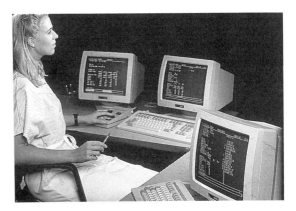

Figure 10.1   VDUs, keyboards and specialised function keys which provide the radiographer–linac interface. (Courtesy of Philips Medical Systems.)

COMPUTER-CONTROLLED LINACS

The advent of microprocessor-controlled, and subsequently computer-controlled, linacs has resulted in many additional features, including asymmetric/independent jaws (see Ch. 2), automated wedges and dynamic diaphragms (see Ch. 8), computer-assisted set-up and multileaf collimators (see Ch. 8). These features have facilitated refinements in technical practice such as customised tumour and isodose shaping.

Historically most linacs were similar in operation and required little staff training. However, complex and manufacturer-specific operating methods now require extensive radiographer training. The associated machine servicing is also complex and many linacs now have some fault analysis software to hasten repair.

COMPUTER VERIFICATION

Computer verification can be defined as a machine parameter monitoring system. Radiotherapy treatment techniques, using all available technology, require the setting of complex machine parameters. Repeated manual setting of the latter can lead to errors. Computer verification aims to reduce machine parameter errors by comparing each daily set-up with a verification prescription previously entered into the machine.

The functions of computer verification

The details of the functions of computer verification are listed below, but it is of interest to note that computer verification is essentially a complex 'select and confirm' system which:

- provides a monitoring system to minimise the risks of machine parameter error
- facilitates the computer-assisted set-up function
- produces a hard copy of the daily treatment conditions for each exposure delivered
- limits the total dose delivered to a patient, to that entered into the patient database.

System components

There is a wide range of systems on the market as each manufacturer has developed their system in isolation. Furthermore, at present each system can only be used on a linac manufactured by the same company, so it is impossible to use only one system when linacs from more than one manufacturer are installed in the department.

Some systems have a fixed format and convoluted input processes, whilst others provide a very flexible system with the opportunity to choose the format and even to customise the language. Customising a system such as this may seem daunting at first, but in the long term there are considerable advantages. These include a linac that uses local department terminology, and the option to use as many of the system functions as you choose.

Hardware

The fine detail of the system hardware will depend on the manufacturer and degree of integration with the linac controls. However, the list below outlines the basic components:

- Data storage system, usually a hard disk, for the storage of patient data sets. This may be integrated into the linac control (Fig. 10.2).
- Printer to produce hard copies of patient data sets and daily ledgers (Fig. 10.3).
- Keyboard and VDU. This may have integrated switching on/off keys (Fig. 10.1).

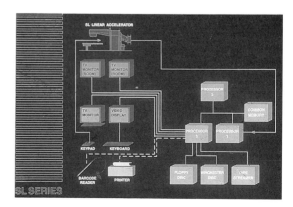

Figure 10.2 A schematic diagram of integrated computer verification and linac computer control. (Courtesy of Philips Medical Systems.)

- Bar code reader for patient identification (Fig. 10.3).
- Remote access terminal; of particular importance if the switching-on terminal is combined with the verification VDU.

An outline of the verification process

Despite the variation in system details the processes involved in preparation of patient data sets and treatment verification are essentially the same.

1. A menu option will permit patient data input.
2. Machine parameters and dose details are entered into the system, either at a terminal or directly from the first patient set-up.
3. Subsequent verification of set-up is achieved by recalling the patient data set from the patient file.
4. The set parameters are compared with the patient data set.
5. If the set parameters match those of the patient data set then the linac can be switched on. If any parameter is incorrect then the discrepancy will be highlighted and the linac will not switch on. Correction of the discrepancy, or overriding

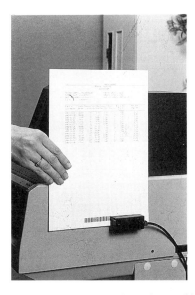

Figure 10.3 A printer with bar code reader provided for the generation of patient data set hard copies and daily ledgers. (Courtesy of Philips Medical Systems.)

the system, will allow the exposure to be delivered.

6. On completion of all the treatment fields a summary of the treatment may be printed on the patient's verification sheet.
7. The next patient may then be recalled from the database.

Tolerances and parameter checks

The process of verification rests on the ability of the system to compare the set machine parameters to those entered into the patient data set and flag up any discrepancies.

The reproducibility of the machine parameters from day to day depends on the treatment technique employed. Thus the discrepancies permitted by the system, between the set and entered value of each parameter, may need to be different for each technique employed in the department.

A set of permitted discrepancies for all the parameters for a given set-up are defined at customising and are known as a tolerance. Up to 16 tolerances may be provided, but in practice not all will necessarily be used. The development of a workable tolerance table is vital for successful use of computer verification. It is important to get a balance between tolerances which are sufficiently tight to reduce errors, and parameter tolerances which are too tight for the set-up and thus cripple the patient throughput. This leads to radiographer frustration and excessive use of the system override function, which totally defeats the purpose of the system. Changes in treatment techniques will require regular tolerance updates. A formal schedule for tolerance review is a vital component of good practice.

Computer-assisted set-up

This feature takes the process of computer verification a step further. The linac will automatically set the parameters defined in the prescription entered to the linac when the radiographer presses a single button on the handset.

At first sight this would seem the ideal way to reduce parameter errors to zero, but in practice this has not been found to be the case. If patient data set errors are undetected, because no cross-checks are routinely carried out, the very errors the system is designed to minimise are repeated daily. At worst this could result in a serious radiation incident. The problem arises from a subtle change in the role of the radiographer and the success of such a system depends on radiographers changing their practice (Short 1992).

Systems of work, computer verification and assisted set-up

Historically the treatment card and plan have always been the primary source of information for the treatment set-up, and radiographers refer to the plan to obtain information about machine parameters and patient position. As computer-assisted set-up regulates most of the parameters the radiographer may not need to refer to the plan for information. However, patient data set errors will go undetected, unless a system of work is devised which highlights the change in the role of the radiographer, i.e. from setting parameters, to cross-checking with the plan parameters set by the machine. Furthermore the routine checks applied to a treatment card must also be applied to a patient data set.

It is advantageous to have devised and documented a system of work prior to the commencement of clinical treatment delivery. This system should form part of the local rules for the linac. Updates and revisions in practice are often required in the first months of clinical use. However, once the teething problems are ironed out, computer-assisted set-up and treatment verification enhance patient throughput and error reduction.

Training for computer-controlled and verified linacs

Although training is more generally discussed in Chapter 26, it is necessary to outline specific training needs for computer-controlled and verified linacs here. The training programmes offered by equipment manufacturers detail the mechan-

ics of the verification system. This working knowledge of the system is really just the beginning of the process of developing a safe system of work. Thus details of the staff training programme employed for computer-controlled and verified linacs are the remit of radiotherapy managers. It is important to note that the future efficiency of the linac depends on the quality of training the staff receive, the organisation (see Ch. 26) of the staff and whether a system specialist is appointed.

Outlined below is a specimen training programme.

1. 6 months prior to clinical use a clinical specialist is appointed.
2. Clinical specialist and another appointed member of staff undergo manufacturer training programme.
3. If necessary other departments using the system are visited, for help with system development.
4. Set out a system of work and document this. At this stage set up a multidisciplinary forum to discuss technical developments if necessary.
5. Produce a manual detailing the proposed methods of use of the linac.
6. Devise a programme for staff training. It is often helpful to include some form of informal assessment.
7. Begin with a small number of patients and only the two radiographers who have developed the system of work. (Allow time for continued system development at this stage.)
8. When the system of work is proven to be effective increase the staffing to three.
9. Commence staff training, once a minimum level of competence is achieved then increase the staffing to four.
10. The clinical specialist will be permanently assigned to the linac whilst others take turns for training. Initially staff will require a minimum of 6 months if training is to give them the required depth of knowledge.

The time spent training the staff must be regarded as an investment which will reap returns of high patient throughput and low error rate.

NETWORKS AND DATA TRANSFER

Data input takes a considerable amount of radiographer time and, if no remote terminal is available, a considerable amount of linac time. Furthermore there is the problem of errors resulting from transcription of information from one system to another (Leunens et al 1992). It is therefore important to consider the number of times data is transferred in the system of work and to minimise this number.

To this end manufacturers are working towards the paperless department, where data is transferred from simulation and planning directly to the linac. These systems are known as networks; the block diagram shown in Figure 10.4 demonstrates the network links required for such systems.

Advantages of a network system

- Reduction of input errors.

- Reduction of radiographer time spent transcribing data.

- Transfer of patient data sets from one linac to another in the event of breakdown etc. Complicated treatment techniques may be transferred with less risk of set-up error.

- Permits transfer of highly complex treatment parameters which could not be input manually, for example the leaf positions for multileaf collimators.

Disadvantages of a network system

- The need to completely redesign systems of work.

- Considerable training implications.

- Systems unique to each manufacturer do not communicate with each other.

- At present there is no single network system which will link equipment from different manufacturers.

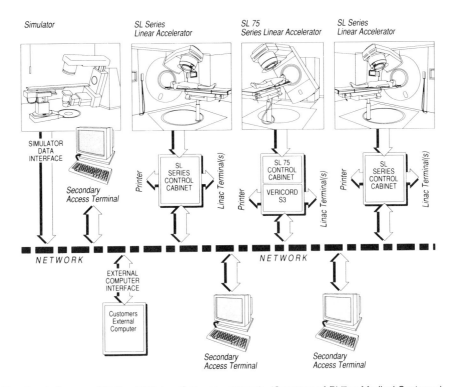

Figure 10.4   Functional diagram of Philips RTNet radiotherapy network. (Courtesy of Philips Medical Systems.)

Future considerations

To facilitate the complex treatment techniques demanded by modern radiotherapy, treatment data will have to be transferred via networks. The role of the radiographer will be to check the validity of the data rather than data input. Comprehensive radiographer training programmes will be required to ensure an effective transition to the new methods of work demanded by these systems.

COMPUTERS AND SERVICE MANAGEMENT

Computer systems are increasingly useful for radiotherapy administration and information generation, as well as in workload management, treatment planning and delivery. The above data can be generated almost as a by-product of a system used for patient booking and scheduling. Linked to an appropriately used clinical information system, this can provide information for use in audit and research.

The number of tasks for radiographers (see Ch. 25) may be reduced via direct links from the simulator or planning department to each linac. For example, there is a reduction in the number of repetitive manual arithmetic checking tasks in the preparation of treatments. However, any such system must have an associated human checking process designed to ensure data validity.

The usefulness of any system depends on three related factors:

1. how easy it is to use
2. how well its capabilities match the needs of the department

3. how well it is used.

Incomplete or inaccurate data is at best useless, and can be dangerously misleading, either in treatment-related tasks, or when used as a basis for management. The security of data, especially patient data, must be ensured by access codes and systems of use.

Some functions of a patient management system are outlined below.

Patient booking and diary system

Computer-generated prediction of the number of machine spaces available, and the times of these on future dates, are available as an electronic diary. Patients may be scheduled to start treatment on a particular date, then the rest of their treatments and appointments are automatically booked and recorded in the system. A printed list of the patients booked for a particular unit can be generated for each day if required. Confirmation of attendance and the type of treatment/exposures given can be entered, thus generating workload statistics etc. Lists of patients on treatment or finishing treatment can be produced. The timing of events, including start and finish times and exposure intervals, can also be recorded if the system can be linked to the treatment unit control via a gateway.

Patient diary and letters

The bookings made can be printed out as a diary sheet for the individual patient. As he/she moves through the booked events, the appropriate letters and follow-up procedures can be generated by the system.

REFERENCES AND FURTHER READING

Bleehen N M et al 1991 Quality assurance in radiotherapy. Report of a Working Party. Standing Subcommittee on Cancer of the Standing Medical Advisory Committee
Blue Book 1991 Radiation oncology in integrated cancer management. Report of the inter-Society Council for Radiation Oncology (USA)
Horiot J C, Johansson K A, Gonzalez D G et al 1986 Quality assurance control in the EORTC co-operative group of Radiotherapy: 1. Assessment of radiotherapy staff and

equipment. Radiotherapy and Oncology 6: 275–284
Leunens G, Verstraete J, Van den Bogaert W, Van Dam J, Dutreix A, Van der Schueren E 1992 Human errors in data transfer during the preparation and delivery of radiation treatment affecting the final result: 'garbage in, in garbage out'. Radiotherapy and Oncology 23: 217–222
Short C A 1992 The safe use of computers in treatment delivery. Radiography Today 58: 19

11

Imaging and radiotherapy

Imaging modalities are increasingly important in radiotherapy planning and in treatment delivery. Prior to treatment planning, the patient may have undergone imaging with conventional X-ray or computerised tomography (CT), magnetic resonance imaging (MRI), ultrasound or radioisotope scans to diagnose and stage their disease. Subsequently, specially set-up CT or MRI scanners may be used to localise the disease and provide information for direct use in treatment planning.

A treatment simulator is used for checking proposed treatments. During treatment special films and/or cassettes are used to produce portal films for retrospective verification and checking treatment field placement. Digital portal imaging devices are available to provide real-time image verification of field positioning during treatment. Aspects of these which are relevant to treatment planning or delivery will be outlined.

The principles and role of conventional radiography

Images of the patient tissues are produced on film (Fig. 11.1A) or on a fluoroscopy screen. Conventional diagnostic X-ray films (Fig. 11.1B) are used in the diagnosis and staging of disease, rather than in the treatment planning process. Xeroradiography (using dry paper and 'reversed' images, rather than film) is used for mammography to detect and localise breast tumours (Fig. 11.2).

Image quality and feature enhancement

Using a conventional X-ray machine, an image is produced which reflects the densities of tissue structures through which the beam has passed,

A

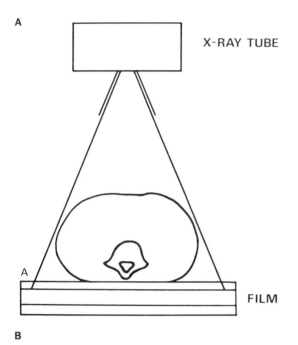

X-RAY TUBE

A

FILM

B

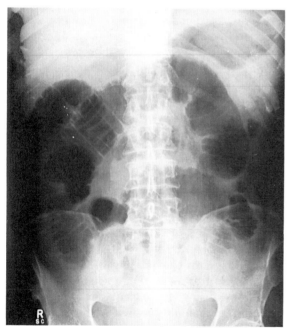

Figure 11.1 **A** The relationship of the X-ray film to the patient and the X-ray source. **B** A plain diagnostic radiograph of the abdomen. (Reproduced from Dixon & Dugdale 1988.)

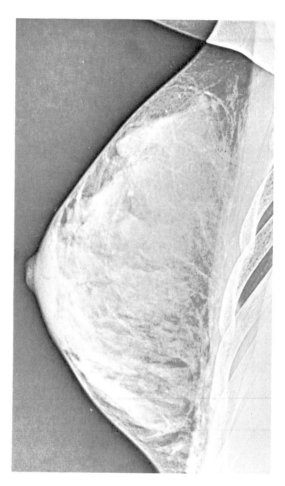

Figure 11.2 A Xeroradiograph of the breast, showing a carcinoma. (Reproduced from Dixon & Dugdale 1988.)

as differing degrees of film blackening. The image will appear blacker where more radiation is transmitted through the patient and reaches the film, so that bone and soft tissue can be differentiated (Fig. 11.3). The X-ray energy may be increased for greater transmission through larger patients to achieve a suitable image.

The contrast of features within the image may be changed by varying the beam energy (at around 100 kV, a small change in energy gives a large change in the relative absorption in bone and soft tissue because the level of attenuation varies with the atomic number of the absorber; see Walter et al 1982). The relative absorption in the different tissues is unaltered by changes in beam intensity, but an increase in the tube current or time (milliampere-seconds, mAs) intensifies the degree of blackening across all features on the image.

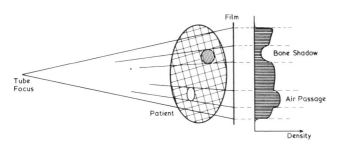

Figure 11.3   The variation in film density from X-rays reaching the film after passing through tissue structures of differing densities within the patient. (Reproduced from Walter et al 1982.)

Digital imaging systems

In computerised digital imaging systems, the image is made up of a number of units of information, called pixels (similar in effect to the dots on newsprint). With a three-dimensional system the unit is a voxel. The image quality is improved with a larger number of pixels per cm². Where the pixel size is 1 mm × 1 mm, any measurement made on the image via the software cannot be accurate to less than 1 mm.

Image enhancement. With digital images, sophisticated means of image manipulation are available. The contrast within the image can be enhanced after the initial image acquisition so that an optimum view is produced. Black and white images feature a number of shades of grey (grey scale) which give definition to structures on the image. The computer facility allows adjustment of the range of greys on the image to change the contrast and highlight particular types of tissue, so that the structures of interest are viewed more clearly. Similarly, colour systems allow choice and manipulation of colours in the image.

The nature and role of computerised tomography (CT)

Computerised tomography scanners are specialised machines in which an X-ray source and detectors spin in a full circle round the patient during the imaging of one tissue slice (Fig. 11.4A). The X-rays reaching the detectors are summated by the computer and converted to record electron densities within the tissue slice

traversed. These images are particularly useful for tumour staging and localisation: normal and diseased tissue have different appearances on images, so that even small tumours are detectable. Each type of tissue can be differentiated using CT data, and soft tissue structures can be clearly seen (Fig. 11.4B).

Images of several slices can be reconstructed by the computer into a three-dimensional image giving a great deal of accurate clinical information, which can be displayed as hard copy or electronic scan data. Whether or not a radical treatment plan can be made depends on the extent and spread of the tumour. Following CT detection of more advanced disease than was clinically estimated, the patient may be judged unsuitable for radical therapy. Patients are therefore more likely to receive therapy appropriate to the true stage of their disease following CT investigation.

In order to use CT images to plan treatment, the images must be produced under conditions valid for the purpose. The scan conditions require that:

• The curved CT table top must be fitted with a flat insert (removable for diagnostic scans) to simulate a treatment table.

• The image produced must not be distorted (diagnostic scans may be), so the equipment must be adjusted to give a truly proportional image.

• There must be a facility for taking 'slices' (sectional images) every 1 cm or less through the region of interest (see Ch. 14).

• The scan time must be fast to ensure that the patient is unlikely to move during imaging.

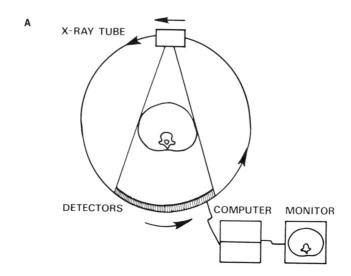

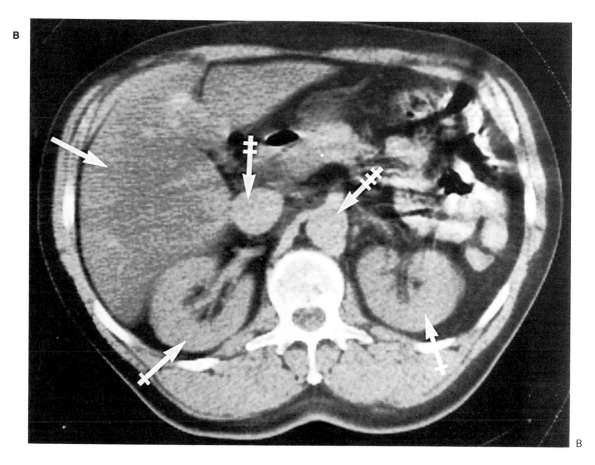

Figure 11.4 A The principle of computerised tomography. **B** A CT cross-section of the abdomen. (Reproduced from Dixon & Dugdale 1988.)

• Patients must not be scanned while holding a deep breath, as anatomical structures will then differ in position from treatment conditions, where normal breathing takes place. (Using surface marks put on at CT scans with breathholding, simulator volume verification has shown centring discrepancies of up to 4 cm.)

• Normal diagnostic preparation of the patient which distorts the anatomy from its normal position or size, e.g. induction of high fluid levels, must not be used for planning scans.

CT units which can provide the appropriate scanning conditions are used to provide three-dimensional patient information for direct use in radiotherapy planning. Tumour volume determination has been shown to be better with CT than with conventional X-ray images, by comparison of both methods within the same series of patients (Rothwell et al 1983). However, CT imaging is limited to the planes orthogonal to the table, or to within 30° of them.

The nature and role of magnetic resonance imaging (MRI)

Magnetic resonance imaging utilises a strong magnetic field and radio waves to produce high quality computer-generated images in any plane (Fig. 11.5). MRI imaging of head and neck tumours has been shown to be superior to CT images for staging disease (Kabala et al 1992) and the multiplaner images give greater accuracy (and flexibility) in radiotherapy planning (McCarty et al 1992). MRI may therefore supersede CT as a means for producing images from which to plan routine or sophisticated treatments, once the facility becomes more widely accessible. Various media may be used to provide markers on the images, for use in relating structures imaged to surface marks.

MRI has no radiation risks to the patient or operator, and is noninvasive in application. There are some hazards but these may be minimised by good practice.

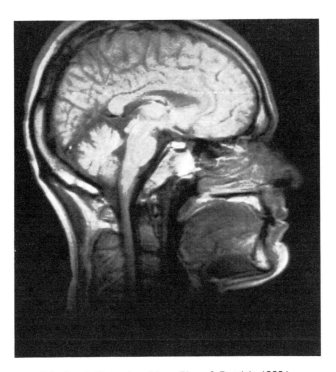

Figure 11.5   A sagittal MRI scan of the head. (Reproduced from Dixon & Dugdale 1988.)

Ultrasound

Sound with frequencies above the audible range is reflected and scattered back from tissue interfaces. The images (Fig. 11.6), initially produced electronically on a video screen, can be used to give information which is useful in treatment planning for external beam applications, and in dosimetry assessment for brachytherapy. Ultrasound imaging may be used for the assessment of chest wall thickness for use in the planning of breast treatments (see Ch. 16). However, CT may also be used for this purpose.

Radioisotope images

Low doses of radiopharmaceuticals having gamma emissions of energy 50–300 keV approximately are used for imaging physiological systems. The isotope is administered to the patient as a component of a radiopharmaceutical which will selectively concentrate in the tissue of interest. After a suitable time interval to allow isotope distribution in the body (up to 4 hours for a technetium bone scan), a gamma-sensitive 'camera' is used to obtain a film image created by emissions from within the body. This type of image is mainly used to detect and localise bone metastases (Fig. 11.7) which can be difficult to detect on an X-ray image. The principles and practice of radioisotope imaging are described in detail elsewhere (Sharp et al 1989).

Radiotherapy treatment simulator

The treatment simulator (Fig. 11.8A, B) is essentially a specialised X-ray machine which simulates all the movements and beam geometry features of radiotherapy treatment machines. It provides simulation of beam divergence, beam direction, f.s.d. settings, field size and light beam shape, using a diagnostic range of X-ray energies. A small focal spot (3–6 mm) is required to project a clear image of fine field-defining wires against the anatomy. A scatter-removing grid, either with

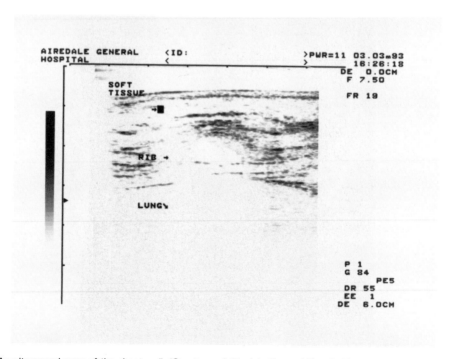

Figure 11.6 An ultrasound scan of the chest wall. (Courtesy of Airedale General Hospital.)

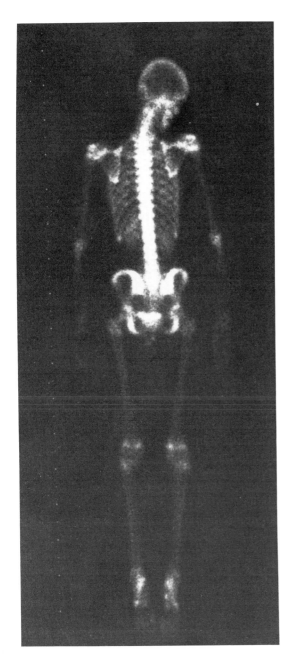

Figure 11.7 A bone scan. (Courtesy of Dr Bury, Leeds General Infirmary.)

a particular field size is set, the field-defining wires will indicate the field limits on the anatomy shown on the image. Some simulators have a CT facility, so that simulator images may be used for tissue outlines etc. However, the quality of image produced is much inferior to that produced by a CT scanner, and regular quality control checks must be performed to check that there is no distortion.

Beam direction and accessories. It is essential to have the same type of beam direction facilities available on the simulator as on the treatment machine, and a couch top and accessories giving compatible patient positioning (see Chs 9, 13 and 14). A system for simulating shielding blocks is also essential for accurate work.

Basic simulation principles

Simulation is used to visualise and adjust the anatomy contained within a proposed treatment portal for a patient set-up, as if for treatment. The patient undergoing treatment planning may be screened using fluoroscopy, during which the patient/couch can be moved, using remote control, until the best set-up to include the desired treatment zone is achieved (Fig. 11.10).

A hard copy image on paper or photographic film is produced of the anatomy contained in a particular treatment field. These hard copy images are subject to some distortion which arises within the screening system, so cannot be used for accurate planning purposes but serve as a record which is easily filed in case-notes. X-ray film is used for accurate images for treatment planning purposes.

Simulator verification of the treatment volume using the proposed treatment set-up is usually performed by taking two orthogonal films, which allow three-dimensional identification of points of interest within the patient (Fig. 11.11). Field check films, using the set-up parameters may be taken as a pretreatment portal check.

Magnification correction

Because of the inverse square law effect of beam divergence, the size of anatomy on the image is related to the distance between the film and the

parallel components (Fig. 11.9) or focused to follow the divergence of the beam, is used to improve image quality.

The field-wire arrangement moves in the same way as the collimators on a treatment machine. If

A

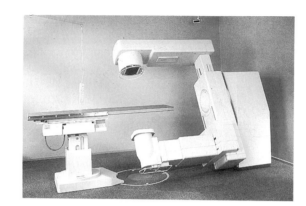

B

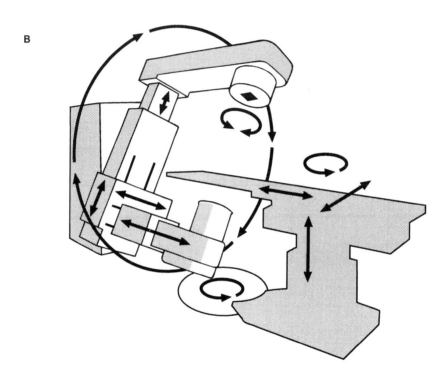

Figure 11.8 A A treatment simulator. **B** Movements of a treatment simulator. (Courtesy of Philips Medical Systems.)

patient (Fig. 11.1A), and to the isocentre position relative to the anatomy. Where films are to be used in planning or in verifying that a plan is appropriately applied to the anatomy, some indication of the isocentre position relative to the patient and the film is required so as to allow calculation of film magnification. Demagnified measurements are then used.

Magnification marker devices. A range of radio-opaque marker ladders (see Fig. 17.3) and rings of known diameter are set at appropriate points on or near to the patient, near to the central axis of the field, e.g. entry and/or exit points, to indicate magnification. These ladders contain metal markers in a particular spatial configuration, e.g. at 1 cm intervals. Measurement of the ring size or separation of the markers on film (see Fig. 17.4) indicates the magnification.

Rangefinder readings for focal film distances can be used to calculate film magnification: for

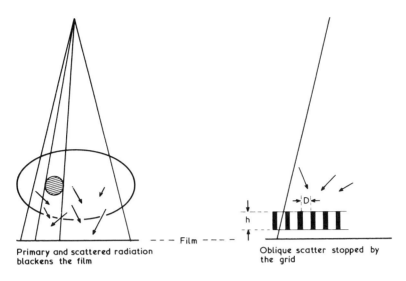

Primary and scattered radiation
blackens the film

Oblique scatter stopped by
the grid

– – – Film – – – –

Figure 11.9   A parallel scatter grid. (Reproduced from Walter et al 1982.)

example, for a 100 cm f.s.d. set-up, a film at 130 cm from the target will have a magnification of:

$$\frac{130}{100} = 1.3$$

Use of contrast. Contrast materials may be introduced into the patient to allow organs such as the kidney to be localised for shielding purposes. There are risks to the patient when using contrast. In imaging the oesophagus, swallowed contrast material may enter the lungs via any fistula, so a doctor should be present to monitor the procedure. The patient may be allergic to injected material. It is necessary to have emergency equipment and drugs close by, and to know the signs of adverse reaction to these contrast agents – the patient may rapidly die if prompt action is not taken. The batch number and details of the agent introduced, needles used etc. must be kept with the simulation record, and

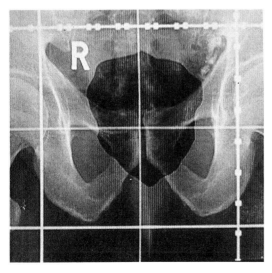

Figure 11.10   A simulator image of field-defining wires on the anatomy. (Courtesy of Varian Oncology Systems.)

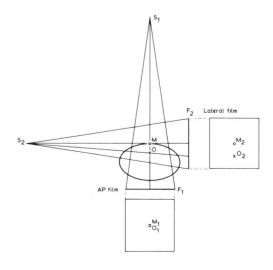

Figure 11.11   The principle of orthogonal films for localisation. (Reproduced from Walter et al 1982.)

in the patient's notes, to comply with product liability requirements.

MEGAVOLTAGE PORTAL IMAGING

Precise localisation and planning procedures do not necessarily lead to precise treatment, since there are many uncertainties arising on treatment (see Chs 12 and 13). Therefore it is necessary to verify treatment field accuracy for radical work, by means of portal images produced by the treatment machine at the time of set-up. It is recommended (Bleehen et al 1991) that portal checks be carried out on the first treatments, in cases where accuracy is required such as head and neck procedures. The timing and frequency of portal checks depends on information regarding reproducibility. Where there is confidence that a technique is acceptably reproducible throughout a treatment course (see Ch 12), a single film or image is meaningful in verifying that the set-up on the accelerator is comparable to that planned on the simulator.

Various megavoltage portal imaging modalities are now available, including both film and electronic devices.

Portal verification with films

There are two types of film available for checking treatment fields or portals. The bony anatomy and air spaces are visible on these films, and are used as landmarks against which to check field edges. The visible anatomy shown within a small field area may be insufficient for the purpose, so a double-exposed film showing the portal within a larger area of anatomy may be used.

Double-exposed portal localisation films

Fast films are used for a small fraction of the treatment exposure to produce an image. The image quality is good at 6 MV and 8 MV, showing soft and bony tissue, air spaces and the shell outline (see Fig. 17.5). The lung treated on breast patients is also visible. The definition of the 'edge' of the treatment field is clearly delineated on the surrounding anatomy. Electron films need

only one exposure to show the applicator position on a larger area of anatomy. Films taken with cobalt are not suitable for accurate checks on field alignment, as the treated field 'edge' is very blurred (Fig. 11.12), although some anatomy is visible.

Film/screen combination and exposures. The film used for portal verification is standard diagnostic fast film, loaded (in the darkroom) into a Kodak portal localisation cassette which has a copper front screen and a lead back screen for image intensification. Each exposure requires 2–6 cGy, 2 cGy being suitable for head and neck fields, 4–6 cGy for the pelvis. The surrounding area may be given a lower exposure than the field area, especially if the eye is included.

(If reloading in daylight, Special Kodak X-omat G film, individually light-tight wrapped, can be used but it requires higher exposures such as 10 cGy.)

Double exposure process. The film has to be taken at the start of the treatment and retrieved before the field dose is given, or taken after the treatment exposure. Images are usually acquired without a wedge. Double-exposed portal films (see Fig. 17.5) are taken using semiautomatic portal film facilities available on most linacs. An exposure of 2–6 cGy is given to the field area, then the collimators are opened to give a larger field size and a further 2 cGy given. The sizes and

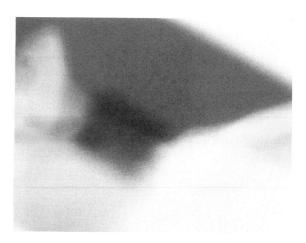

Figure 11.12 A double-exposed portal film of a larynx treatment using cobalt.

exposures can be programmed so that the colli-mators open automatically, decreasing the time and effort required for each film compared with manual changing of collimator sizes.

Size of background area. The field size used for the background anatomy depends on local policy, and the accelerator used. Software allows a choice between a set addition to axis length, or a full 40 cm × 40 cm, and a choice of dose.

The dose given to the wider field area is considered to be a necessary part of the treatment process, and to be clinically insignificant, even for the eyes.

Treatment verification films

For checking complex leaded parallel opposed fields such as mantles (see Fig 18.7), Kodak X-omat V film is used (a single film in a light-tight pack), left in position for the whole daily dose to that particular field. The film is placed on the treatment couch, directly beneath the treated area of the patient since it is not bulky enough to affect the set-up. The useful exposure range is from 40 to 150 cGy (exit dose). The image quality is improved by using a 1 mm steel sheet (plus paper for warmth) on the patient side of the film, or by using a Kodak verification cassette (Fig. 11.4). The latter increases the image quality by use of a copper front screen but requires the use of a cassette holder.

Artefacts will appear on the image if the film is kinked at any stage. The film can be fogged if left in a hot place such as on a radiator, but will not be fogged by scattered radiation. Should a veri-fication film be accidentally left in the treatment room, providing it is not directly in the beam, it will not become damaged or fogged from use of the linac, as a portal film will. A single verifica-tion film can therefore be used to record several small fields, or one field day after day on different (appropriately labelled) areas of the film. This is advantageous since the film size is large and the cost is approximately four times higher than for a diagnostic film of the same size.

Portal versus verification films

The use of verification film is less time-consuming than using portal films, since there are no extra trips into the room to retrieve the film. However, verification film provides a poorer quality of image. These images may not give enough information with small fields, and the exposure requirements preclude the use of the double exposure technique. However, a verifica-tion film provides adequate information for man-tle and dogleg fields.

Because the patient is required to hold an exacting position for a mantle set-up, the extra time required to perform a portal film may be unacceptable, and radiographers entering the room may lead to patient movement, especially since the patient is used to being able to move out of position once an exposure is finished.

Limitations of film

There are limitations in using film, which must be developed and so can only be viewed after a treatment has been administered. Either the pa-tient attends for a treatment film prior to treat-ment starting, or any correction must be made subsequent to at least one treatment. Any ran-dom error large enough to need correcting (see Ch. 12) cannot therefore be corrected using film. A further limitation is that either an 'average' image treatment is recorded with verification film, or a portal film representing the set-up at the start or finish of one treatment exposure is obtained. Films must be labelled effectively, but the information which can be given on a small label is limited.

Standardising film or image magnification

The magnification of each accelerator film should be the same as the planning simulator film, so that comparison for the purpose of checking against the 'plan' is simple. A simple but effective distance-setting device is provided by a cane, which is a few centimetres longer than the chosen isocentre-to-film distance, marked around its girth at the correct distance from the end. The mark is aligned with the overhead or sagittal laser, and the film or detector is set to touch the unmarked end (Fig. 11.13). This cane is easier to use than a ruler in the half-light used for setting up.

Cassette stands and supports

Cassettes or verification films may be supported by a mobile cassette stand (Fig. 11.14) which is adjustable for height and angle. Some stands have angulation scales to allow the film to be aligned orthogonally in the beam. However, where a scale is not available, the film can usually be aligned by eye (and by using the magnification stick) to within a few degrees. Any inaccuracy in the image from a misalignment of 10° or so will be insignificant relative to the dimensions being assessed. It is desirable to have enough cassettes and stands to meet the needs of various machines.

Alternatively, a linac accessory cassette holder is available for some makes of equipment, which attaches in the manner of a backpointer (see Ch. 9), and gives accurate film–beam alignment.

Another similar device, requiring no manual effort in use, is commercially available for fixation to the linac gantry. This device is merely a slim, U-shaped support arm which lies flat against the gantry when not in use, and features motorised movement into position when required. There is no bulky cassette support, the cassette being secured into place via a small magnet at the centre of the arm.

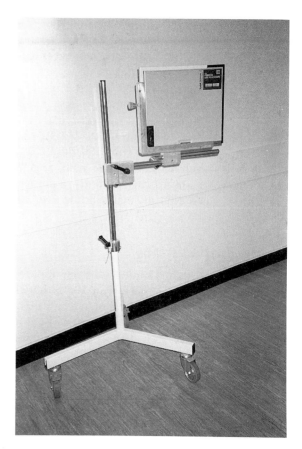

Figure 11.14 A portal cassette in a mobile cassette holder.

Image compatibility

Images on verification film are not totally compatible with either portal or simulator films using short exposures. Another difficulty arises because of the differing radiographic appearance of some anatomy on images produced at differing energies, such as employed on the simulator and on megavoltage machines. Reference points for use in comparisons must therefore be chosen carefully.

Field central axis and edge definition. A problem may arise, with either films or digital imaging, from not being able to see the central axis point unless a custom-made device, similar to a front pointer, is attached to the treatment head to indicate the central axis. A lead wire cross may be placed at the central axis point on the patient, but does not give very accurate results especially when on a sloping surface. Software may provide

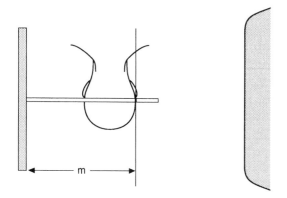

Figure 11.13 Use of a cane as a film distance-setting device.

centre crosses or grids on screen to help with determining reference points and image magnification.

On most machines the field edges are sharp on the films or images. However, on certain machines (Philips SL-75 series) the beam is unstable for the first few monitor units and the field edges are blurred on one axis, necessitating the use of up to 5–10 monitor units to establish the Y-axis field edges. The SL series give sharp edge images as do Varian Clinacs. Electronic portal imaging devices must be regularly calibrated to ensure that there is no distortion across the image at any gantry position, and that magnification factors or corrections are consistent. The field edges are degraded during image enhancement processes, and may be indistinguishable unless the edge is defined on the screen using a separate software facility.

Electronic portal imaging devices

The advent of digital imaging systems for linear accelerators has vastly increased the potential for not only studying accuracy trends and patterns for techniques used, but also for making instant corrections for errors seen on screen at the start of and during treatment. Corrections for patient movement, and for organ movement, may be possible via studies to assess organ movement during each treatment fraction, and during a treatment course.

Most systems operate via a fluoroscopic screen viewed by a closed-circuit television (CCTV) camera (Fig. 11.15) through a mirror system. An alternative system (Meertens et al 1990) uses arrays of liquid crystal detectors, building up an image line by line. All systems provide some image enhancement facilities, and all produce images which are useful for the purpose for which they are required. The images are generally of a comparable quality to those obtained with portal films. Images can be filed and retrieved with patient and treatment information annotated on the image.

User requirements

A number of features are required to make a system usable in routine clinical practice:

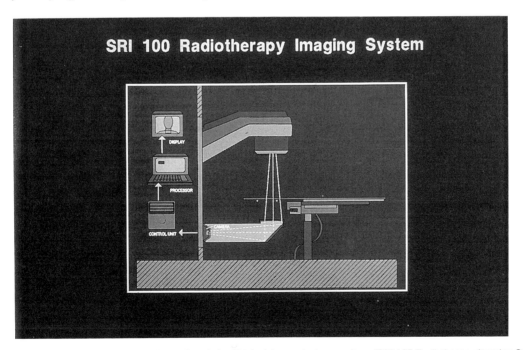

Figure 11.15 An imaging device employing a closed-circuit television and mirror system. (SRI 100 Radiotherapy Imaging System, courtesy of Philips Medical Systems.)

- user-friendly controls and software
- fast image acquisition
- clear field edge definition
- onscreen facility to compare the image with a reference image
- onscreen field overlay facility
- onscreen ruler facility to measure distances and discrepancies
- invert/reverse image facility to allow direct comparison between opposed lateral or opposed vertical fields
- onscreen magnification indication and correction facility
- image analysis software
- detector height indicator, where height is adjustable
- fast, paper-based hard copy print facility
- facility to transfer images to an off-line workstation
- a compatible laser backpointer system where non-isocentric set-ups are used
- minimal bulk to allow the radiographer access to the set-up and to the patient
- a retractable or detachable system, which is quick to operate and avoids the need for lifting heavy components. This is essential to retain full use of the linac and couch movements for setting up a range of techniques.

User requirements for interventional corrections. In order to achieve correction by set-up intervention at the start of a treatment, a good quality image must be produced by a few monitor units. Also, user-friendly quantitative analysis software allowing the operator to identify the actual size of any correction to be made, e.g. 0.5 cm correction in couch height, is required, otherwise several attempts will be made before the correction is achieved. The interventional correction of errors is not likely to be simple, since movements in two planes may be involved, or a patient rotation correction may be required (see Ch. 13). To assess field accuracy, a comparison with another image on screen (either the simulator film, or an accepted treatment set-up check image) is a prerequisite (see Ch. 12).

Types of image

A single image may be produced by a minimum of 2 cGy (Theraview) or a dose corresponding to the time taken to acquire it (Philips, 4 seconds; Varian, several seconds). Following the first image a sequence of images may be automatically acquired during the exposure. Several images may be viewed consecutively as a movie loop sequence, which shows intratreatment movement. Software provided with digital imaging devices allows an average image to be created from the sequence, if required.

Double-exposed images can also be acquired, for the same purpose as when using film.

Image analysis and manipulation

The software allows contrast enhancement for particular tissue types within the treatment field, and manipulation of the image library of a patient in order to compare and contrast these on the screen or on printouts (Fig. 11.16). Software facilities for assessing and quantifying changes in field angle or positioning on multiple images are required, for analysis of accuracy trends in one patient and within a series of patients treated with a given technique (see Ch. 12).

Advantages and limitations of electronic portal imaging

Where an electronic portal imaging device (EPID) is available, there are potential savings in time and in film costs. The cost of a paper printout is about one-tenth of the cost of a film. Also there are no staff costs in transporting a cassette for processing, and reduced use of processing facilities (health and safety gains). Image acquisition is less labour intensive than using film and the availability of an instant onscreen image is more relevant for a treatment set-up check than a film developed later. However, where there is a policy to intervene to adjust a set-up, an appropriate explanation must be given to the patient, and a potential for considerable addition to set-up times must alter patient scheduling and daily treatment

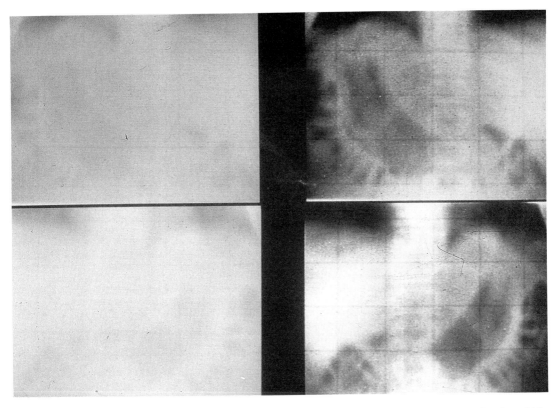

Figure 11.16   Corresponding anterior and posterior portal images, before and after image enhancement, showing grid for measurement and analysis for functions. (Courtesy of Philips Medical Systems.)

capacity. This facility demands additional skills of radiographers in decision-making, or adds a further organisational difficulty if a doctor has to be present to make the decisions. Once a set-up is deemed unacceptable, an informed decision on how the set-up should be corrected must be made.

An EPID can be used instead of simulation for emergency treatments to the chest or spine, to confirm the adequacy of a marked area and facilitate adjustments, saving time for the patient and the staff, where treatment outside normal working hours is undertaken.

Analysis of treatment accuracy trends (see Ch. 12) on a series of images/patients can be undertaken more easily with the appropriate software (Fig. 11.16) than manually, using film. This function will become more and more important, with shaped and reduced treatment volumes (see Ch. 23), in order to allow appropriate safety margins. EPIDS may also provide a means of assessing in vivo exit dosimetry across each field (Van Dam et al 1992).

There are some limitations in flexibility with EPIDs. For example, the presence of the device may restrict the range of techniques which can be undertaken, hence the need for a detachable unit. Not all fields can be imaged due to physical restrictions, for example superior head fields. However, these cannot be imaged by other means either.

The linac gantry must be modified before it can accept an imaging device, and this may change the operating characteristics of the linac. The devices are not routinely movable from one unit to another, as calibration must be undertaken for each unit, even where devices are physically compatible with more than one unit. At present, most EPIDS are adapted for use with a particular linac or make of linac.

REFERENCES AND FURTHER READING

Bleehen N M et al 1991 Quality Assurance in Radiotherapy, Report of a Working Party. Standing Subcommittee on Cancer of the Standing Medical Advisory Committee

Bomford C K, Dawes P J D K, Lillicrap S C, Young J 1989 Treatment simulators. British Journal of Radiology Suppl 23

Dixon, D, Dugdale L M 1988 An introduction to clinical imaging. Churchill Livingstone, Melbourne

Evans P M, Gildersleve J Q, Morton E J 1992 Image comparison techniques for use with megavoltage imaging systems. British Journal of Radiology 65: 701–709

Griffiths S E 1990 Radiotherapy quality control: portal and verification films. Radiography 56: 17

Kabala J, Goddard P, Cook P 1992 Magnetic resonance imaging of extracranial head and neck tumours. British Journal of Radiology 65: 375–383

McCarty M, Leslie M, Baddely H, Saunders M, Dische S 1992 Staging of head and neck cancer using magnetic resonance imaging. 50th Annual Congress of the British Institute of Radiology, Abstr

Meertens H, Van Herk M, Bijhold J, Bartelink H 1990 First clinical experience with a newly developed portal imaging device. International Journal of Radiation Oncology, Biology, Physics 18: 1173–1181

Mizer S, Rodgers Scheller R, Deye J A 1986 Radiation therapy simulation workbook. Pergamon, New York

Rothwell R, Ash D V, Jones W G 1983 Radiation treatment planning for bladder cancer: a comparison of cystogram localisation with computed tomography. Clinical Radiology 133: 103–111

Schad L R, Gademann G, Knapp M, Zabel H J, Schlegel W, Lorenz W J 1992 Radiotherapy planning of basal meningiomas: improved tumour localisation by correlation of CT and MR imaging data. Radiotherapy and Oncology 25: 56–62

Sharp P F, Gemmell H G, Smith F 1989 Practical nuclear medicine. Oxford University Press, London

Van Dam J, Vaerman C, Blackaert N, Leunens G, Dutreix A, Van der Scheuren E 1992 Are port films reliable for in vivo dosimetry? Radiotherapy and Oncology 25: 67–72

Walter J, Miller H, Bomford C K 1982 A short textbook of radiotherapy, 4th edn. Churchill Livingstone, Edinburgh

From principles to practice

SECTION CONTENTS

12

Treatment accuracy and reproducibility

INTRODUCTION

With new imaging technology, tumours can be accurately staged and visually localised in three dimensions, so that we can produce a theoretical treatment plan to treat all of the tumour tissues at a particular site, and shield or exclude other uninvolved tissue lying in close proximity to the target tissues. Treatment is planned from images taken at one patient attendance, then delivered via another piece of equipment each day for some weeks.

It is assumed that the plan is achieved and that the delineated target tissue is irradiated, without deviation, for each of the 20 or more separate treatments comprising a course. However, for this assumption to be valid, well researched methods and verification procedures should be used at every stage of the planning and treatment process. Radiotherapy practice is a rapidly developing field. Processes which were previously accepted are gradually changing as new technology and the results of widespread practical research are applied.

The practices involved in the actual delivery of a prescribed treatment, and verification of the accuracy of delivery, have received relatively little attention in radiotherapy journals, until quite recently. Numerous variations in practice are in use in centres around the world. Each centre has evolved its own methods of practice, some of which are found in other centres. In many instances, the basic method appears similar but will often be found to vary in detail. Our experience, gained both from our own studies, and from our knowledge of the work of others, shows that the details of the methods used will determine the accuracy and reproducibility of treatment. This chapter outlines the main factors underlying the reliability of treatment methods, and discusses how to assess the accuracy and reproducibility of a set-up method.

The weak link: the treatment delivery process

Potentially the weakest link in the whole radiotherapy process is the treatment itself as many factors influence set-up accuracy. Treatment is said to be reproducible if the target anatomy is successfully irradiated on each treatment. Other factors potentially affect whether the dose received is the same, to within a few percent, as the dose prescribed.

The quality of treatment delivery depends on the skills and knowledge of the staff concerned. The delivery of each treatment fraction is a complicated series of processes (see summary in Ch 26). Each process is based on a principle. If any of the principles are flawed, perhaps because of an assumption that equipment accuracy is perfect under every condition of use, or that patient marks always relate consistently to the target anatomy, then treatment will not be delivered as planned.

In subsequent chapters, the basic principles of various commonly used techniques are outlined, with advantages and disadvantages in terms of potential accuracy. General principles for achiev-

ing the best results with current knowledge and equipment are given. Before considering individual setting-up methods, some of the uncertainties in treatment delivery are discussed and the treatment process presented as a three-dimensional problem which must be overcome in practice.

The challenge for radiotherapy practitioners

The target within a living person

The challenge for those designing and applying treatment methods arises from the patient's being a living, mobile and to some extent fluid, three-dimensional entity within whom there is a discrete tissue portion requiring irradiation (Fig. 12.1). The flexibility of the body and the mobility of the skin and internal organs present uncertainties in the accuracy of treatment delivery. In addition, involuntary movements such as breathing occur continuously, and the emotional state of the patient may affect the tissue geometry through muscle tension.

The radiation beam zone

The radiation beams chosen to form routine external beam treatment plans, are a fixed physical entity within a disc-shaped space or zone, of which the machine isocentre is the centre (see Fig. 2.3). A treatment beam of the required cross-sectional size at the isocentre can be chosen,

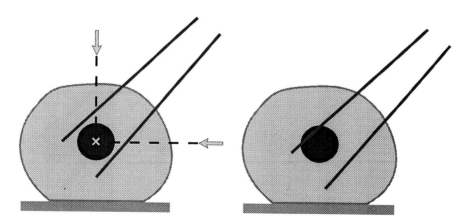

Figure 12.1 A discrete portion of tissue within the patient has to be set correctly with respect to the isocentre, in three dimensions.

for application along any radius, by selecting appropriate diaphragm and gantry settings. Shielding may be introduced to shape the beam, or wedging to change the dose distribution produced by each beam (see Ch. 8). All beams have a fixed three-dimensional shape, the cross-sectional size of which increases with distance from the X- or gamma-ray source (Fig. 12.2) because of the inverse square law effect. However, when incident on a patient surface with irregular contours, the field shape on the skin changes with variations in f.s.d. (Fig. 12.3).

The radiation beams and the patient

Subject only to the mechanical accuracy of machine parameters, the chosen beams will pass through the zone and geometrically interact with each other in the same way, whether or not a patient is introduced.

Which tissue is irradiated within the patient will depend on his/her three-dimensional posi-

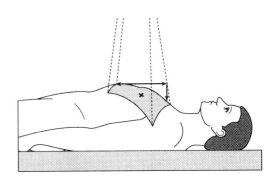

Figure 12.3 Shape variation when field is incident on a sloping patient surface.

tion within the beams, and this cannot be reproduced by using a single two-dimensional mark on the skin (except for treatment of the surface). The detailed dosimetry in the patient varies with the three-dimensional shape and density both of tissue and of any other material, such as wedges or bolus, which is introduced into the beams.

Uncertainties in treatment delivery

Perfection in directing beams at the target tissue will rarely be achieved. There are several reasons for this, including limitations in equipment accuracy and use, tissue changes within the patient and variability of the patient's exact position from planning to treatment and from treatment to treatment. Since the assessment of the geometrical constancy of tissue is currently not well advanced, it is assumed throughout the text that the dimensions of the target tissues, and their configuration relative to bony anatomy, remain constant, except where specific discussion of the issue is made. (At present, research is being conducted to assess ranges of movement of internal tissues and organs.)

Constancy of relationship between reference marks and target tissue

All setting-up methods rely on the use of marks or tattoos on the surface of the patient (either on the skin or on a closely fitting shell) for centring or applying treatment beams, to treat tissues at

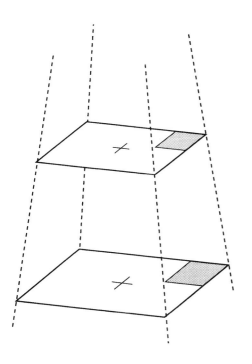

Figure 12.2 The cross-section of a field, increasing uniformly in area with distance from the X-ray source.

various depths in the body (Fig. 12.4). A well researched method will ensure that the position of the skin or shell which bears the surface marks is constant in relation to the target anatomy. The three-dimensional patient positioning and support methods used will affect this constancy (see Ch. 13).

A reproducible treatment position which is both tolerable to the patient and effective for the technical processes is required throughout planning and treatment.

Equipment limitations

A viable setting-up method must also take into account the limitations in equipment accuracy, the effect of particular methods of use of equipment and the effect of any additional procedure, such as the insertion of shielding or bolus material into the treatment beam.

The nature of set-up variations

Set-up variations and their effects may be either systematic, that is, repeated on each treatment, or may be random in occurrence, changing from day to day.

Where variations in field placement are regu-

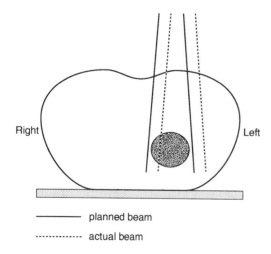

———— planned beam

············· actual beam

Figure 12.4 A beam applied by alignment with marks on the anterior surface of the patient only, resulting in irradiation to the left of the planned beam position.

larly seen, the contributory error factors can be isolated and the treatment method modified to improve accuracy. For readers new to this subject we would emphasise that the term 'error' does not reflect inattention, but is used in the quantification of treatment variations which only become apparent when studies are conducted of treatment methods.

Any particular treatment method will result in similar accuracy when set up by different staff groups, all of whom will be diligent in their use of the method. All treatment fields appear correct at the time of set-up because they can only be assessed with relation to surface marks and machine parameter displays. An account of the findings from various accuracy studies will help to illustrate the problem.

Studies of set-up accuracy and common findings

A study using treatment verification film, conducted by Byhardt et al in 1978, provided information on the differing field placement accuracy achieved at various body sites in one centre at that time. The pelvis and abdomen gave rise to the largest inaccuracies (up to 4 cm), but other sites such as the head and neck, were more precisely treated. Byhardt et al suggested that error patterns are related to the setting-up practices used, such as the use of skin marks, and that error patterns would vary from centre to centre. This was one of the first published studies. Our own studies have consistently shown that errors occurred either randomly, varying from day to day, or were systematically repeated every day. The errors did not get larger with time and were not related to the renewal of marks. Nor were errors usually seen to be related to the side of the couch used by the patient for access, although in one study there was a correlation suggesting that this may play a part (presumably because the patient's skin was pulled slightly in one direction). This was also seen by Richards & Buchler (1977) for pelvic fields.

The volume of literature which now exists is greater and a review reveals that most authors:

• identify field placement discrepancies of varying degree and type

- find a random variation in edge position of ±3 mm even in the head and neck (Rabinowitz et al 1985; Kihlen & Ruden 1989)
- find that the use of verification film allows significant errors to be identified by measurement, and that the use of films leads to greater precision (Marks et al 1976; Hulshof et al 1989)
- agree that most significant errors tend to be systematic and can be corrected by a single intervention (Hulshof et al 1989; Leunens et al 1990; Mitine et al 1991).

However, the possibility of progressive changes with weight loss during treatment should be considered according to the site treated and technique used. Electronic portal imaging has now widened the possibilities for study and routine treatment monitoring. The concepts are similar to those involved when using film, except that if an error is seen within two monitor units on a treatment, there is a possibility of intervention and correction before treatment continues. Intratreatment movements can also be monitored using a dynamic system.

The accuracy with which doses received correlate to the expected dose is less easy to assess on a regular basis. However, a study by Leunens et al (1990) used semiconductor detectors to measure entrance doses on head and neck patients, finding a standard deviation of 2.8% for the series. Two treatment techniques were identified which led to erroneous dose delivery, also a systematic deficiency in a treatment planning algorithm. The causes of all errors could be identified and eliminated for subsequent treatments. This study demonstrated a reliable process useful as an addition to quality assurance programmes.

Geographical miss and the effect of complex field shapes

When part of a tumour falls outside the high dose zone on one or more treatments, whether due to an inadequacy in clinical tumour localisation or to an inaccuracy or some variation later in the process, a geographical miss of the tumour is said to have occurred. This results in part or all of the tumour receiving a lower dose than that intended, which may in turn lead to treatment failure or tumour recurrence. The more complex the field shape, the more difficult it is to achieve accurately (see Chs 13 and 18).

Assessment of accuracy and reproducibility and portal (field) placement

To assess the accuracy with which treatment fields are placed in relation to the target volume, as delineated on planning films, a means of checking the daily treatment field orientation is required. Some of the factors which affect which tissue is actually irradiated are difficult to assess daily, particularly organ movement. The effect of others may be partially assessed.

Checks via portal verification

Routine use of portal or field films or electronic portal imaging devices provides verification, on a two-dimensional image, of the anatomy actually irradiated by a field (see Ch. 11). For a series of patients treated by a particular method, daily or less frequent visual checks, from portal films or digital images, can show the accuracy trends for that treatment method, so that practice can be monitored and analysed, and accuracy predicted for each technique.

Timing of checks and corrections

The appropriate timing and frequency of films or imaging used for routine checking of field accuracy depends on the reproducibility of the technique being checked. For a reproducible technique, where the significantly large errors are systematic, one correct film is meaningful and any adjustment necessary can be checked by a further film to assess its effectiveness.

Therefore, before a routine film checking system can be effectively used, the reproducibility of each technique should be assessed, at least by taking three port films of the same field during a treatment course, for several patients, analysing these, and observing whether inaccuracies seen on one film are repeated on the others. This will allow decision rules to be formulated for making corrections. (This is discussed further later.)

Magnification correction and film or detector distance setting

It is important, when assessing accuracy, to make measurements on the images and to correct them for any magnification. Measurements of field displacements should be corrected for the relevant depth in the patient, since the error and its magnification will increase with depth, just as the field size does (Fig. 12.4). For example, an error of 15 mm may be measured on an image taken at 150 cm target-to-film distance, for a field used isocentrically. The inaccuracy at the isocentre depth (100 cm) in the patient will then be 10 mm.

The process is simpler if the magnification of all images is the same. This can easily be arranged by assessing a film or detector-to-isocentre distance, usable on both simulation and treatment for a particular type of set-up, then using this distance routinely (see Ch. 11).

Assessing a trend from several films

If three or more treaments with a particular field (without set-up modification between films) are recorded on the portal images, field placement accuracy on each of these can be compared with a simulator image (see Fig. 13.6).

Once suitable images are available, the field edges should be defined by software or marked by eye (with the latter it is preferable for one person to mark all films, then for another to check to provide consistency in the measurements). Where software is used, a check should be made that the field edge definition is geometrically correct, as the outer portions of the image are often degraded during image processing.

Stable anatomical points, preferably bony, can be selected and marked on each image, so that comparison of their positions relative to points on the field edge can be made by measurement, overlaying images or taking multiple tracings by lining up the key points then recording the edge

position (see Fig. 13.6). Alternatively, the field edges can be aligned and the discrepancy in anatomical positions recorded. However, this method is inferior for many applications especially where 'edges' are defined by manually placed shielding blocks.

For any study series it is useful to note, at the time when the images are taken, any additional information which may be relevant. For example, it should be noted if there is anything unusual about the set-up process, such as a greater degree of difficulty in positioning the patient, a lack of continuity in the staff team or treatment performed on a different treatment unit due to breakdown etc. These factors can affect the outcome and such information can be vital during a retrospective analysis where there is a need to establish causes of variations.

Check protocols

Our aim is to achieve reproducible treatment techniques with relatively small errors which rarely need correction. Once the consistent error pattern for a particular method is known, then a protocol for the timing and frequency of portal check images can be used with confidence. For example, for a reproducible technique the protocol may be one check at the start, then a correction if required, followed by a further check. Subsequent images should not reveal any further error large enough to need correcting. The reasons for this will become clear later in this chapter.

Dynamic imaging and intervention

Viewing the treated anatomy via a dynamic series of images allows continual assessment of the adequacy of fit of the field to moving anatomy. Before dynamic set-up intervention and correction can be undertaken, further decision rules must be formulated. These must take into account the size of errors to be interventionally corrected, and how (and when) adjustments should be made, since a simple couch movement may not be the answer. A great deal therefore has to be learned.

This type of intervention has two drawbacks: one is the extra machine time required, which must affect patient throughput rates and waiting lists, and the other is the patient's potential anxiety at treatment having to be 'corrected'. However, there is a need to correct as soon as possible for obvious dosimetry reasons.

Random and systematic errors and their identification

A systematic error (repeated on each occasion) is likely to have additional random variation from day to day, so a statistical analysis of measurements from a series of films is required, to determine the relative magnitudes of random and systematic error in any one treatment technique/method. The analyses should also allow the identification, by deduction and investigation, of factors causing errors so that knowledge of how to correct or prevent errors is gained. (For example if an error is due to patient rotation, moving the couch is unlikely to fully correct the beam direction in the patient.)

Measurement and statistical analysis of error

When measurements from a series of films of one field are analysed, each 'error' will be found to have both random and systematic components. The two may be distinguished from each other, as demonstrated by Figure 12.5, where the edge positions of three treatments are seen relative to the planned field edge position. If the central treatment field edge represents the average or median field edge position, then the distances between this median edge and other treatment field edges represent the random positional variation. This random variation can be quantified by calculating the standard deviation of the field edges about the median. The distance between the median edge and the planned edge position represents the systematic (constant) error, which in this figure is larger than the random error.

From the information thus obtained, decision rules on which to base corrective action can be formulated, covering both how and when to correct. This process also allows an assessment of

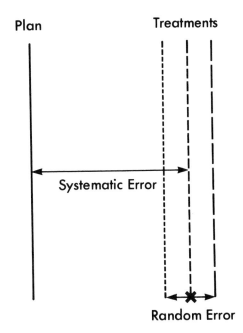

Figure 12.5 Three field edges compared with the planned edge, showing systematic and random lateral shift error.

the accuracy routinely achieved for each technique, useful when defining the necessary margin widths during planning (see Ch. 14).

Set-up error: reduction and correction

If the random error is large in comparison to the systematic error, a modification to the technical method is required (or a correction at the beginning of each treatment).

Many random effects may be reduced in magnitude by improving methods. If the inaccuracies found when using a particular technique are random, then there is little benefit from making a weekly check followed by a correction, since the error has been shown to vary in a random way. Many random effects can be reduced to an acceptable magnitude by small changes in methods.

If the systematic error is large relative to the random error, then the majority of treatments will be corrected by intervention on or following the first treatment (Mitine et al 1991). An inaccuracy which is consistent from one check to the next can be eliminated by a single correction. Because there are statistical variations in the errors there are, however, occasional rogue instances where further action is required.

Each systematic error, once identified and quantified for each technique or patient, can therefore be eliminated. Thus techniques producing largely systematic error are reproducible techniques which, once modified, become accurate techniques.

Causes of set-up error

The two error components may arise either from separate factors within a technique, e.g. a random error due to patient positioning variation plus a systematic error due to an equipment inaccuracy, or both may have the same cause. For example, a lateral field shift effect (see Fig. 13.6) may be caused solely by lateral rotation of the patient. Patients generally 'relax' on treatment sessions subsequent to the planning session, so that a

relatively constant changed position occurs throughout treatment, leading to a systematic error. Patient rotation can be stabilised to reproduce the exact rotation present during treatment planning (see Ch. 13), so that this systematic error effect is removed. However, the accuracy with which this stabilisation of rotation is achieved is finite, so a small random variation in the position still occurs from day to day.

Errors from equipment, dosimetry calculations and computer programs

Similarly, random and systematic error in equipment settings, or in dosimetry calculations, can occur. These may vary considerably between centres, depending on the numbers and experience of staff (Dutreix 1984), and are related to the quality assurance programmes undertaken: 'A top level centre with effective quality assurance programmes will have fewer unidentified systematic errors within its processes. A systematic error which is not identified or corrected becomes a mistake'.

In recent years two incidents have occurred in the UK where several patients were injured by serious systematic errors in dosimetry resulting from errors in the dose rate factors programmed into planning computers. In two other incidents, lethal doses were received by patients owing to equipment malfunctions (one to inadequate computer control/interlock of beam current and target movement, the other to interlock bypassing).

Dose variations may be discovered by the use of detectors placed on or in a patient during treatment. Quality assurance programmes should include the conduction of such dosimetry checks at intervals for each type of technique, either on patients or using a phantom.

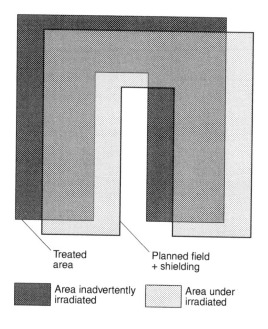

Treated area

Planned field + shielding

Area inadvertently irradiated

Area under irradiated

Figure 12.6 Areas outside the target area which have been unintentionally irradiated, areas within the target area which have been 'missed' on some occasions, and areas adjacent to shielding receiving under- or overdosage because of field placement variation.

The dosimetric effects of set-up variation

Areas around the field edges receive varying doses with field placement variation. Some portal imaging software systems present the overall picture as an 'image of regret', showing areas irradiated unintentionally and areas of underdosage within the target anatomy. Where there is shielding or compensation within the field, the area receiving incorrect dose increases and may comprise the whole area (Fig. 12.6). A larger dose variation occurs with an uncorrected systematic error than with a random error, but with random error the dose variation may be spread over a larger portion of the target area.

Progress towards greater accuracy via sequential studies

The accuracy studies conducted at Cookridge Hospital over the last decade have shown that continual progress towards the achievement of accuracy is possible. A brief outline will illustrate the process.

Sequential studies were conducted by using films taken on the treatment machine itself during each of several treatments for each patient. Films were stored then analysed retrospectively to give a true picture of the trends within an unaltered treatment course. (Patients were not routinely monitored in this way, so normal practice was studied.)

First studies and improvements

Firstly we studied the accuracy resulting from three treatment methods designed to achieve the same result in the abdomen and pelvis (Griffiths & Pearcey 1985; Griffiths 1986). Each method showed a different pattern of errors. Different factors contributed to the shift for each technique. Some errors arose from the way the equipment was used for a particular method and were random, therefore uncorrectable. One technique was therefore discontinued. The most accurate and reproducible method was adopted for all patients, but was modified to reduce effects from its main inaccuracy factors (see Ch. 18). Accuracy was improved, as demonstrated by a subsequent study of a second series of patients treated using the modified method (Griffiths et al 1987).

Further studies and findings

Some lateral shift inaccuracy remained, so we continued to investigate modifications to pelvic field set-up methods, in order to gain further improvements. A study was conducted using the simulator to produce hard copy images of the same patients, set-up using different methods to achieve the same plan. (Ethical approval would be required for this method now, following the 1987 regulations minimising patient exposure.) We demonstrated that centring the field by using a field centre tattoo rather than a skin mark (see Ch. 13), on patients who were set-up in either the prone or supine position, but using lateral tattoos and lasers to stabilise rotation, gave a very high degree of accuracy (Griffiths et al 1991) in the lateral direction. By contrast with results for patients who were set-up using a comparable method in earlier studies, the systematic error was reduced by two-thirds, and the random error at 1.5 mm had been halved (and was half that quoted in other literature).

This type of work has firmly established the principles of checking treatment field accuracy and modifying practice accordingly. However, there are other techniques which call for improvement, and many centres are only at the start of this learning process.

REFERENCES AND FURTHER READING

Byhardt R W, Cox J D, Hornburg A, Liermann G 1978 Weekly localisation films and detection of field placement errors. International Journal of Radiation Oncology, Biology, Physics 4: 881–887
Dutreix A 1984 When and how can we improve precision in radiotherapy? Radiotherapy and Oncology 2: 275–292
Griffiths S E 1986 Reproducibility in radiotherapy. Radiography 52: 167–169

Griffiths S E 1989 Hit or miss – is perfection achievable in radiotherapy? Radiography Today 55: 24–26
Griffiths S E 1990 Radiotherapy quality control: portal and verification films. Radiography 56: 17
Griffiths S E, Pearcey R G 1985 The reproducibility of large lead protected radiotherapy fields to the abdomen and pelvis. Radiography 51: 247–250
Griffiths S E, Pearcey R G, Thorogood J 1987 Quality control in radiotherapy: the reduction of field placement

errors. International Journal of Radiation Oncology, Biology, Physics 13: 1583–1588

Griffiths S E, Khoury G G, Eddy A 1991 Quality control in radiotherapy during pelvic irradiation. Radiotherapy and Oncology 20: 203–206

Hulshof M, Vanuytsel L, Van den Bogaert W, Van der Schueren E 1989 Localization errors in mantle field irradiation for Hodgkin's disease. International Journal of Radiation Oncology, Biology, Physics 17: 679–683

Kihlen B, Ruden B I 1989 Reproducibility of field alignment in radiation therapy. Acta Oncologica 28: 689–692

Leunens G, Van Dam J, Dutreix A, Van der Scheuren E 1990 Quality assurance in radiotherapy by in vivo dosimetry. 1. Entrance measurements, a reliable procedure. Radiotherapy and Oncology 17: 141–151

Marks J E, Haus A G, Sutton H H, Griem M L 1976 The value of frequent verification films in reducing localisation error in the irradiation of complex fields. Cancer 37: 2755–2761

Mitine C, Leunens G, Verstraete J, Blackaert N, Van Dam J, Dutreix A, Van der Scheuren E 1991 Is it necessary to repeat quality control procedures for head and neck patients? Radiotherapy and Oncology 21: 201–210

Morgan A The effect of shielding trays on surface absorbed dose outside primary megavoltage radiotherapy beams. Personal communication

Rabinowitz I, Broomberg J, Gotein M, McCarthy K, Leong J 1982 Accuracy of radiation field alignment in clinical practice. International Journal of Radiation Oncology, Biology, Physics 8: 165–175

Richards M J S, Buchler D A 1977 Errors in reproducing pelvic radiation portals. International Journal of Radiation Oncology, Biology, Physics 2: 1017–1019

13

Patient positioning

PATIENT POSITIONING AS A BEAM DIRECTION PROCEDURE

Beam direction procedures are sometimes viewed as involving only the setting of certain parameters such as gantry and couch angles. If these parameters are set as detailed on the treatment plan, or as indicated by beam direction devices attached to the patient such as a shell, the geometrical beam direction through space or through the shell will indeed be correct, the degree of accuracy depending on the devices (see Ch. 9) and the method used.

However, whether the beam direction through the patient and the target tissue is correct will depend on the three-dimensional position of the patient on planning and on treatment. Beam direction is therefore a complex process involving parameter setting and appropriate patient positioning for each treatment method. The procedures described in this and following chapters are designed to ensure accurate beam direction in the patient.

Consistent patient positioning throughout planning and treatment

The position of the patient for treatment should be determined at the first stage of planning, such as on CT or simulation, taking into account the technical restrictions of the equipment to be used throughout the process. The position should be reasonably comfortable for the patient but compatible with treatment requirements.

For all techniques used, the appropriate support devices, such as headrests, chestboards, armpoles, footrests or firm foam blocks in a range of standard shapes, should be available in each planning and treatment room. The use of soft pillows or cushions is not recommended where accuracy is required, but may be appropriate for large field palliative treatments. The use of a thin foam mattress under the patient will compromise accuracy (Griffiths et al 1991), but should be considered for patient comfort where palliation is undertaken, to enable the patient to lie still for the treatment exposure.

Depending on the technique being used and the degree of accuracy required, the type of couch section/s supporting the patient on planning should have the same degree of rigidity as the couch sections to be used during treatment.

Any patient position adopted for planning should be reproducible by means of reference marks giving adequate three-dimensional information. Some patients have spinal curvature or other conditions which make it difficult to adopt the standard treatment positions. They may require extra supports or an unusual position. If they are manipulated into an unnatural position on planning, it is less likely that their position will be well reproduced on treatment. Written comments about whether a patient appeared to be straight or flat after positioning at planning, will supplement the information available to treatment staff. Ideally simulator staff should be able to see the first treatment set-up for complex work or unusual set-ups.

Comprehensive principles for positioning the patient are described below, and are generally applicable to most techniques. Additional issues for particular techniques are described in the appropriate chapters.

Three-dimensional patient positioning

There are two main criteria for achieving correct three-dimensional orientation of the patient on both the treatment and planning table:

- straightness of the longitudinal or caudocephalic axis
- degree of lateral rotation of the part of the body to be treated.

In order to set the patient correctly in the beam in all three dimensions, two other factors are important:

- the method used to centre the patient in the isocentric axis laterally and longitudinally
- the method used to set the patient at the correct height in relation to the isocentre.

All of these procedures are subject to inaccuracy depending on the method used. Treatment fields will always appear to be correct on setting-up according to surface marks and the specified machine parameters.

Three-dimensional patient position on the table

Precise reproduction on each treatment of a patient's planning position requires the use of appropriate patient support devices, lasers, skin marks and tattoos, and efficient communication and transfer of positional information from planning to treatment staff. This information, including supports used, and measurements from tattoos and/or anatomical points to the treatment centring point, should form part of the prescription or a written protocol.

Straightness in the longitudinal axis

The straight axis of the patient used during planning should be reproduced on treatment. If the patient is skewed on treatment, fields applied will be rotated with respect to the planned target anatomy. The errors resulting from field rotation increase with field size, f.s.d., and field complexity as demonstrated by Figures 13.1A, B and 13.2 where the effect of the same error is shown for different fields.

Patients may be aligned and simulated lying straight, and the sagittal laser axis marked intermittently, e.g. with up to three well spaced tattoos (Fig. 13.3). The longitudinal field axis may be used instead of a laser, but because the projected centre cross-axis may not run exactly straight (Fig. 9.13), this practice may lead to slight discrepancies when the patient is aligned for treatment. By aligning the patient's marked axis with the laser on each treatment, the position is well reproduced. Patients with shells may have the laser line marked on the shell, and may be positioned each day so that the laser runs along this line and straight down the sternum or spine.

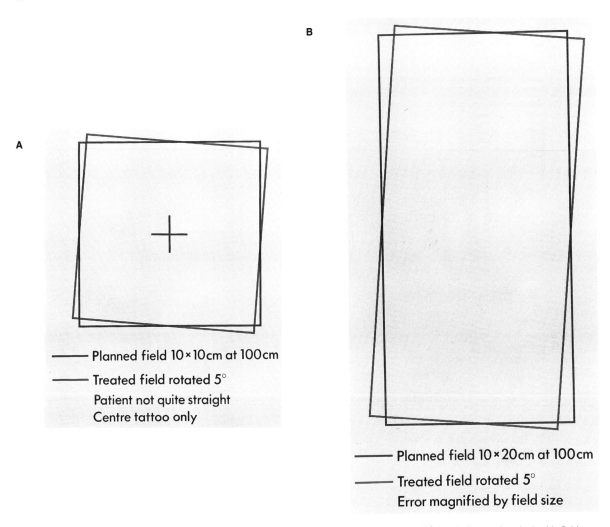

Figure. **13.1 A, B** The increasing effect of the same degree of treatment field rotation (5° in relation to the plan) with field size (f.s.d. is 100 cm).

Tattoos placed on the lateral aspects of the patient, in line with each other longitudinally, can help in reducing local anatomical skew, but strategically placed midline tattoos (as described above) are superior for overall patient straightness as the skin bearing the lateral tattoos can be very mobile in the longitudinal direction (Fig. 13.4). It is consequently sometimes difficult to align lateral tattoos in the longitudinal direction, while keeping the patient straight and flat, so skill and judgement is required in deciding which to use for each technique.

Stabilising lateral rotation

It is known from studies using treatment verification film that patients show differing degrees of lateral rotation or 'roll' from treatment to treatment and from planning to treatment. Lateral rotation causes misdirection of treatment beams, so that when a field is set correctly at the surface, the anatomy at a depth in the patient is laterally misaligned (Fig. 13.5). The size of the shift is proportional to the amount of roll compared with that on the original simulation or treatment, and

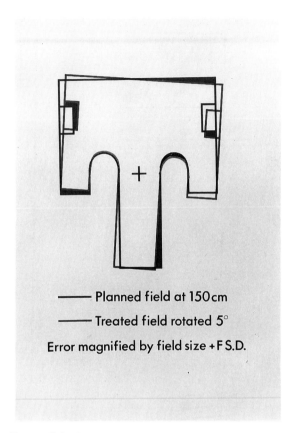

——— Planned field at 150cm

——— Treated field rotated 5°

Error magnified by field size +F S.D.

Figure. 13.2 The same rotation as shown in Figure 13.1 causes larger and multiple errors on a large field with complex shielding and a longer f.s.d. (150 cm).

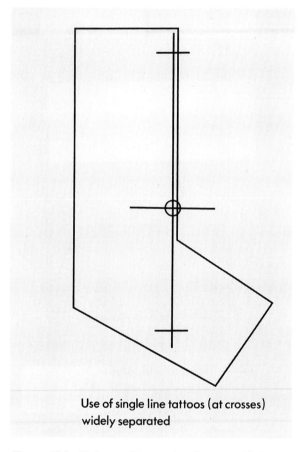

Use of single line tattoos (at crosses) widely separated

Figure. 13.3 Well-spaced tattoos for alignment with the sagittal laser.

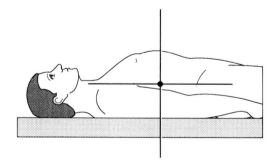

Figure. 13.4 Alignment of a lateral tattoo with the lateral laser.

increases with depth from the surface. A discrepancy of 1 cm in height between the tattoos produces a lateral shift of 7 mm at the centre of an average-sized patient.

On a film or image of the treatment, lateral rotation is seen as a lateral shift of the field across the patient. It can be minimised (Fig. 13.6A, B) by using lateral tattoos, equidistant from the table top, placed on the patient during planning. By realigning the marks for each treatment, usually using lateral lasers, the lateral roll at planning is reproduced and the treatment beams are correctly aligned right through the patient.

If the patient has rolled since being positioned, on checking the patient set-up between fields, the field will appear to have moved off-centre. The patient should be rolled back until the field is again centred. The lateral laser position may be rechecked, but will usually be correct unless gross

movement has taken place, since the movement of each marked point corresponds to that of the others.

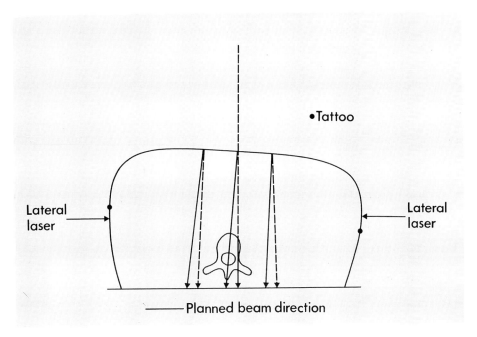

Figure. 13.5 Lateral patient rotation causes misdirection of the treatment beam.

Treatment fields will appear to be correct on setting them to two-dimensional surface marks.

if viewed as setting a light beam to a mark (the target anatomy being hidden from view).

Centring the target anatomy in the treatment beam axes

Once the patient is correctly positioned on the treatment table, the target anatomy must be centred correctly in relation to the machine isocentre in three dimensions, laterally, longitudinally and vertically.

Centring the target anatomy in the isocentric axis laterally and longitudinally

Centring the patient in the longitudinal and lateral directions is achieved by aligning surface marks with the light field and centre cross, or with a lateral laser cross. The type of surface mark used (Griffiths et al 1991), and the way that the marks relate to the target anatomy each day, affect the accuracy of the field alignment. Details in the method used will change the accuracy achieved. The pitfalls may be obscure because treatment centring appears to be a simple process

Variations in shape of field and shielding outlines marked on skin

Marks for aligning the field or shielding positions are often drawn on the patient's skin during simulation, with dye such as gentian violet. The use of such marks is not recommended where accuracy is important (Byhardt et al 1978) as they tend to distort easily, and may never be the same shape as intended once the patient has moved. This is demonstrated by the observed variability from one day to the next of the shape of the shielding blocks required to fit the marks on a patient's skin (Griffiths & Pearcey 1985; Griffiths 1986, 1989). It may be equally apparent that the field light does not fit a particular marked field outline in the same way each day, as the shape of the marks varies. The potential effects of this for fields of complex shape, and some methods of avoiding error, will be further discussed in Chapter 18.

Movement of marks with position, and relationship with target anatomy. The topographical

A

No lateral tattoos

B

Lateral tattoos used

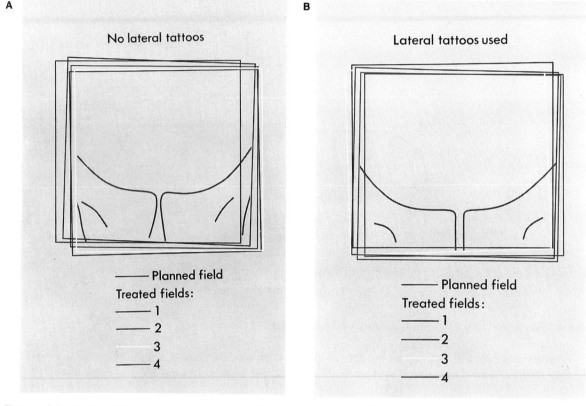

————— Planned field
Treated fields:
————— 1
————— 2
3
————— 4

————— Planned field
Treated fields:
————— 1
————— 2
3
————— 4

Figure. 13.6 Treated fields compared with the planned field, showing lateral shift. **A** Without the use of lateral tattoos and lasers the error is largely systematic, all treated fields being well to the right of the planned field. **B** With the use of tattoos and lasers there is small random error only, so that the treated fields are slightly to left and right of the plan.

relationship of any type of surface marks to the internal target anatomy changes with patient position. For example:

• Changes in head height owing to use of a pillow or varying head supports can substantially alter the position of marked or tattooed skin on the chest and abdomen.
• The skin on the trunk moves when the arms are moved.
• Weight from the arms or hands resting on the trunk can distort the shape of the abdomen and cause movement of the skin.
• Tight clothing has to be loosened or removed to avoid shape distortion and dragging of the skin.
• Care has to be taken to ensure that the skin is not dragged in one direction by its contact with

the surface of the table when the patient gets on the couch, or during positioning.
• Where planning takes place with the patient on a rigid surface but he/she is then treated on a less rigid surface, positional changes may take place which lead to a centring inaccuracy, owing to altered surface contours and a changed relationship of marks to the target anatomy.

An example of the type of error which may occur owing to mobility of surface marks is the 1 cm longitudinal shift of the treatment field with relation to the target anatomy shown in Figure 13.7. This figure represents the edges of three anterior fields, recorded on successive pelvic field treatments of a patient, related to the demagnified edges of the simulated field and bony anatomy.

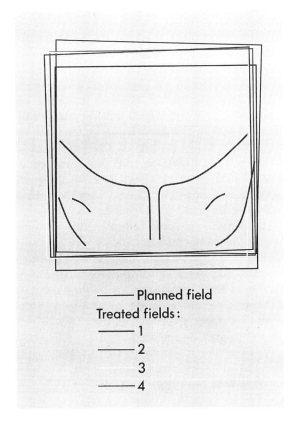

Planned field

Treated fields:

———— 1
———— 2
3
———— 4

Figure. 13.7 The mobility of surface marks with relation to internal anatomy causing a superior shift of all treated fields from the plan. (See text.)

Tattoos

Tattoos as centring points. The use of tattoos, for centring and directing treatment from the skin surface, is recommended for increased field placement accuracy (Griffiths et al 1991). Studies show that tattoos over stable points are more accurate than thick field marks for use in centring treatment fields. Finely marked points may yield similar accuracy, providing that they can be kept or renewed accurately throughout the course.

Correct identification of the tattoo for centring. An approximate measurement from the tattoo to an anatomical landmark such as the suprasternal notch (SSN) should be given on prescription data, to allow a check to be made that the tattoo has been correctly identified. This information is also useful with ink marks, especially when they fade or are smudged onto an adjacent area, but is only

an approximate guide, since two people will not measure in the same way. Where there are two tattoos or similar marks present on the same area of the body, the information helps to avoid centring on the wrong point, since one of the marks is identifiable by measurement as being the treatment centre or reference point. Making a second tattoo in any area is to be avoided. A new treatment centre may be referenced by measurements from an existing tattoo. A photograph of the treatment field or centring point on the body surface may be helpful to confirm the approximate area treated, especially when adequate staff continuity is difficult to achieve.

Retrospective reconstruction of treatment via tattoos. A tattoo will remain throughout a course and may later serve as a reference point for a previous treatment. A check film taken using the tattoo and compared with a previous portal film can demonstrate whether a skin tattoo still represents the centre of anatomy treated at an earlier date (weight changes in the patient will affect the position of the tattoo).

Tattoos as reference points. An existing tattoo on a stable point may be used as a reference point, with measurements to the required centring point (Fig. 13.8).

Centring may then be achieved by moving the couch the appropriate distance after setting up on the reference point, but the accuracy of this practice depends on how the couch movement is measured. Couch movement scales may be unreliable for the distances involved, and should be tested under treatment conditions such as with a body weight on the couch. Measuring horizontally along the patient's skin, or using a ruler laid on the couch top and a laser to measure the movement, are accurate methods (Probst 1991).

If, after measurement and movement, the field centring point is marked on the skin, a visual check on whether the patient has moved during treatment can be made between fields (slight movement is not always detectable via closed-circuit TV). The mark could be used to confirm the centring point each day, however the distance should be checked, measured, and the skin remarked each day, especially on a mobile abdomen or breast.

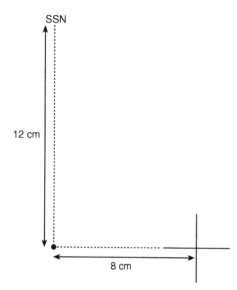

Figure. 13.8 A tattoo used as a reference point for the treatment centre. The reference tattoo is approximately 12 cm inferior to the SSN. The treatment centre is 8 cm to the right of the reference tattoo.

Centre measurement information should be clearly annotated to ensure that couch movements are made in the required direction from the reference point. Directional errors are less noticeable with small movements, since treatment will still appear to be centred on the relevant part of the body. For example if 0.5 cm to the left is marked instead of 0.5 cm to the right, this is more likely to go unnoticed than an error with a 5 cm movement. If a centre is marked with a directional error, checking information each day will reveal the error and prevent repetition.

Tattoos for straightness. When using midline tattoos for ensuring patient straightness, the further apart the tattoos the more accurate the result, since tattoos which are close together give little information for whole body alignment.

Lateral tattoos. Tattoos for identifying lateral laser points may be used to set or centre fields in the longitudinal direction, if they are longitudinally aligned with the treatment centre and each other at planning (see Fig. 13.4).

Accuracy, positioning and marking considerations for pelvis and abdomen

Pelvis patients may be positioned supine or prone. The supine position gives rise to less lateral rotation (Griffiths et al 1991), but if lateral tattoos are used to reduce roll, accuracy will be equal for both positions.

Lines marked on the skin for field and shielding outlines are particularly mobile on the buttocks, owing to variation in tensing and relaxing of the muscles. Using such marks for field centring leads to inaccuracy in the caudocephalic centring, particularly on thin or emaciated patients (Griffiths et al 1991). Use of alternative centring and shielding systems should be made, especially for complex fields (see Ch. 18).

The central or near-central tattoo is on a potentially very mobile surface on a supine patient. On heavyweight patients in the supine position, additional centring procedures such as the use of the sagittal laser for midline reference and a longitudinal reference measurement from a mark at a stable level such as the pubis or even the thigh, may be required.

For patients lying in the prone position, a tattoo over the spine or sacrum, used alone, will allow accurate field centring.

COUCH HEIGHT SETTING: THE THIRD DIMENSION

The accuracy of many treatments depends critically on the factors associated with couch height. There are various pitfalls, of which the radiographer/planner needs to be aware, in the method of measuring the couch height (patient factors), and in setting height (equipment factors).

All processes used in couch height setting should be evaluated. The tumour is at risk of a partial geographical miss from any couch height discrepancy, especially where lateral or oblique fields are used. The requirement is usually to set the treatment (tumour) centre level in the patient at the isocentre height, which involves determining the height of this point above the couch. Thus a height above couch measurement (see Fig. 15.10) is obtained for use in couch height setting on each treatment.

Rounding the required setting up or down to the nearest 0.5 cm on planning, plus a slight discrepancy owing to other factors, may add up to a systematic inaccuracy of 0.5 cm or more which makes a significant difference to the dosimetry in the target volume (Fig. 13.9A, B).

Couch top factors

Couch top sag is potentially a major problem (see Fig. 9.9B). It is sometimes assumed that sag

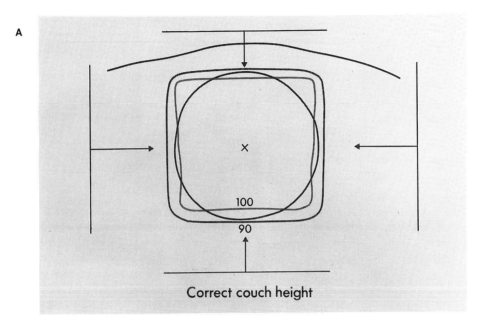

A

100

90

Correct couch height

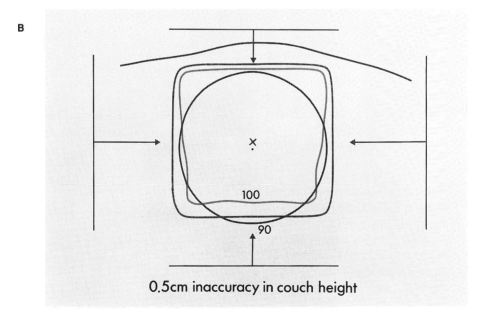

B

100

90

0.5cm inaccuracy in couch height

Figure. 13.9 **A** The dose distribution for a four-field treatment (to a circular cross-section target volume) with a correct couch height. **B** The effect of a 0.5 cm couch height inaccuracy is that the lower edge of the target volume falls outside the high dose zone.

effects will be constant on a given type of top from day to day and on different machines, i.e. that planning can be carried out on a tennis racquet type top so long as treatment is given on a similar top. However, couch sag varies daily for the same patient in the same position on the same top (Quinn 1992). The maximum sag is under the centre of the patient, and has been measured at an average of 1 cm when using a tennis racquet section for supine pelvic treatments (see Fig. 9.9C). This is a potential setting inaccuracy likely to be repeated on every treatment, plus or minus daily variations.

Couch height scales and their limitations

Analogue (mechanical) couch height scales can be unreliable, and newer equipment has only an electronic (digital) readout of couch height. A backup check via some other scale or measurement should be available. Scales or readouts are usually checked daily, but have been seen to vary with a patient on the couch. They also represent the theoretical height of the couch without sag or flex rather than an accurate indication of the height of the patient.

Lateral laser and vertical rule method

Couch height can be accurately set by use of a lateral laser (or the field centre line for a horizontal field) to indicate the isocentre height on a vertical scale standing on the flat (rigid) table top (Fig. 13.10). The scale must be placed at the centre of the laser cross, as the longitudinal limb of the cross does not run parallel with the table top (even a rigid couch top flexes with patient weight). The accuracy achieved will depend on the accuracy of the laser at the point where the scale stands. (The lasers may not run horizontally across the room, and the couch top may tilt slightly towards one side.) These factors should be checked out for each piece of equipment so that their effects can be taken into account.

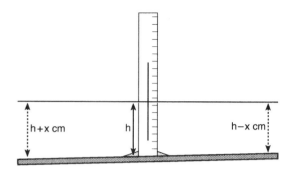

Figure. 13.10 Use of a vertical scale standing on a rigid couch top at the isocentre position, with the lateral laser or field centre, to set the required height above couch. (Not appropriate for couch sections which allow sag.)

Tattoos for height setting

A possible method for setting the height is by use of the lateral tattoos on the patient, where these have a known relationship to the isocentre height. However, as with any other method, it should be well researched in the centre of use to establish its adequacy.

Using the rangefinder to set height

In certain circumstances, the rangefinder may be used to set the couch height by raising the couch until the appropriate reading is seen on the patient surface. This method is only viable either where the tumour is effectively at the relevant surface, e.g. breast, or where the patient surface to be used is not subject to daily variations in contour, since this would lead to similar daily variations in the couch height set.

Where the tumour is attached to the surface, as in breast treatments, height setting at a stable point on the surface is valid. In other circumstances where the patient shape is 'fixed' by the surrounding bony anatomy, the surface may be used for measurement. (See also Chs 2 and 9 for rangefinder design factors affecting setting accuracy.)

REFERENCES AND FURTHER READING

Byhardt R W, Cox J D, Hornburg A, Liermann G 1978 Weekly localisation films and detection of field placement errors. International Journal of Radiation Oncology, Biology, Physics 4: 881–887

Griffiths S E 1986 Reproducibility in radiotherapy. Radiography 52: 167–169

Griffiths S E 1989 Hit or miss – is perfection achievable in radiotherapy? Radiography Today 55: 24–26

Griffiths S E, Pearcey R G 1985 The reproducibility of large lead protected radiotherapy fields to be abdomen and pelvis. Radiography 51: 247–250

Griffiths S E, Pearcey R G, Thorogood J 1987 Quality control in radiotherapy. The reduction of field placement errors. International Journal of Radiation Oncology, Biology, Physics 13: 1583–1588

Griffiths S E, Khoury G G, Eddy A 1991 Quality control in radiotherapy during pelvic irradiation. Radiotherapy and Oncology 20: 203–206

Probst H 1991 B.Sc project work, Cookridge Hospital, Leeds

Quinn G 1993 An investigation into radiotherapy treatment couch sag. Radiography Today 59: 9–12

14

Planning the treatment

Before radiotherapy can be given, the size and location of a tumour must be known, so that a treatment plan can be made. The planning process includes several procedures, many of which are dependent on each other and which together form the theoretical basis for delivery of the desired dose to the target tissue. Planning methods and procedures are continually updated and improved as new knowledge and technological advances in the fields of diagnosis, localisation (imaging), planning, and treatment delivery emerge.

There are, however, limitations to the accuracy with which the theoretical plan may be applied to the patient. These stem from approximations made in the planning process, from machine accuracy limitations and from the patient as a mobile body of complex shape. Thus on some occasions the plan may be seen not to fit the patient and so the planning process may be partially repeated and the plan subsequently modified. The plan may therefore be perceived to be a theory which can only work to a degree consistent with the limits of practicality, and which is judged by the outcome of quality checks and verification procedures when it is applied to treat the patient. The plan for each patient must enable accurate set-up processes to be used and therefore issues of equipment usage must be considered during plan design.

Those planning processes which have the most direct influence on the accuracy of treatment will be considered in some detail. Other linked processes such as the construction of beam direction shells, shielding blocks, compensators etc. are described in other literature, and will only be referred to where they relate to issues discussed. Similarly the process of field planning will not be described in detail.

PRINCIPLES OF TREATMENT PLANNING

Steps in the planning sequence

Treatment planning consists of several basic principles, applied in sequence after tumour diagnosis and staging:

- Selecting an appropriate technique.
- Selecting a patient position compatible with the treatment site and the technique envisaged, including the type and arrangement of any supports or accessories.
- Collecting information about the size, shape and location of the tumour, with the patient in the selected treatment position.
- Collecting information about the size and shape of the region of the patient which contains the tumour and geographically relating the tumour to this and to critical organs in the proximity.
- Applying information about the available treatment machines and radiation sources/beams to the patient, to plan a detailed technique for dose prescription and delivery.
- Performing check procedures on the plan and patient to verify the adequacy of the plan when applied to the patient.

Within the planning programme, the construction of beam direction shells and manufacture of shielding blocks also take place as required.

Selecting an appropriate technique

The site, size, shape and stage of the tumour as assessed on completion of diagnostic procedures including clinical, surgical and radiological findings determines the type of technique and whether or not radical treament can be delivered. If a large target volume is identified, this will influence the technique and the dose given. A large volume may render a tumour unsuitable for treatment by a technique which is designed to give radical high dose treatment.

Where a radical treatment is appropriate, the technique chosen is dependent on various factors. These include the size and location of the tumour and the practices of the department or individual consultants for treating particular tumours. The site of and proximity of a tumour to critical organs influences the degree of treatment complexity required to achieve a radical treatment. The expertise of staff involved and the available planning facilities affect treatment practices; for example, sophisticated computer planning systems show 'hot spots' and 'cold spots' on plans which appear adequate on less sophisticated systems. Efforts to perfect the distribution often lead to greater complexity. Techniques used depend to some extent on the practical limitations of the available treatment machines and couches, since designs used by the various manufacturers allow differing degrees of freedom in set-up.

Some simple radical or palliative treatments can be delivered without the need for complex planning procedures (see Ch. 15). Others, particularly those to organs lying deep in the body require the application of many of the processes outlined in this chapter.

Selecting a patient position

The position to be adopted for the first stage of planning must be the one which will be used during treatment (see Ch. 13). Therefore this position must be:

- acceptable to the patient, who must be immobile for the duration of each procedure
- reproducible from one occasion to another
- compatible with applying treatment beams to the region to be treated
- compatible with any special requirements for the treatment machine likely to be used.

An exact duplicate of any immobilisation device used during planning must be available and known to be viable for treatment use.

Collecting information about the size, shape and location of the tumour

The process of localisation results in the size and geographical position of the target tissue, in three dimensions, being identified and related to marks, body landmarks and/or a beam direction shell. The reliability of the information is dependent on the patient's position during the procedures being exactly as it would be for treatment.

Localisation procedures, for tumours suitable for the application of radical treatments, are used to assess the exact tumour size and position. Computerised tomography (CT) has become the radiological medium of choice for tumour assessment, although magnetic resonance imaging (MRI) is increasingly used, especially for neurological sites and for limbs since the images available for these are exceptionally detailed compared with those using other modalities (see Ch. 11). Ultrasound is also occasionally used for specific purposes such as assessing chest wall thickness in breast planning (see Ch. 16).

The use of simple radiological means such as fluoroscopy and radiographs produced on a radiotherapy simulator is common. This, together with clinical findings and/or diagnostic radiographs, presently appears to be adequate for identifying the target tissue for some routine treatments.

Localisation using CT scans

For many patients, planning is now started on a CT scanner (see Ch. 11). The scanner (and the patient) must be specially set up for radiotherapy planning scans (described in detail by Ash et al 1983) for information to be valid under treatment conditions. The superior accuracy of localisation using CT planning compared with conventional radiography has long been proven (Rothwell et al 1983).

A description of the planning process used for treatment to the bladder will illustrate the main steps.

The patient is asked to empty the bladder immediately before scanning. He/she is then positioned straight and flat on the CT table, usually lying supine, so that the sagittal laser (see Ch. 15) runs through the suprasternal notch, the xiphisternum, and the centre of the symphysis pubis. A thin wire along the laser path taped to the skin of the abdomen and pelvis will show the surface midline on all slices (Fig. 14.1).

Cross-sectional views (slices) of the area of interest plus margins, superiorly and inferiorly,

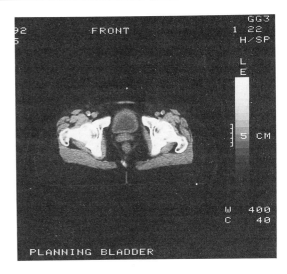

Figure 14.1 CT slice showing wire marker coincident with the sagittal laser on the anterior skin.

are taken. The pelvis is scanned to produce a scout view, giving a view similar to an anteroposterior radiograph, on which lines are displayed showing where the centre slice has been taken (Fig. 14.2). The centre of the likely target tissue in the longitudinal direction is determined from the slices and marked on the skin while the patient is still in position. This point is marked and measurements relating it to identifiable points on the surface anatomy (and to the

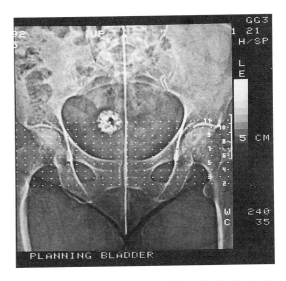

Figure 14.2 Anteroposterior scout view of patient and slices taken.

midline point on a specific CT slice) are noted for use in finding the mark at simulation.

The lateral laser points (see Ch. 13) should also be marked, then tattooed when a height above table is established, i.e. they should ideally be made at the height of the treatment centre.

The images are copied onto floppy disc or serial-linked for viewing on the treatment planning VDU. The body surface, tumour and critical organs may be outlined within each slice (Fig. 14.3). The summation of the slices containing tumour together with those immediately superior and inferior, gives the volume length including a margin (see Fig. 14.4). The largest cross-section of tumour, plus safety margin, is delineated within the body outline on the central slice, to use with beam data for dosimetry planning. The images are scaled down in size relative to the actual anatomy, so that measurements on them can be converted to actual size using a ratio factor. Once the centre of the target volume is established relative to the mark made at CT, the centring point should be identified, verified by simulation, then tattooed.

Delineating the treatment volume and margins

The definition of treatment volumes has become more precise following a report on dose prescrip-

tion from ICRU 50 (1992) which recommends new definitions. Various concepts are involved, firstly the clinical concept of tumour volume. The gross tumour volume (GTV) is 'the volume occupied by a mass of cancer tissue' and does not exist in a patient who has had a complete surgical resection.

The target volume is a related oncological concept. The clinical target volume (CTV) contains the tumour volume plus an 'oncological safety margin' containing clinically undetectable cancer cells. Delineation of the target volume and the thickness of this safety margin depend on the tumour characteristics. Regional lymph nodes at risk may be included as additional target volumes.

To ensure that the target volume is actually irradiated, a planning safety margin must be added. This margin is an attempt to allow for movement with respect to e.g. bony anatomy, or from changes in shape of the target volume, and from inaccuracies in patient or beam positioning. The planning target volume (PTV) includes the target volume plus the planning safety margin. A margin corresponding to the width of the penumbra for the beams to be used is added to the planning volume size to give field sizes (Fig. 14.4).

The relative size of the tumour and the two margins depends on the site, and on the precision with which radiation can be delivered. A bronchial tumour, situated within tissue which moves during breathing, needs a large planning safety margin even with an accurate setting-up method. Any improvement of reproducibility of patient position and accuracy of treatment delivery which can be achieved (see Chs 12 and 13) will reduce the size of the planning safety volume required for each site. It is advantageous to reduce this volume, in order to minimise irradiation of healthy tissue and because a greater dose can be tolerated by smaller volumes (see Ch. 23).

Subsequent reference to the 'target volume' should be taken to either refer to the PTV as defined above, or to the tissue intended to be included within anatomical/field boundaries defined clinically or on simulation, depending on the context.

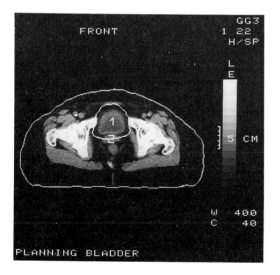

Figure 14.3 Slice with body surface, target volume (1) and facility to outline a second volume of critical tissue if required (2).

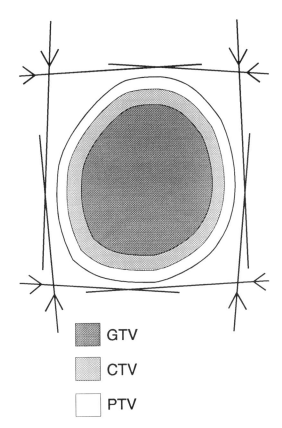

GTV

CTV

PTV

Figure 14.4   Relationship to the tumour (GTV) to margins (CTV and PTV) and to field sizes.

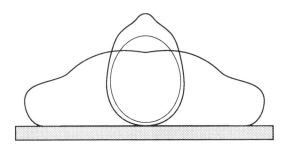

IA

Treatment volume

Irradiated volume

Figure 14.5   Gross planning volume and tissue irradiated by the four fields used. (Courtesy of P. Williams.)

Figure 14.6   Irregular body shape in the region of the neck, necessitating the use of outlines at various levels.

Geographically relating the tumour to the surrounding tissues and surface

In order that dosimetry can be predicted throughout the region (Fig. 14.5), the shape and composition of the tissue through which radiation beams will pass during treatment delivery, and where the tumour lies in relation to the surface, must be known.

Accurate outlines of the body surface in the treatment region, with the patient in the treatment position, are required. Outlines are usually taken round the body at the centre of the target area, and at the superior and inferior extremities of the target area when the body shape is irregular (Fig. 14.6). An extra outline at the largest part of the patient within the region of interest is required to check that beams will give adequate cover. For example, for a breast patient, an outline at the largest part of the breast should be taken whether or not this corresponds to the centre of the treatment region.

Outline methods

There are many ways of producing an outline of the body surface. Some are less accurate than others, and few are ideal.

Mechanical devices.

1. Flexi-curve. The simplest method for a small area is to use flexicurve, which is a strip of material easily moulded to the body surface. However, alteration of its curves may occur during the process of transferring them to paper, and the length of the outline is too limited for most uses.

2. A mechanical device placed on the treatment or planning couch, over the patient at the

region of interest. A series of radially arranged rods are pushed gently in to touch the patient (Fig. 14.7), so that a number of points from the outline can be transferred to paper and joined together. Alternatively a pointer can be moved around the patient's outline, with a pantograph arrangement to simultaneously draw the outline on paper.

Gantry rotation of linac or simulator. Similarly, an isocentrically mounted treatment machine can be moved around the patient so that rangefinder readings can be taken at the surface after every ten degrees of machine rotation, to give information for reconstructing an outline.

Contours of shell. Surface outlines for head and neck treatment may be taken from the inside of a beam direction shell in the plane of interest.

Each of these methods has drawbacks:

• A limited number of points gives only an approximation of contour.

• Demands for machine time may preclude the use of a machine to take outlines.

• The pantograph method is subject to inaccuracy since the device is cumbersome and the pointer may distort flabby surface tissue.

• All these methods limit the available cross-sectional outline to that around the patient, orthogonally to the table.

• An accurate indication of the table height at either side of the patient is required to establish a baseline beneath the patient.

• Distortion of the patient from the true treatment position may be necessary to obtain the outline with a pantograph, which reduces the value and accuracy of the outline.

• The efficacy of the shell contour method depends on how closely and reproducibly the shell fits the patient.

Electronic contour methods employing lasers and digital images. Newer methods of producing patient contours include laser devices mounted on the simulator head (development work is presently underway at Cookridge Hospital, Leeds), and CT images produced under treatment conditions. Both of these methods rely on computer reconstruction of data to give three-dimensional contour information throughout the region of interest.

These methods are superior since:

• There is no risk of distortion of the patient surface when imaging the contour.

• There is a possibility, with appropriate software, of obtaining outlines in any plane.

• Data can be directly transferred to the planning computer without risk of manual transcription error.

• A continuous indication of the contour is given instead of only one or two outlines.

In the event of a treatment centre being moved or defined after the outline process, data at the field centre position are automatically available. The data are also suitable for use in compensator construction using a computerised cutting device.

Regular quality assurance checks are required to ensure that any system is operating correctly, including calibration to ensure that no distortion of tissue shape is occurring.

Tissue thickness or field separation measurements

For some treatments a body outline is unnecessary. For these treatments simple measurements of body thickness at appropriate points may suffice for determining the dosimetry, e.g. for

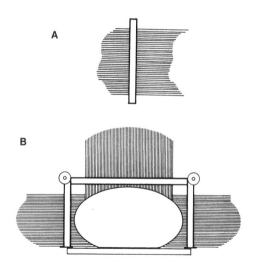

Figure 14.7 Radial rod outline device. **A** Round the ear. **B** For complete body contours. (Reproduced from Walter et al 1982.)

parallel opposed fields (see Ch. 15). These thickness measurements are called separations (the distance separating the surfaces where fields are applied, usually taken only at the field centres).

Combining treatment beam and patient information

Two-dimensional planning

The beam planning process involves the application of isodose data (see Ch. 7) for one or more treatment beams to the cross-section of the tissue geography. Information about the treatment region is often represented as a two-dimensional cross-sectional diagram through the plane to be used for treatment plan generation (Fig. 14.3), i.e. the central treatment plane. The cross-section of the PTV, representing the largest dimensions of

the tumour plus margins, is delineated proportionally within the patient outline.

Dosimetry data for appropriate beam widths are applied to the tissue outlines, using computer planning software so as to encompass the planning volume. The beam lengths are determined from the length of the treatment volume, identified from CT slices etc. during localisation. A printout of the treatment plan thus obtained is generated as a two-dimensional diagram (Fig. 14.8).

The dosimetry from the chosen beams may be predicted at tissue levels other than the central plane, on similar diagrams, but the whole picture cannot be represented so this method is known as two-dimensional planning. More sophisticated methods are available to allow three-dimensional planning to be undertaken where it would be advantageous, for example with irregular volume shapes (see Ch. 23).

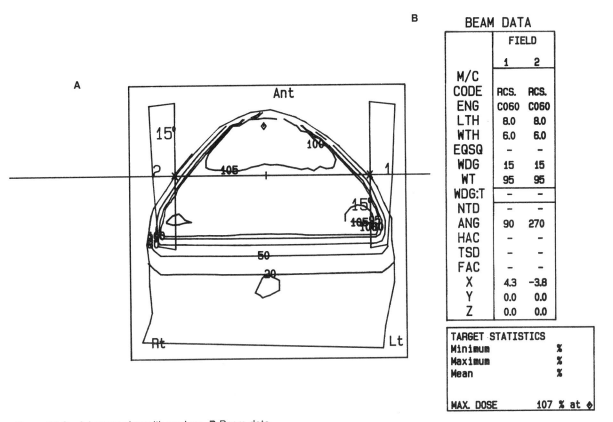

Figure 14.8   A Larynx plan with wedges. **B** Beam data.

Selecting the treatment beams

The application of beam or source data to the patient geographical information is required to produce a plan of the radiation modalities and settings to be used for treatment, and to predict a dose distribution in the region. The number and position of beams used determines the total volume of tissue irradiated (Fig. 14.5), and thus the integral dose received by the patient.

Historically beam arrangements were selected laboriously using hand planning. This is achieved by overlaying isodose curves onto a cross-section of the body contour and noting the percentage of the central axis dose maximum for each beam at each point of interest (Fig. 14.8). Where more than one beam is used, the dose contribution from each is summated at each point. The points of equal dose can be used to predict an isodose zone in the tissue. The basic principles used in hand planning are now employed in computerised treatment planning systems, which carry the relevant machine data, allowing more speed, sophistication and optimisation in planning beam arrangements and dose distributions.

Shaping the high dose zone

The shape of the isodose zone for the clinically relevant dose level (the zone within which the dose is uniformly high) is required to conform to the shape of the delineated target volume (Figs 14.5 and 14.8). The shape of this isodose zone can be altered by changing the number, arrangement, wedging, and dose weighting of the applied beams. Beam parameters are chosen to give the optimum isodose distribution throughout the planning volume. Any nearby critical organs may complicate the process, as the field arrangement may be restricted by the need to avoid irradiating them. Shielding may be introduced into one or more beams to protect uninvolved tissue, a process now commonly used. When special beam arrangements or shaping are used to achieve an irregularly shaped high dose zone, the technique tends towards conformal therapy where the high dose zone is tailored to fit exactly to the tumour shape (see Ch. 23).

Wedging

When beams are incident on a sloping tissue surface as, for example, two opposed fields to the anterior half of the neck, wedges (or compensators) will be required to produce an even isodose distribution. Without modification to compensate for the 'missing' anterior tissue, the beams would give higher doses anteriorly, since the beams are less attenuated before they reach the midline. The effect is slightly offset by the increasing f.s.d. more anteriorly (Fig. 14.8), reducing the radiation intensity at the skin surface.

Alternatively, the desired effect can be produced by constructing and using suitable compensators, but this is more time- and resource-consuming and would not normally be undertaken where the shape of a wedge provides adequate compensation.

Similarly, where two beams are applied obliquely to each other, progressively higher summated doses would occur across the zone where the beams merge, necessitating the use of a wedge on at least one field. A wedged pair at right angles is a useful arrangement for treating a wedge-shaped volume of tissue (see Ch. 8).

With a wedged beam, the attenuation in the wedge results in a lower dose being delivered than for the same monitor units for the same field unwedged. A wedge factor may be applied during monitor unit calculations to compensate for the attenuated dose. Alternatively, there may be an automatic correction for the attenuation if the data held by the planning computer result from measurements of isodose curves for wedged fields (see Ch. 8).

Tissue compensators. Remote compensators (see Ch. 8) may be used instead of wedges to compensate for complex body shapes etc. Appropriate attenuation factors are then required in the dose computation.

Weighting

The proportion of dose from beam to beam can be altered, allowing manipulation of the shape or position of the isodose zone produced by a given combination of beams. For example, using four fields where the tumour lies anterior to the centre of the body cross-section, if there is a greater dose weighting for the fields applied posteriorly than for the field applied anteriorly (see Fig. 15.8), this will result in a more uniformly shaped distribution for the four fields than if equal weighting is used.

The relative weighting of wedged fields is higher than would be required for the same field unwedged if the planning software holds wedged dosimetry measurements or uses the application of a wedge factor.

Dose specification and normalisation

In dose planning and prescription, a system is required to annotate and calculate the dose level at the tumour in proportion to that applied by each beam. An acceptably shaped isodose line is chosen as defining the dose received by the tumour. This isodose line (see Fig. 15.8) results from summation of the contributions from each beam, and may be of the order of 190% of the central axis dose of one beam at the dose maximum. In this case, 100% represents the given or applied dose of one beam.

Alternatively, the isodose at the tumour may be designated as representing 100% of the required tumour dose (Fig. 14.8), thus each beam will give an appropriate percentage of the tumour dose, i.e. the contributions to the tumour dose from the applied beams will total 100%. In this case the dose is said to be normalised to give 100% at the tumour volume. In either case the dose prescribed at the tumour will be the same, e.g. 45 Gy, and the proportionality of this dose to the applied doses from constituent beams will also be the same. Only the annotation is different. Any point can be chosen for normalisation to 100%.

Optimisation

If a standard beam or, in brachytherapy (see Ch. 5) source arrangement, does not give a distribution of the required shape or uniformity, a computer program can optimise the plan by arranging a distribution which gives the required shape. This involves optimisation software manipulation of beam parameters or sources until the required conformity is achieved. Inverse planning (see Ch. 23) is another method of optimising the dosimetry, utilising compensators to change the intensity across the beam.

Inhomogeneity corrections

A requirement for an accurate treatment plan is the appropriate use of tissue inhomogeneity corrections and/or compensators, to obtain optimal dose distributions and protect against unexpected 'hot spots' where a higher dose occurs because of nonuniformity of tissue density and shape.

Compensation for reduced density of lung tissue is often used in plans to the chest.

Combined modalities

Dual modality treatments, using two photon beams of different energies, or a photon plus an electron beam or brachytherapy (see Ch. 23), are occasionally used to achieve a particular dose distribution. For example, the combination of a 250 KV and a 100 KV X-ray beam is sometimes used to treat skin lesions which are too thick to be effectively treated by a 100 KV beam alone, where the proximity of underlying bone prevents treatment wholly by 250 KV. If the isodose curves for a 6 MV beam plus a 14 MeV electron beam applied from the same point are summated, the distribution obtained will be unique to that combination, and may occasionally have a practical application.

For two-phase treatments, often used in the head and neck region (see Ch. 17), a plan for the first phase, using one modality such as 6 MV photons, can be summated with a plan for the second phase, using a different modality such as electrons. An overall dose distribution is then predicted incorporating both phases.

A combined dose distribution from external beam plus brachytherapy treatment (see Chs 21 and 23) may be obtained when suitable software is available.

Three-dimensional planning

In two-dimensional planning the largest cross-section of the tumour is used to determine the beams used and their parameters. It is assumed that the tumour lies within an approximately cylindrical high dose zone produced by those beams (see Fig. 23.1). The change in body contour through the length of the treatment zone will change the dose distribution. In addition, the tumour cross-section is likely to alter, so that the high dose zone includes excessive normal tissue at the volume 'ends'. Reducing this effect requires the use of a system capable of using three-dimensional patient contour, tumour shape, and beam geometry to produce a suitably shaped (conformal) three-dimensional dose distribution (see Ch. 23).

Noncoplanar planning

Conventionally, treatment beam axes are planned in one plane. This is akin to the spokes of a cartwheel where the hub represents the target volume. This limits the possibilities for achieving ideal treatments to certain sites. New technology and methods allow field axes to be angled out of the plane. This is achieved by using couch rotations in addition to gantry rotations. Examples of use are angled couch breast techniques (see Fig. 16.8) and stereotactic treatments (see Ch. 23).

Checking and verification of the plan

Printouts of the plan, giving relevant parameters and information, are produced so that the planner and the radiotherapist can check for adequacy of predicted dose distribution, and for calculation of doses to critical organs. The plan forms part of the prescription and setting-up information for the radiographer to use.

The field placement can be verified by carrying out simulator verification procedures. The treatment fields can be checked on the patient for adequate cover (e.g. breast), or screened to check the position of critical organs such as the spinal cord and to check shielding block placement. Most fields can be recorded on an image and checked for accuracy. These images should then be used as a reference against which to check the accuracy of at least the first treatment, using portal imaging (see Chs 11 and 12).

A further check is available for isocentric set-ups, involving measurement checks of certain distances on the patient at each set-up against those shown on the plan. Measurements may be made by using the rangefinder to check treatment centre-to-skin distances (see Fig. 15.11). Discrepancies of more than 1 cm could indicate a significant problem with the plan or a change in patient shape.

Some potential sources of inaccuracy during planning

- Transcription errors (Leunens et al 1992)
- Computer algorithm deficiencies (Leunens et al 1990)
- Incomplete, conflicting, inadequate or misleading data on the treatment sheet or plan
- Incorrect or incompatible data, e.g. where X and Y axes or scales differ from machine to machine
- Magnification related problems
- Tissue inhomogeneities, tissue movement

The subject of computer planning, and planning processes, is too large to discuss further in this text. Some additional reading is suggested below.

REFERENCES AND FURTHER READING

Ash D V, Andrews B, Stubbs B 1983 A method for integrating computed tomography into radiotherapy planning and treatment. Clinical Radiology 34: 99–101
Dobbs J, Barrett A, Ash D 1992 Practical radiotherapy planning, 2nd edn. Arnold, London
ICRU 1992 Prescribing, recording and reporting photon beam therapy. Report 50. International Commission on Radiological Units and Measurements, Washington DC
Leunens G, Van Dam J, Dutreix A, Van der Schueren E 1990 Quality assurance in radiotherapy by in vivo dosimetry. 1. Entrance dose measurements, a reliable procedure. Radiotherapy and Oncology 17: 141–151

Leunens G, Verstraete J, Van den Bogaert W, Van Dam J, Dutreix A, Van der Schueren E 1992 Human errors in data transfer during the preparation and delivery of radiation treatment affecting the final result: 'garbage in, garbage out'. Radiotherapy and Oncology 23: 217–222

Mould R F 1985 Radiotherapy treatment planning, 2nd edn. Adam Hilger, Bristol

Rothwell R I, Ash D V, Jones W G 1983 Radiation treatment planning for bladder cancer: a comparison of cystogram localisation with computed tomography. Clinical Radiology 43: 103–111

Walter J, Miller H, Bomford C K 1982 A short textbook of radiotherapy, 4th edn. Churchill Livingstone, Edinburgh

15

Basic principles of external beam techniques

TYPES OF FIELD ARRANGEMENT

1. Single Fields. Where a single beam is used, this is usually directly applied to a tumour at or near the surface of the patient. The beam is centred via the use of marks or tattoos on the patient's skin so that the tumour on or beneath the marked skin area is contained within the beam.

2. Parallel Opposed Fields. Two fields with co-incident central axes may be applied from opposing directions, so as to encompass a volume of tissue extending virtually from one surface of the patient through to the opposite surface. This method is used to treat risk areas occupying a large volume or a central location in the patient, and may be applied isocentrically or at standard f.s.d.

3. Multifield Treatments. Where a high dose is required for a relatively small tumour volume, especially where the tumour lies deep in the body, two or more fields with noncoincident central axes may be directed at the tumour. This method ensures a high dose where the beams meet in the patient, giving a high dose to the tumour zone while giving lower doses to the skin and other tissue traversed by each of the beams.

These methods may be used alone or with others to form the basis of commonly used treatments for various sites of the body. The basic principles will be described here, together with some applications. Each type may be used in an increasingly complex manner. More complex or specialised applications will be described in later chapters.

SINGLE FIELDS

The principles

A single field may be used to treat a tumour which is near enough to the body surface for enough dose to be received without overlying or underlying tissue being overdosed by the treatment beam. It is the simplest type of technique but nevertheless various factors are critically important. The principles covered here apply equally to electron single fields, but with the latter, additional, more complex issues are involved, considered separately in Chapters 5 and 21.

Field planning

Choice of modality or beam energy

The dosimetry effect required for a particular patient is achieved by choosing an appropriate beam energy or modality. A short f.s.d. superficial X-ray beam will result in a high surface dose with a rapid fall-off thereafter. A high energy electron field will give a maximum dose at a particular depth dependent on the beam energy used (Ch. 21). The appropriate beam modality therefore depends mainly on the thickness of, or depth in the body of, the tumour.

There may be a need to establish the depth at which a critical underlying structure, such as the lung, lies so that a beam energy can be chosen which will treat the tumour but not the underlying structure. The dose to the skin may also be taken into account when choosing a modality. However, in practice the ideal choice of energy may not be an option because of limited machine availability, so the final choice may be a compromise.

The field size and shape is chosen according to the tumour size, so that the tumour plus margin of risk will be encompassed by the useful beam (Fig. 15.1).

Marking/simulation

If the tumour is at, or palpable from, the body surface, a skin area of appropriate size and shape is marked using clinical judgement, for example for skin tumours or underlying painful areas.

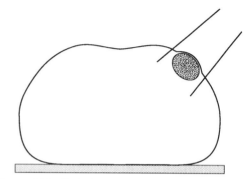

Figure 15.1 Single field encompassing tumour plus margin.

Simulator screening is used to determine field position where necessary, for example for a bone tumour or secondary deposit in the spine. Where possible the patient should lie prone for a spine field to be applied, since screening from the anterior surface of the patient may give a false impression of the size of field required due to beam divergence and consequent field magnification (Fig. 12.2), depending on the depth of the tumour in the body. A tumour lying approximately at the centre may be imaged from either surface.

Planning for single fields which form part of more complex treatments, such as boost fields, will be discussed with the techniques which they supplement.

Setting up

The method of set-up for single fields is usually very simple. Distance setting is achieved by setting the required rangefinder reading on the surface, or via an applicator set to touch the skin (Fig. 15.3). The edges of a field light or applicator are aligned with marks on the surface of the patient. Some difficulty may arise where the applicator obscures marks as it is brought close to the patient. However, achieving the expected dosimetry across the field may be dependent on beam direction, especially at short f.s.d.s.

Beam direction

Single fields are usually applied directly to the contour of the patient, i.e. if an applicator is used

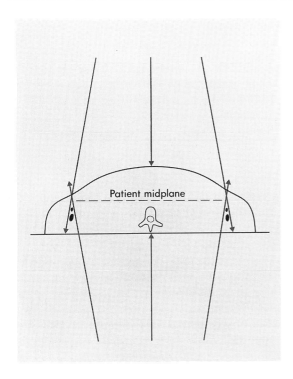

Figure 15.2 Beam divergence effect on field size through the patient, for parallel opposed pair. Tissue which is included in the overhead beam may not be included in the under-couch beam.

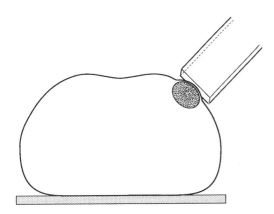

Figure 15.3 Use of a front plate or applicator face to align the beam orthogonally to the patient.

this should be aligned so that its surface is as flat as possible across the treatment area, to give a relatively uniform f.s.d. across the field. The same general effect is required without an applicator,

where the beam may have to be aligned by eye, or by the use of a front pointer with a flat plate attached to simulate the applicator face (Fig. 15.3).

Alternatively a reflective sheet aligned with the patient surface may be used with an optical front pointer to direct the beam (see Fig. 9.16), or by using a fixed patient position, gantry, collimator and floor angle.

Accuracy, reproducibility and patient position. Patient position does not play an important part in many of these set-ups, but is important for the accurate application of through-the-couch fields, or special set-ups using set gantry and floor angles. Single fields applied as boosts often require identical patient positioning to that used for the main phase of treatment and here reproducibility of the set-up (see Ch. 12) may be critical to avoid geographical miss and achieve the correct dose distribution.

It is easy to 'hit' a tumour near the surface if a generous field is simply applied to obtain 'best fit' to skin marks, often used for simple palliation of a surface painful deposit. However, where the lower thoracic or lumbar spine is treated from under the couch, using anterior marks, the use of lateral laser marks to properly align the patient is necessary to ensure that the spine will be central in the field (see Fig. 13.5). In the case of the upper spine, it is sometimes possible to check the alignment by palpating for spinous processes through the couch and checking visually that these are central in the light field.

Beam alignment on the patient surface. Where an area has been marked to allow for the effect of divergence of the light field across an irregular contour (see Fig. 12.3), set-up is achieved by using angles used at planning, or by rotating the gantry, couch and collimators until the light field is the same shape as the marks and the beam alignment appears reasonable.

The accuracy with which the cross-sectional plane of a field is aligned with the patient contour is more critical at shorter f.s.d.s, where a small difference in distance at different points in the field makes a significant difference to dosimetry across the field. At short f.s.d.s, small changes in distance have a relatively greater effect on dose rate because of the effect of the inverse square law on radiation intensity. Where a longer f.s.d. is used the alignment is less critical.

Avoidance of critical structures. For some sites, it may be desirable to direct the beam slightly away from critical structures which are not involved by the tumour, such as the eye (Fig. 15.4) or the spinal cord. In these cases appropriate instruction about beam direction should be given on the prescription, although most radiographers would enquire (or proceed to aim away from the eye) if no instruction was given. Radiation protection of the patient, or critical organs is part of the beam direction process on each treatment.

Where a single field is used as part or whole of a radical treatment, any special requirements should form part of either a departmental protocol or each prescription.

Compensation for irregular shape

For low energy X-rays, applied at short f.s.d., an irregular contour results in a large variation of dose distribution across the field, due to the different f.s.d.s within the field and relatively large inverse square law effects. The dose at any point and the overall range of doses may be estimated by applying a distance correction factor at each point, whether greater than or less than the correct f.s.d. For example, using an applicator calibrated for an f.s.d. of 10 cm, if the contour results in an f.s.d. of 10 cm at the centre but 11 cm at the periphery, then the dose received at the periphery is lower than that at the centre by a factor which is easily calculated:

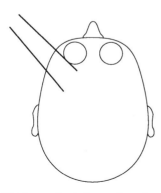

Figure 15.4 The beam directed away from the eye.

$$\frac{10 \times 10 \text{ (square of calibrated f.s.d.)}}{11 \times 11 \text{ (square of actual f.s.d.)}} = \frac{100}{121} = 0.8265$$

The effective machine output at the periphery is reduced to 0.8265 of that at the centre. The dose received at the periphery is thus only 82.65% of that received at the centre.

But for the same discrepancy at 100 cm f.s.d.:

$$\frac{100 \times 100}{101 \times 101} = \frac{10\,000}{10\,201} = 0.9803$$

The effective machine output at the periphery is reduced to 0.9803 of that at the centre. The dose received at the periphery is 98.03% of that received at the field centre.

This formula may be applied to calculate the dose variation across the field to assess its acceptability or to determine the required dose adjustment. Where an applicator is prevented from fitting closely to the area because of the tissue shape, the whole field is applied at a somewhat greater f.s.d. and a similar correction to the machine output is calculated. The formula can be applied to correct a standard output to that for the predominant f.s.d. across the area so that the treatment time is calculated to give the prescribed applied dose.

Use of bolus to even out contours

Where the range of doses across an irregular contour is unacceptable, the treatment surface may be made flat by the use of contoured bolus. Any air space within the field, such as an orifice or crater, may be filled with wet gauze to act as bolus within that space. When bolus is considered with high energy beams, the significance of the loss of skin-sparing effects must be evaluated against the desired treatment outcomes.

Irregular field shape

Where the field area is an irregular shape due to shielding, the output for the altered shape must be calculated or measured so that, again, the treatment time used results in the correct dose being received. Shielding and shaping lead cut-outs are constructed and fields set up so that wherever possible the beam centre remains central to the area treated.

Sites treated

Any site where a single field will suffice, but particularly skin lesions.

Treatment of skin lesions by superficial X-rays

The treatment of basal cell carcinoma (BCC) by single fields is one of the most successful radical radiotherapy treatments, 95% or more tumours being cured where the field cover is adequate (a margin of 0.5 cm round the obvious lesion to allow for microscopic disease infiltration is required).

Accuracy and immobilisation

Failure is almost always due to inadequate coverage, or to the patient's moving during treatment which gives the same effect. Therefore it is most important that the radiographer keeps the marks in good order, sets the field accurately, and watches the patient closely to detect movement. The applicator is set firmly on the skin to help to avoid movement of the area during treatment. The patient is immobilised as far as possible by the strategic placing of heavy sandbags and supports.

Shielding

Protection of organs adjacent to treatment areas is important. For example, it is routine for radiographers using superficial X-rays for skin lesions to place 1 mm thick lead shields over the eyes when treating close to the eye, to protect them from scatter or the primary beam. Any adjacent treatment areas are also protected by 1 mm lead sheet shielding (Fig. 15.5A). Because the absorbed dose from low energy X-rays is increased in bone, cartilage and adjacent soft tissue elements, these tissues should be protected where possible. Small pieces of lead can be cut to shape and wrapped or specially coated to prevent lead being absorbed by the patient, and used for insertion into nostrils or under the lip to protect the nasal septum or the gums from treatment applied to overlying tissue.

Where lead cut-outs are used, these should be moulded to the patient's shape in order to avoid stand-off of the applicator. A plaster cast of the features may be required onto which the lead is shaped to the contour of the treated area.

Internal eyeshields. Special gold-plated eye-shaped shields, shaped to fit the anterior eyeball, may be sterilised (with a suitable fluid such as chlorhexidine in methanol and rinsed several times) and inserted under the eyelid to give maximum protection to the eye while the eyelid is treated (Fig. 15.5). This requires use of a local anaesthetic liquid in the eye, the effects of which last several hours, so the patient must have that eye sealed behind an eyepad to prevent injury from foreign bodies etc. whilst the eye is insensitive. This means that the patient may not drive home, and must be given appropriate instructions prior to the first anaesthetic.

Machine output

Protection procedures include checking or selecting the correct filters and energy, where a choice is available, and taking account of the fact that interlock systems may occasionally fail. Superficial X-ray apparatus is prone to some fluctuation in beam current (mA). The radiation intensity, and therefore dose rate is highly variable with small changes in beam current.

Correctly treating the patient involves checking the mA meter reading at the start of and frequently during each treatment. Any fluctuation must be immediately corrected. A consistent change in the operating beam current indicates at the least a need to recalibrate the equipment (normally calibrated each morning prior to treating patients) and may indicate a problem with the X-ray tube.

PARALLEL OPPOSED PAIRS

The dosimetric principles

Parallel opposed fields are used to treat a complete thickness of tissue such as anteroposterior chest or abdomen. The isodose distribution for a parallel pair applied either at normal f.s.d. or isocentrically, though not homogeneous, is high throughout the central region of the patient (see

A

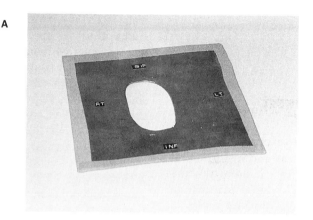

B

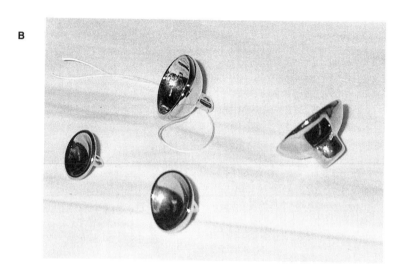

Figure 15.5 **A** Lead cut-out. **B** Lead eyeshields.

Ch. 7). There is some variation in dose in the build-up region near the surface, allowing skin-sparing with megavoltage beams. The dose maximum occurs below the surface and is relevant at spinal cord depth, which may be the dose-limiting factor.

Planning and simulation

Localisation of the target tissue may be determined from imaging procedures, or from clinical knowledge of the disease and the sites at risk. The position and size of the fields to be used are usually determined on the simulator by screening the patient and adjusting the field size and position until the target tissue is encompassed.

Bony landmarks are often used as a reference for adjacent soft tissue structures.

Where beams are vertical, the patient is usually treated lying either prone or supine. Simulation is carried out from above only, and skin marks or tattoos are made only on the uppermost surface. (Some simulators allow screening from under the couch, but it is not possible to mark the patient through the couch, and, if it were, any marks would be distorted on each treatment by contact with the couch during patient positioning.)

Beam divergence effects. The assumption is often made that both fields will encompass the tissue as it is seen when screening from above, which may be correct for an isocentric set-up or for tissue at the midplane of the patient.

However, for set-ups at normal or extended f.s.d., the over-couch field appears much larger at the distal side of the patient than when applied for the under-couch field, due to the beam divergence over a 20–25 cm thickness of the patient (Fig. 15.2). Also, because the beam divergence is in opposite directions for the two fields, structures below the midplane and near to edges or proposed shielding may be excluded from the under-couch beam.

For these reasons and others related to equipment, where accuracy is critical the patient is often prone for one field and supine for the other during simulation and treatment for each (see Ch. 18). Similarly, when planning head and neck areas laterally, it is advisable to simulate from both sides of the patient.

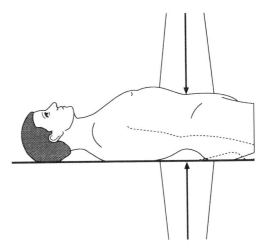

Figure 15.6 Irregular contour under the patient's spine, ignored during set-up.

Setting up

Distance setting

For an f.s.d. set-up, the normal f.s.d. is set at the central axis of each field or at the point where the tissue thickness equals that used in the dose calculation. The applied dose is calculated according to the thickness of tissue, usually that at the field centre.

Uneven patient contours. Where there is a contour slope (see Ch. 8), the thickness used to calculate dose may not be that at the field centre, so the point used for distance setting must be adjusted to take account of this. For an isocentric set-up, the couch height should be set at a level equal to half the total tissue thickness at the central axis position.

Where there is a gap between part of the treated region and the couch top, this may, or may not, be taken into account when measuring the thickness of tissue treated and may or may not affect the distance-setting procedure. For example the hollow under the lumbar spine on a supine patient undergoing a vertical parallel pair treatment to that region (Fig. 15.6) will usually be ignored. In this example if the centre of the under-couch field fell on the hollow curve and the normal f.s.d. were to be set to the skin surface, then an unexpected increase of dose would arise for two reasons:

1. The points of applications of the fields would be closer than calculated, so the combined dose within the region would be higher.
2. The radiation intensity across the under-couch field would be higher because the patient surface would be closer to the radiation source than it should be.

Beam direction

Patient positioning is important in the application of parallel pairs, particularly where shielding, wedging, compensation or small field sizes and margins are used. In these situations, a reproducible patient position (see Chs 12 and 13) is critical for achieving the required accuracy of treatment. For most parallel pairs the patient is positioned using lasers and tattoos to straighten and prevent lateral rotation (see Fig. 13.5). Fields may then be directed by centring the patient in relation to the isocentre in all three dimensions and using fixed gantry angles. The system of skin reference marking used will affect the centring accuracy. The potential causes of inaccuracy in field centring are outlined in Chapter 13.

The position of the patient is rechecked after treatment with the first field, the patient repositioned if necessary, then the gantry is rotated through 180°, the f.s.d. set and any diaphragm angle reversed. Where beams are lateral, the patient alignment may be checked by using a backpointer or laser at the centre of the opposing field.

Set-up methods for oblique fields. Oblique parallel pairs are almost impossible to set up unless planned isocentrically. This is because couch movements in two directions are needed to set the second field. The anterior field is planned by screening and can be set up again using the same mark and gantry angle. To set the second field (Fig. 15.7A), the couch must be moved X cm vertically and Y cm horizontally to get the correct centring and f.s.d. This involves taking an outline and calculating X and Y for the set up. However, once an outline or a separation measurement is obtained, an appropriate couch height can be set (Fig. 15.7B) and it is simpler to set up both fields isocentrically, solely by gantry rotation after centring for the first field. It is often faster to set up isocentrically, thereby efficiently utilising machine time. An accurate method of setting couch height must be used, especially for oblique or lateral fields, avoiding the use of sagging couch sections (see Ch. 9) and using the principles outlined in Chapter 13.

Compensation for irregular shape

Where there is any significant variation in patient contour across the treated region, such as a slope on the chest (see Fig. 12.3), this will cause dose variation across the region. Depending on the magnitude of the dose variation and the desired clinical outcome, some form of tissue compensation (see Ch. 8) may be required in order to produce a more even dose distribution. For example, for a low dose two-fraction palliative bronchus treatment, the variation in dose may be accepted. Or, an attempt to build the patient surface to a more uniform shape using bolus on the skin, either for the whole area, or for the upper half of the field to the centre level, may be made. This will adequately prevent an excessive dose being received by the spinal cord in the thinner region. The extra skin dose received is usually irrelevant in a low dose situation.

Where a high skin dose is unacceptable, and/or greater precision in dose planning is required, remote compensators or wedges may be used on one or both fields. The principles for this are as for planned multifield treatments. The type of compensation used depends on the departmental practices and the need to preserve skin-sparing effects.

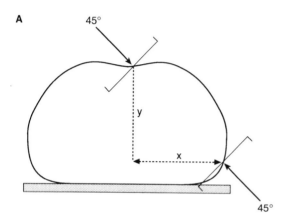

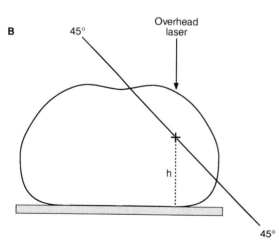

Figure 15.7 Set-up parameters for an angled parallel pair. **A** f.s.d. set-up. The anterior field is set at 100 cm f.s.d. To set the posterior field, the couch is moved across x cm and dropped y cm and the gantry rotated through 180°. **B** Isocentric set-up. The height above couch, h cm, is set and the laser centred over the isocentric position, then the gantry set for either field.

Sites treated using parallel pairs

Parallel pairs may be used on any part of the body where they fulfil the clinical need, but are commonly used for large volume treatments to the chest, abdomen and pelvis. They may also be used for treating the whole brain/head, or for limbs. Oblique parallel fields are often used as the basis for breast techniques. Parallel pairs form part of other, more complex treatments detailed in other chapters.

MULTIPLE FIELD TREATMENTS

The dosimetric principles

Two or more fields can be directed at a tumour so that the tumour receives a high dose, surrounding normal tissue receiving a relatively low dose (Fig. 15.8). Computer summation of the isodose distributions from the constituent fields is performed for either isocentric or normal f.s.d. fields. Isocentric treatments are usually performed for sites within the trunk, but where a beam direction shell is used on the head or neck, either type of set-up may be planned. There is little dosimetric advantage for either method but isocentric treatments are simpler to plan and execute and are therefore the norm. For either method the dose received by the tumour volume will depend on the use of well-researched methods of treat-

ment set-up. (Prior reading of Chapters 9, 12, 13 and 14 is essential in relation to this type of treatment.)

Tumour volume

Conventionally this type of technique was generally chosen only for tumours confined within small, regularly shaped volumes of the order of $10 \times 10 \times 10$ cm^3 or less, since much larger volumes would require a dose reduction incompatible with giving radical treatment. Radical treatment of tumours which are larger in one or more dimension is achieved by shaping the high dose volume irregularly to closely fit or 'conform' to the risk zone. Thus the actual volume irradiated falls within normal limits. The methods of achieving this are discussed in Chapter 23.

This chapter is concerned mainly with conventional techniques where some simple shielding of uninvolved tissue is used with a conventionally produced treatment plan and delivery method (particularly for head and neck sites which are discussed further in Chapter 17). However, the two varieties of technique represent the opposite ends of a continuum to which many principles outlined here apply equally.

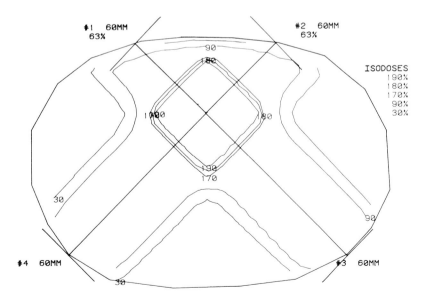

Figure 15.8 Planned central plane dose distribution for a four-field isocentric beam arrangement. (Reproduced from Walter et al 1982.)

Planning and simulation

Many of the planning principles and processes were outlined in Chapters 11 and 14, such as localisation, obtaining geographical patient data and formulating a suitable plan.

Beam arrangement

The beams are conventionally coplanar in arrangement, that is, in a plane orthogonal to the couch (Fig. 15.8). At present developments in noncoplanar planning are taking place which are considered in Chapter 23. Asymmetric or offset diaphragms may be used to change the divergent angle of the beams, for example to avoid treating a critical structure.

Compensation for irregular contours

Compensation for patient shape is undertaken as an integral part of the computer planning process, since the contours are used to produce the plan. The process involves applying different wedging, weighting and positioning of fields, or constructing individual compensators so that an acceptable dose distribution is obtained on the plan. The safe use of compensators requires use of an appropriate factor to account for absorption in the compensator.

Simulation

Simulation processes used are dependent on site and on whether or not detailed localisation data from CT (diagnostic or simulator) are available. If CT planning has been performed, the function of simulation is to verify couch heights, field parameters and shielding, i.e. the treatment set-up, against the bony anatomy. Here orthogonal films or field check films may be used. Alternatively, where confidence in methods has been established, this verification may be sought from portal imaging on treatment.

Where planning is to be performed from routine simulation alone, orthogonal localisation films, with appropriate skin markers, are taken for most sites. Contrast media may be used to establish bladder, oesophagal or rectal positions

and volumes on the films. At a second session, verification procedures are performed as for CT planned patients. For head and neck sites and the breast, the set-up and field marking processes may all be carried out by simulator screening, changing set-up parameters until the target anatomy is encompassed in the fields.

Beam direction

Beam direction is achieved by a combination of reproducible patient positioning through planning and treatment, together with accurate tumour centring in three dimensions (see Ch. 13) and the use of fixed gantry angles or arcs.

Patient positioning

Details of patient positioning as used for CT and/or simulation, should be either standard as in a written protocol, or given on the treatment plan and the prescription. A reproducible position is essential for correct beam alignment in the tissue, and to ensure a consistent relationship of the surface marks to the target volume. Details of the issues in positioning the patient have already been described in Chapter 13, including the mobility of marks on the trunk with changes in position of the head or arms. Fixing the head and arm position improves comfort and helps to stop the patient rolling from side to side during treatment, particularly for treatments to the chest where the arms may be raised so that they are not in the treatment beams.

For treatments to the trunk, patients should be aligned with the laser and well-spaced midline tattoos or landmarks, as on planning. If the patient is allowed to lie slightly askew, the central axis of all fields and therefore the treated volume will be rotated with respect to that planned (Fig. 15.9). The use of lateral tattoos for alignment with the laser is recommended to prevent variations in lateral rotation (see Fig. 13.5).

Treatment centres and tattoos

For patients planned from CT (see Ch. 14), the tattoo over the target region made on scanning

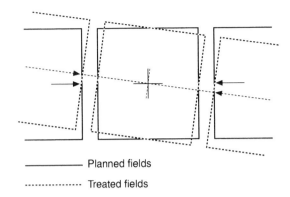

————— Planned fields

--------------- Treated fields

Figure 15.9 Effect of patient skew for a three-field arrangement, all fields rotated with respect to the plan.

may be near to, but not at, the exact treatment centre. For example:

X SSN

X upper abdominal tattoo

+ treatment centre

X pelvic tattoo

Therefore horizontal longitudinal and lateral measurements from the tattoo to the treatment centre are required in order to identify the treatment centre. These should be displayed on a clear and simple diagram on the plan and used daily in centring, together with a horizontal ruler or a reliable couch scale (see Ch. 13) to centre the treatment beams.

Setting the couch height

The methods of determining and setting couch height for isocentric treatments should be well researched and shown to be accurate, on the equipment actually used (see Ch. 13 for more detail), if the target volume is to be wholly included in the treatment beam.

Measurement methods. Having determined the treatment volume and its centre, the couch height to set for treatment can be taken from either of two measurements: from the treatment centre to

the table top (Fig. 15.10), or from the treatment centre to the surface of the patient (Fig. 15.10). Each method has advantages in some situations and disadvantages in others.

For a patient lying supine directly on a hard top, measurement taken from the table is often more reliable than a measurement taken from the body surface, for example, where the pelvis is being treated, since the surface in contact with the table is relatively stable. The anterior abdominal wall is very mobile and a change in bowel contents etc. may give a change in shape. If this surface is used to determine the couch height setting, inaccuracy may result. If the position of the tumour is more likely to relate to the patient surface, e.g. breast, then the measurement used should be that from a stable reference point on the surface. If the surface is stable, such as the sacral area or a beam direction shell, this may be used for distance setting. If some unpredictability of the target height above the table is introduced, for example from a wedge under the chest or use of a sloping chest board, then the height must be set using the surface of the patient.

Equipment factors. Because sag of couch sections (see Fig. 9.9) is a potential cause of setting inaccuracy, a protocol for use of couch sections must be followed, especially where four fields, including a through-couch vertical field, are used. There are several important factors linked to this. It is presently not possible to find a standard couch section for accurate use for all fields, unless the posterior field is treated through the full thickness of the couch, and attenuation

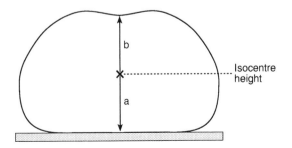

Figure 15.10 Measurements which can be used to set the height above couch are the table-to-treatment centre distance, a, or the surface-to-tumour centre distance, b.

accounted for in the plan. This preserves the validity of surface marks and also ensures that the couch height is accurately set for all fields (particularly important for any nonvertical field). However, the build-up effect of the table thickness may or may not be acceptable, dependent on the dose which the posterior skin would receive. If this is unacceptable, then the anterior and lateral fields should be applied using the rigid couch, then couch sections removed for the posterior field treatment, with the minimum possible disturbance to the patient's position, which should then be rechecked. The couch height for the posterior field is then set using a rangefinder reading equal to the posterior t.s.d. (treatment- or tumour-skin distance) at the couch surface, which eliminates inaccuracy from sag, but any inaccuracy of surface marks resulting from changed patient position must be accepted.

Suitable couch sections are required for treating posteriorly directed oblique fields, for example the custom-made carbon panels now available.

Daily distance checks and their significance

It is important also to check the measurement from the surface to the treatment centre (t.s.d.) for every field, daily, to check for constancy in set-up and to monitor patient shape (Fig. 15.11).

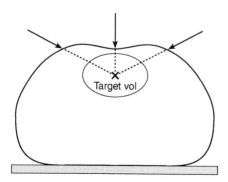

Figure 15.11 Tumour-to-skin distances for a bladder treatment. It is unlikely, on the overhead field, that a variation of 1.5 cm could arise within the 1 cm of tissue between the target volume and the skin surface.

Acceptable variations in t.s.d. and relationship with patient shape. For any field, t.s.d. measurements should correspond to those on the treatment plan, to within plus or minus 1 cm. If the t.s.d. measurement is accurate to within 1 cm, any dose variation owing to this variation of thickness of tissue traversed by the beam is small and therefore acceptable.

However, a discrepancy in t.s.d. signals a variation in patient shape or position from that which was expected on planning and may affect the height of the treatment centre in the body. A discrepancy of 1 cm on an oblique reading is more acceptable (and more likely) than on a vertical reading. For a vertical field or measurement the sum of the t.s.d. measurement and the planned centre height above couch should equal the patient thickness shown on the plan to within about 1 cm (Fig. 15.10).

Unacceptable variations and importance for couch height accuracy. A consistent discrepancy of 1.5 cm or more on the t.s.d. over two treatments should be reported and investigated since it may mean that a reassessment of the couch height measurement is necessary. A variation of 1.5 cm in the measurement for an overhead field would clearly indicate the need for investigation to establish whether the height above couch is correct (Fig. 15.11). In this situation there are far greater risks of undertreatment from a couch height discrepancy, especially for lateral or oblique fields, than from dosimetry discrepancy due to varying t.s.d. A further outline plus simulation, or planning CT scan may be necessary to confirm the tumour height above the table.

Sites treated and related issues

Multifield techniques may be used in any site with a suitable volume for radical treatment, but particularly in the bladder, prostate, oesophagus, bronchus, head and neck, and brain. Some of these common sites present important issues.

Pelvic sites

Patients having treatment in pelvic sites such as for bladder tumours, often have three or four isocentric (or f.s.d.) fields applied (Fig. 15.8), usually lying supine.

Bladder. Since the position and size of the bladder walls varies with the volume of urine in the bladder, a protocol for emptying the bladder is appropriate for ensuring that the target tissue is irradiated each day. Where the bladder is the treated organ it must be emptied within 5–10 minutes of treatment to ensure that anatomical conditions are similar to those on planning and that the tumour/bladder wall is not pushed out of the high dose region by urine.

Prostate. Where the prostate is the treated organ, patients do not have to empty the bladder, in fact a full bladder can be beneficial as it may push the bladder wall and rectum out of the high dose region. (If there is a spigotted indwelling catheter, this should be released if the bladder is uncomfortably full, as the discomfort may alter the treatment position.) The condition of the bladder is not thought likely to distort the position of the tumour relative to the surface mark as the prostate and other structures in the lower pelvis are thought to be relatively fixed.

Chest

The bronchus and oesophagus are often treated by three-field isocentric techniques (see Fig. 15.12), with the patient lying supine. Here a complication may arise owing to the need to angle the target volume with respect to the horizontal, and a need to angle the collimators.

Angled collimators. For treatment of the oesophagus, the collimators are usually angled on posterior oblique fields so that the treatment volume follows the tilted path of the oesophagus. According to whether the upper or lower oesophagus is treated, the collimator angles may be in either of two directions. All fields may be angled, and the angle of each may differ. Unambiguous instructions and diagrams for the angled fields should be given on the treatment prescription, so that there is no likelihood of reversed collimator angles being used inadvertently. A lateral projection of the angle of the tumour volume in relation to the couch top is the clearest way to define the field orientation (Fig. 15.13).

ARC THERAPY

Arc therapy is an extension of multiple field therapy. The gantry is rotated isocentrically round the patient during the treatment (Fig. 15.14). Irradiation may be either intermittent during gantry movement, so that several small arcs are irradiated, or continuous during the whole movement. The aim of this technique is to give a lower dose to tissue traversed by beams aimed at a central tumour. This may spare any critical structure such as lung from high dose delivery, but a larger volume of tissue in total receives radiation. There is some marginal improvement in dose distribution for certain types of tumour volume/site, but it is not a routine

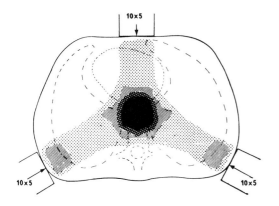

Figure 15.12 A three-field isocentric plan for treatment of the oesophagus. (Reproduced from Walter et al 1982.)

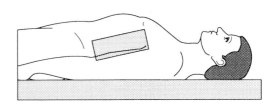

Figure 15.13 Diagram to indicate an target volume angled, with respect to the horizontal, requiring collimator angling for treatment of the lower oesophagus.

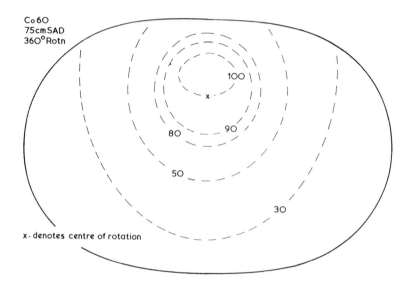

Figure 15.14 Dose distribution using arc treatment. (Reproduced from Walter et al 1982.)

technique. This is partly because arc therapy is time-consuming in application, and the patient may move during the longer exposure period. It is now employed for special applications such as stereotactic or conformational therapy (see Ch. 23).

COMBINED TREATMENT MODALITIES

Any of these basic techniques may be used in conjunction with other treatment modalities, commonly brachytherapy, for example in treatment of the cervix (see Ch. 23).

16

Breast techniques

The role of radiotherapy treatment in breast cancer

Breast conserving techniques (tumour excision with consecutive radiotherapy) used for early breast cancer give local control equal to that of mastectomy (Van Dongen et al 1992). Chemotherapy and hormone therapy are used to control the disease systemically where indicated.

Radiotherapy to the breast or chest wall and adjacent areas at risk is usually given with radical intent to prevent local recurrence. Surgical sampling in the axilla may be performed to assess node involvement in high risk patients, control of disease in the axillary nodes being an important factor in survival.

Treatment is critically planned and delivered so as to minimise radiation dose and subsequent damage to the underlying lung. Gross oedema of the arm is a complication which may follow axillary surgery and radiotherapy, but which can be minimised by early referral to support services specialising in its prevention and control.

In breast cancer, the body region requiring treatment is one of the most complex shapes encountered in radiotherapy practice. Quality assurance programmes are required to prevent treatment variations which would lead to suboptimal local control levels: 'If the tumour is not controlled, the survival and quality of life of the patient will be endangered' (Bartelink et al 1991b).

TECHNICAL PRINCIPLES OF BREAST TECHNIQUES

Areas irradiated

The breast, or postmastectomy chest wall, is usually treated using two opposed fields applied tangentially so as to skim the anterior surface of the lung. The depth of lung allowed within these tangential fields is normally up to 2 cm, occasionally 3 cm when unavoidable owing to patient shape and the position and extent of tissue requiring irradiation (Fig. 16.1). Where the axillary and supraclavicular nodes are at risk, these are usually included in additional fields (Fig. 16.2). Occasionally the ipsilateral internal mammary nodes are irradiated using a matched parasternal field.

Dose, fractionation and beam energy

A modal dose of 45–50 Gy, in 1.8–2.0 Gy fractions, to the whole region is recommended. (This may be followed, where indicated, by a low energy boost of 20 Gy.)

Cobalt is suitable for small breasts where the separation between the medial and lateral border is less than 20 cm. Breasts where this dorsal separation is 20 cm or more require a photon beam of energy 6 MV or more (Bartelink et al 1991b). With such beam energies the dose received in superficial regions has to be considered in relation to the disease present. A tangential pair of fields applied at 6 MV (without bolus) will produce a skin dose which is of the order of 60–70% of the prescribed tumour dose.

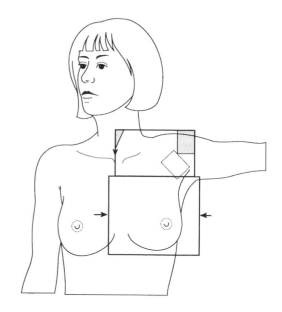

Figure 16.2 The field arrangement to cover the breast, supraclavicular and axillary nodes.

Electron beams are not suitable for direct application to the breast area because of poor cosmetic outcome. Brachytherapy techniques for the chest wall are in use in some centres (see Ch. 21).

Skin dose requirements and use of bolus

For mastectomy patients and those where the skin is seen to be involved, bolus may be used to ensure that 95–100% of the tumour dose is received by the skin lymphatics. Because of the oblique angle of the fields, a 1 cm sheet of bolus wrapped around the chest wall will become effectively 1.5 cm (see Ch. 8) along the path of the beam, giving full build-up conditions for a 6 MV beam.

The use of bolus leads to telangiectasia and poor cosmesis. Where the skin is not at risk, such as in a patient who has had breast-conserving surgery or lumpectomy, the volume for treatment extends from 0.5 cm below the skin surface and bolus is not required (except sometimes for the scar area).

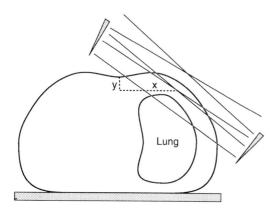

Figure 16.1 Isocentric tangential fields to the chest wall, with their dorsal edges aligned so as to skim the lung. Only a small thickness of lung is included in the fields. The isocentre coordinates x and y are shown related to the tattooed reference point over the sternum.

Technical methods

The methods of applying tangential fields to the chest wall vary. In turn, the way that axillary and supraclavicular fields are applied varies with the method used for the tangential fields, and with the practices used by a particular radiotherapy centre or radiotherapist. There are various recommended techniques used to achieve the same effect, some more complex than others. Some of these methods will now be discussed, starting with the most widely used.

Isocentric tangential pair to the breast area

Patient position

A reproducible patient position is required for successful application of isocentric breast techniques using fixed gantry angles. Usually the patient lies supine, either flat on the table or with a rigid wedge support under the chest. The slope of support wedge used for a particular patient is chosen so that the sternum lies horizontal, which allows a simpler technique to be used, and also reduces the lung volume irradiated in the caudo-cephalic (CC) dimension (Bartelink et al 1991b).

Arm position. The ipsilateral arm should be abducted to at least 90°, and preferably both arms for improved stability and symmetry (essential for bilateral and potentially bilateral treatments). The arm/s are supported by placing the hand on a strategically placed handgrip which should be adjustable, and the specified setting used each time the patient is positioned. The arm support should be fixed so that it ensures reproducibility of the abduction of the arm. This is an important factor in reproducibility of the set-up, reducing the mean CC shift from 15.5 mm (using a movable support) to 5.5 mm (using a fixed support) in a study by Mitine et al (1991).

Head and chest position. The head is supported at a comfortable height level with or above the shoulder. The patient is aligned, using the sagittal laser (Fig 16.3), so that the sternum is parallel with the longitudinal plane which runs through the isocentre. Lateral rotation is controlled using cross-firing lasers.

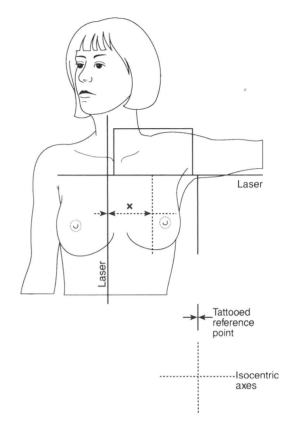

Figure 16.3 The patient aligned so that the lasers run parallel with the isocentric axes. The isocentre position lies x cm from the reference tattoo on the sternum.

Reproducibility. Using these positioning methods results in a reproducible set-up (Mitine et al 1991; Van Tienhoven et al 1991b; Westbrook et al 1991) without the use of more sophisticated and expensive immobilisation devices such as body shells. These groups found that set-ups were reproduced to within 5 mm of the simulated position, in the ventrodorsal direction, and that breathing does not significantly affect the set-up (Van Tienhoven et al 1991b). A reproducibility study using body shells (Valdagni & Italia 1991) reported 1.8–2.0 mm mean deviation in the CC direction, where Mitine et al reported 5.5 mm, but 15% of patients had to have a new shell mid-course because of changed breast morphology or errors noted on films.

However, fields will not be perfectly consistent on the anatomy each day and local protocols for dealing with variation should be prepared.

Marking and simulation procedures

Approximate field positions are marked on the patient clinically prior to confirmation on simulation, or are marked at simulation. The latter requires the use of a simulation technique which produces a plan for gantry angle, isocentre position in the patient and field size.

Set-up parameter determination. Markers are placed on the skin at the medial and lateral borders, in the central transverse treatment plane. The approximate isocentre depth and distance from the midline are selected using the outline in the central plane, together with approximate field sizes, either by practised judgement by eye or from an outline on paper showing the marker points. The patient is appropriately set up to the isocentre coordinates (Fig. 16.1). Gantry angles are determined by moving the gantry until the two markers are coincident on the dorsal field border, for each field.

Field cover. The field cover of the breast is checked at the superior, inferior, medial and lateral borders according to the limits required, usually extending 1 cm or so outside the edge of the breast. Fields should cover the breast anteriorly during all phases of the breathing cycle, with 2 cm clearance (Bartelink et al 1991b) to allow for penumbra effects, patient movement and extra clearance to allow cover if the breast swells during treatment. The depth of lung included is measured (Fig. 16.1). If the cover, lung depth or matching with other fields is inappropriate, then the set-up is suitably adjusted.

The patient is marked so that the set-up can be reproduced for treatment, using an isocentre reference point on stable skin overlying the sternum (Fig. 16.3), rather than on mobile breast tissue (Gagliardi et al 1992). The couch height will be set using this reference point, then the couch moved laterally for a measured distance X cm. Lateral laser points are marked or tattooed on skin overlying ribs, rather than on the breasts.

Treatment plan production and dosimetry considerations

While the patient is in the treatment position, contours of the region are taken at least at the central level and preferably at several levels. A plan for treatment is then produced with or without compensation for lung volume (Fig. 16.4A,B) and irregular tissue shape. A 3–7% correction to compensate for increased transmission through lung tissue may be applied (Mijnheer et al 1991). Because of the shape of the chest, the use of 15°–30° laterally orientated wedges is usually required, chosen for the individual patient. It is desirable to ensure that the variation between minimum and maximum doses in the target volume is no greater than 15% (Bartelink et al 1991b). Tissue compensators may be considered.

The final plan should include a description of all set-up parameters, the anatomical position of reference points, details and settings of positioning supports. The above principles are applied for any of the isocentric set-up types described below.

Anterior supraclavicular fields and field matching

Anterior fields may be used to treat lymph node chains in the region of the supraclavicular fossa (SCF) and lower deep cervical nodes. The angle of edge divergence of a 10 cm long SCF field is approximately 3° with an effect of 2.5 mm at 5 cm below the skin surface (Fig. 16.5A). The effect of this small divergence may be removed, if desired, by turning the couch through 90° and angling the gantry so that the inferior field edge is vertical (Fig. 16.5B). The head of the humerus, and also the larynx, is usually shielded (Fig. 16.2). The gantry may be angled laterally or asymmetry used so that the field is directed away from the spinal cord.

Matchline position. Where SCF fields are added to breast fields, complications due to field matching occur, as described below. The SCF field directly irradiates underlying lung and therefore should not extend inferiorly any further than necessary for matching. Its lower border usually forms the matchline and runs through the upper axilla. It should be placed so that tangential fields can be matched with the arm clear of the beams.

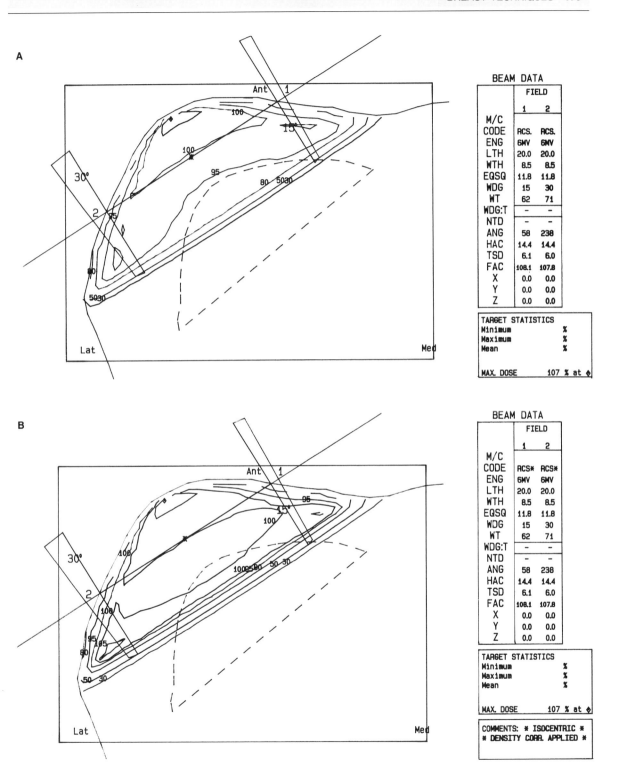

Figure 16.4 The dosimetry for tangential wedged fields. **A** without lung correction. **B** with lung correction.

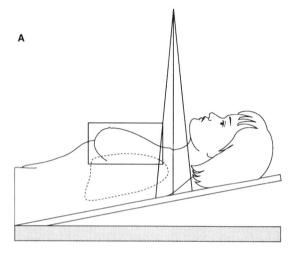

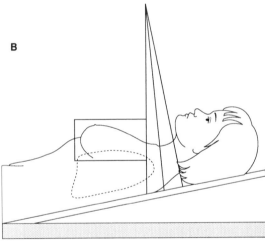

Figure 16.5 **A** The SCF field matched on the skin surface and diverging into the tangential fields at a depth. **B** The gantry may be angled (approximately 3°) away from the lung so that the inferior field edge is aligned with the tangential fields.

The patient must have sufficient mobility in the arm to achieve the required position. Physiotherapy and exercise may be required.

Matching tangential fields to an anterior supraclavicular field

Effect of patient movement between fields. It is important that the patient keeps still throughout the treatment of all matched fields, since the matchline is drawn on the skin. If, for example, the arm or the whole patient is moved between fields the matchline will move without necessarily moving all underlying structures and underlap or overlap of fields can then occur below skin level.

Match zone dosimetry. The upper border of the tangential fields must be matched to the lower border of the SCF field in a way which gives a uniform dose to the whole region, including the matchline. Since SCF and axillary fields are only applied where the axillary lymph nodes are at risk, it is particularly important that the axilla should receive an adequate dose. Where the lymphatics of the skin of the whole region are considered to be at risk, even dosage is also required at the medial extremity of the matchline.

This ideal is difficult to achieve because of the divergence of the lateral fields. Either cold spots occur at the medial and lateral aspect of the matchline, in triangular areas lying outside the entry ports of the tangential fields (Fig. 16.6), or field entry ports are abutted to the matchline and divergence into the SCF field occurs. Various methods of matching which fall between the two extremes or eliminate divergence are in common use. Most methods have limitations and difficulties.

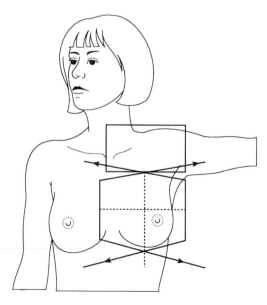

Figure 16.6 Tangential fields (straight couch) matched to cross the matchline at the isocentric axis. Some divergence into the SCF field occurs.

Asymmetry. Using asymmetric 'half-blocked' fields with nondivergent edges at the upper border of the tangential fields and at the lower border of the anterior supraclavicular field, is potentially a good method as all three light field edges are simply fitted to the matchline and no divergence into other fields occurs (Fig. 16.7A, B). However, whether this technique can be applied depends on the equipment available, since many linacs have no asymmetric diaphragm facility, or only have the facility on the opposite pair of diaphragms to those required for wedged tangential fields. Where the facility is available, or using half-blocked fields (Siddon et al 1981), the maximum field length is likely to be 20 cm, and less than this when wedged. Asymmetric fields may also be used to give nondivergent edges through the lung (Fig. 16.7C).

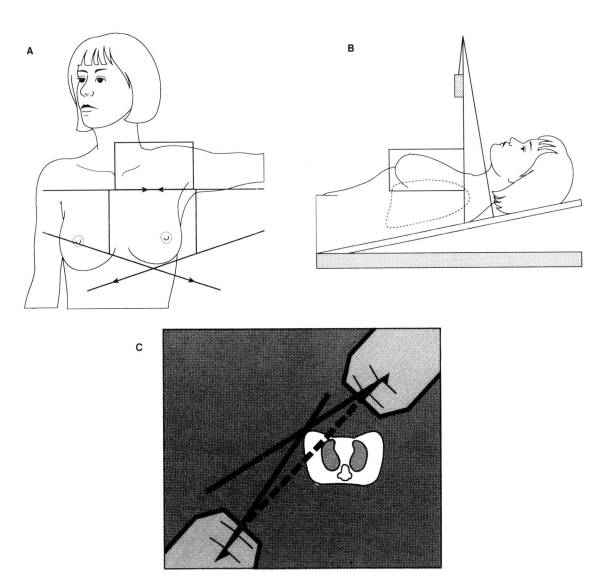

Figure 16.7   A Use of asymmetric (half-blocked) tangential fields to achieve a non-divergent edge along the matchline. **B** Use of a vertical half-blocked SCF field to achieve matching with the superior vertical edge of the half-blocked tangential fields. **C** Use of asymmetric fields to give nondivergent edges through the lung. (Courtesy of Philips Medical Systems.)

These principles apply whether the patient is supported on a sloping chestboard or flat on the couch.

Matching methods in common usage

When matching to an SCF field is required, the upper border of the chest wall fields should be aligned with the horizontal arm of the laser. This ensures that the divergent effects of the medial and lateral fields affect the junction line equally (and helps to reproduce the arm position and therefore field fit).

Patient on slanting chestboard

When the patient is supported so that the sternum is horizontal, the long axes of the tangential fields are horizontal (i.e. with no collimator rotation) and the matchplane is vertical (Fig. 16.7B). There are different methods of matching when using such fields.

Couch angled. This is a widely used practice where fields are angled towards each other in more than one plane (noncoplanar). By twisting the couch in opposite directions for each field, the divergent superior borders of the tangential fields can be arranged so as to run exactly along the inferior border of the SCF field (Fig. 16.8). Where the tangential fields are around 20 cm in length, the divergent edge angle is 6°, so the angle of couch rotation is approximately 6° for each field. These fields are planned as though there were no couch rotation, and no significant discrepancy in dose is likely as a result of this.

Couch straight. Where divergent fields are used with a straight couch, it is difficult to achieve a perfect match by any conventionally accepted method, and a variation in dosimetry along the matchline must be expected. The best match is achieved by positioning the slanting edge of the tangential fields so that they cross the matchline at the isocentric plane (Fig. 16.6). This method gives a lower dose level at the extremities, i.e. in the axilla, but is within 5% elsewhere. However, there will be a slight overlap of the distal light beam above the matchline, which is acceptable over the treatment region, but may seem unac-

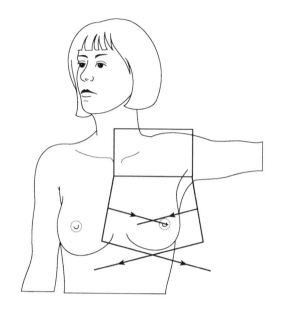

Figure 16.8 Use of couch twist to achieve alignment of the divergent superior edges of noncoplanar tangential fields with the matchline.

ceptable where it splashes onto the arm from the medial field. In order to avoid this, a gap is sometimes left between the tangential fields and the anterior supraclavicular fields, but even a 0.5 cm gap results in a lower dose in the junction region, e.g. 55% of the tumour dose.

Patient flat on table

Where the patient lies supine and flat on the treatment table, a collimator angle is used to simulate the angle of the sternum, for both tangential fields (Lichter et al 1983). This arrangement results in the need for shielding at the superior aspect of the fields, to avoid overlap with the SCF field at depth (Fig. 16.9). This is a more complex method which is not as widely used.

Problems with tangential fields

Many treatment planning systems require the isocentre to be below the build-up depth in tissue or bolus in order to produce a dose distribution in the central cross-sectional plane. A problem in

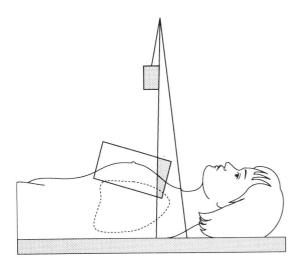

Figure 16.9 Field matching arrangement for a patient lying flat on the couch. Collimator rotation is used on the tangential fields to minimise lung irradiation at the inferior border. This necessitates the use of shielding blocks at the superior border to achieve matching with the SCF field in the vertical plane.

achieving this can arise for mastectomy patients because of the limited thickness of the chest wall (Fig. 16.10). Using a symmetric field, the field width required to give adequate cover of the chest wall and anterior axillary fold may result in

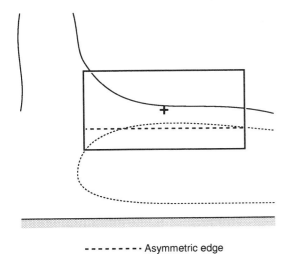

- - - - - - - - Asymmetric edge

Figure 16.10 Asymmetric tangential field planning allows the isocentre and anterior and posterior field limits to be placed appropriately to minimise the irradiation of the lung, while achieving the required beam cover.

inclusion of an unacceptable depth of lung. Use of asymmetric fields can prevent this planning problem, and/or give a nondivergent edge through the lung to minimise lung irradiation.

Potential tangential field set-up problems

On the first treatment, fields may not fit well in relation to the external anatomy, especially where they have not been checked on a simulator, or where any changes to setting points or parameters have been made after simulation. Checking the fit of, and the t.s.d. reading for both fields first is advisable on the first treatment, although the time that this takes can lead to patient stress and movement. There are more problems with lateral field fit than with medial field fit, so routinely starting with the lateral field set-up allows identification of problems before any field is treated.

Assuming parameters are correctly set, the following problems may occur:

1. The medial or lateral field edge falls well within or outside planned position.

Causes: lateral rotation of the patient, discrepancy in couch position laterally, or discrepancy in couch height possibly because of patient relaxation.

Correction: The couch height and lateral measurement should be checked; if found to be correct then the patient position requires adjustment. The patient should sit up, then lie down again with the head facing slightly to the appropriate side to correct the rotation.

2. The lateral field edge runs at an angle to planned position.

Causes: The patient's back is too relaxed and/ or the arm position needs adjusting.

Correction: The arm position should be adjusted and if the problem is not resolved, the patient should tense the back a little (patients are usually more tense when planned).

3. The length of either field appears short, giving inadequate cover at one or both ends.

Causes: The patient's arm is pulled up too high, distorting the patient shape.

4. A discrepancy in t.s.d. reading greater than ±1.5 cm.

Causes: Small discrepancies are to be expected with oblique field and irregular contour; a larger discrepancy indicates a plan or set-up inaccuracy.

Correction: The set-up and patient position should be checked; if not resolved, a check outline and replan may be necessary.

5. Noticeable patient roll or shift during treatment.

Causes: Inappropriate support and/or patient position.

6. Either field not covering the breast anteriorly.

Causes and correction: As treatment progresses, the breast often swells a little. Unless the fields allowed generous cover, the width may then need to be increased in order to cover the breast. Increasing the field width would increase the lung depth treated so an alteration of the isocentre position is preferable to maintain the same dorsal limit. This may involve taking a new outline and printing out a revised plan.

One simpler solution is to use asymmetry to increase the anterior half of the field width to cover. Where a large increase in field width is required, and/or where the t.s.d. readings are unacceptable, a new outline etc. may be indicated. However, the plan is often produced on the central cross-sectional contour only and, because of the variation in contour of the breast region, is only an approximate guide to measurements and dosimetry. Local tolerance and decision guidelines should be set.

Posterior axilla top-up field

The posterior axilla top-up field is the only field which is not critically matched to others, but the dose from it is summated with that from the SCF field. Therefore the tissue thickness at the central axis of the axilla field must be accurately measured, which is difficult to achieve when the patient is lying on a slanting surface except by appropriate use of scales and/or lasers (Fig. 16.11). Although the total dose from the top-up field is relatively low, if it is given on a thrice-weekly schedule a thickness variation of 1.5 cm or more can significantly affect the fraction dose on the top-up field days.

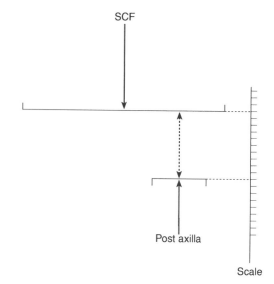

Figure 16.11 The anterior SCF and posterior axillary fields are planned as a parallel pair to the tissue thickness at the central axis of the axillary field. The thickness can be checked at set-up by subtracting scale readings.

Boost dose to tumour bed (breast conservation patients)

Brachytherapy (see Ch. 20) is the recommended boost method (Bartelink et al 1991b), since this minimises the volume treated, but may not always be available. The results of the current EORTC trial on the role of the boost, when complete, may lead to either reduction or increase of the requirements for boost doses.

Single-field boosts may be applied using cobalt, caesium, or electron beams, depending on the tumour bed depth and the importance of subsequent cosmetic appearance. The energy is chosen to adequately treat the tumour bed area, without giving a high dose to underlying lung. Megavoltage photon beams irradiate a large lung volume when directly applied to a small thickness of breast. The field may however be directed obliquely to the chest wall (Fig. 16.12), avoiding direct travel into the lung.

Internal mammary node treatment

Occasionally an indication arises for treatment of the internal mammary (IM) nodes via a vertical field to the ipsilateral and contralateral chains.

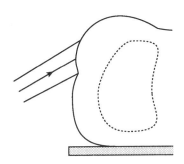

Figure 16.12 A boost field to the breast can be positioned to avoid directly irradiating the lung.

Usually a cobalt or 4–6 MV field is matched to the medial tangential field. The field is planned together with the tangential fields, and the required gap or overlap of the light beams on the skin is measured from the plan (Fig. 16.13). Use of a lower energy beam for the IM field than for the tangential fields may be preferred in order to give a lower dose to the mediastinum. However, where a different machine is used for the IM field, this compromises field matching because the patient has to be moved between fields.

It is not possible to achieve treatment of these nodes without hot spots or cold spots occurring in the match zone or without treating an excessive lung volume. Some type of compromise is required, usually that the light beam for the medial tangential field may overlap a few millimetres into the IM field. Where the overlap is greater than this there is a risk of overdose and damage to the matchline tissue.

Nonstandard techniques

Lateral decubitus position

The application of planned tangential fields to patients with very large breasts, lying supine, can be problematical because either the breast position is not sufficiently reproducible or the fields used to encompass the lateral aspect would include too much lung. A technique using vertical photon beams is described (Fourquet et al 1991) where the patient lies first on one side, then on the other with the breast supported, so that it lies flat on the support. The other breast has to be held out of the way by the patient for the 'medial' field. Reproducibility is difficult to achieve but the technique has been successfully used.

Tangential pair at normal f.s.d.

To set up nonisocentric tangential breast fields, a device such as a bridge, or some ingenious method, is required to set the f.s.d. correctly. Fields may be applied at normal f.s.d. with the aid of a device for beam direction and distance setting, using marks on the patient denoting the superior and inferior edges of each field, and medial and lateral field borders. The most commonly used device is a 'bridge' consisting of two parallel plates with a distance between them corresponding to the maximum thickness of the region to be treated (Fig. 16.14).

Principles of the bridge technique

The plates may be mounted on the machine in the manner of a backpointer, or may be constructed into an individual bridge. Using either of these, the lower edges of the plates are set on the patient's marks during the setting-up process. The patient lies with the ipsilateral arm up to allow treatment to the chest wall without irradiating the arm (Fig. 16.14). If the axilla is to be included, the field lengths are extended and the lateral, superior, field border will include several centimetres of arm. It is important that the mark is accurately renewed. It is difficult to include the SCF nodes, which lie 2–3 cm deep, so a separate top-up field to the SCF is required.

Dosimetry. The dosimetry assumed is that for a parallel pair treating a uniform volume of the same thickness as the plates plus evenly packed bolus. Alternatively, treatment may be planned using wedges as missing tissue compensators.

Reproducibility. The reproducibility and technical sophistication of the method is limited compared with isocentric, planned techniques with matched fields, where lung irradiation can be minimised.

Machine-mounted bridge method

With a machine-mounted bridge the plate nearest the isocentre is fixed at the isocentric distance, the

A

B

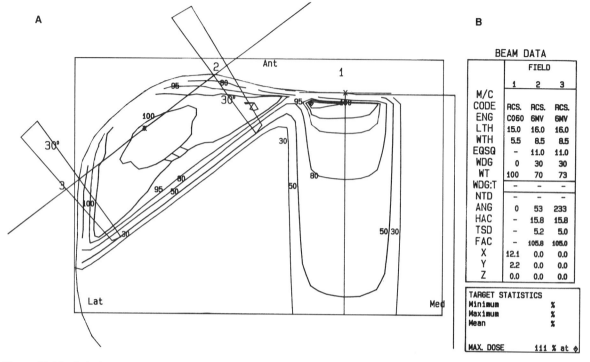

	FIELD		
	1	2	3
M/C CODE	RCS.	RCS.	RCS.
ENG	C060	6MV	6MV
LTH	15.0	16.0	16.0
WTH	5.5	8.5	8.5
EQSQ	–	11.0	11.0
WDG	0	30	30
WT	100	70	73
WDG:T	–	–	–
NTD	–	–	–
ANG	0	53	233
HAC	–	15.8	15.8
TSD	–	5.2	5.0
FAC	–	105.8	105.0
X	12.1	0.0	0.0
Y	2.2	0.0	0.0
Z	0.0	0.0	0.0

BEAM DATA

TARGET STATISTICS
Minimum %
Maximum %
Mean %

MAX. DOSE 111 % at ◊

Figure 16.13 **A** An internal mammary field abutting a tangential pair. **B** Beam data.

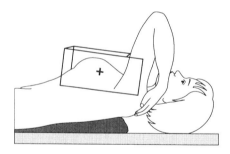

Figure 16.14 Patient rolled on support cushion for a non-machine-mounted bridge with parallel plates for beam direction of opposed fields applied to the breast. The contours of the breast are bolussed to fill the bridge to achieve parallel pair dosimetry. (Nonstandard technique.)

more distal plate being adjustable so that a specified plate separation for the patient can be set. The patient may lie flat on the couch for this technique.

For either field, the gantry is angled until the lower edges of both plates fit to both medial and lateral field marks on the patient. According to local preference, either fixed gantry angles may be used each day, which means that the patient must be 'fitted' to these, or variable angles are used to 'fit' the patient position. The light beam cover, especially of the breast and axilla, is used to verify the adequacy of the set-up.

Individually tailored bridge method

This method requires the patient to be rolled to one side, so that the bridge is horizontal, leading to major disadvantages since the patient position is rarely reproducible and the marks are liable to distort. Any twist of the bridge on the patient may lead to irradiation of the head by the lateral beam.

The f.s.d. and field centre are set on the bridge, and the gantry and couch rotated until the treatment plane defined by the bridge is orthogonal to the central ray, for each field.

REFERENCES AND FURTHER READING

The majority of articles listed were published in a special issue of *Radiotherapy and Oncology* with the title 'A consensus meeting – quality assurance in conservative treatment of early breast cancer'.

Bartelink H, Van der Schueren E, van Glabbeke M, Pierart M 1991a The conservative management of breast carcinoma by tumorectomy and radiotherapy: an EORTC phase III study (22881/10882). Radiotherapy and Oncology 22: trial protocol only

Bartelink H, Garavaglia G, Johansson K A, Mijnheer B J, Van den Bogaert W, Van Tienhoven T G, Yarnold J 1991b Quality assurance in conservative treatment of early breast cancer. Report on a consensus meeting of the EORTC Radiotherapy and breast cancer cooperative groups and the EUSOMA (European Society of Mastology). Radiotherapy and Oncology 22: 323–326

Fentiman I S 1991 Quality control in breast cancer treatment: what information can the surgeon provide? Radiotherapy and Oncology 22: 226–230

Fourquet A, Campana F, Rosenwald J C, Vilcoq J R 1991 Breast irradiation in the lateral decubitus position: technique of the Institut Curie. Radiotherapy and Oncology 22: 261–265

Gagliardi G, Lax I, Rutqvist L E 1992 Radiation therapy of stage I breast cancer: analysis of treatment technique accuracy using three dimensional planning tools. Radiotherapy and Oncology 24: 94–101

Grimaud E, Chavaudra J 1991 Breast cancer treatment: which inhomogeneities have to be taken into account? Radiotherapy and Oncology 22: 237–238

Kirby M C, Williams P C 1991 Portal imaging for the verification of breast treatments. Radiotherapy and Oncology 22: 314–316

Leunens G, Verstraete J, van Dam J, Dutreix A, Van der Schueren E 1991 In vivo dosimetry for tangential breast irradiation: role of the equipment in the accuracy of dose delivery. Radiotherapy and Oncology 22: 285–289

Lichter A S, Fraass B A, Van der Geijn J 1983 A technique for field matching in primary breast irradiation. International Journal of Radiation Oncology, Biology, Physics 9: 263–270

Mijnheer B J, Heukelom S, Landson J H, van Battum L J, van Bree N A M, Van Tienhoven G 1991 Should inhomogeneity corrections be applied during treatment planning of tangential breast irradiation? Radiotherapy and Oncology 22: 239–244

Mitine C, Dutreix A, Van der Schueren E 1991 Tangential breast irradiation: influence of technique of set-up on transfer errors and reproducibility. Radiotherapy and Oncology 22: 308–310

Redpath A T, Thwaites D I, Rodger A, Aitken M W, Hardman D J 1992 A multidisciplinary approach to improving the quality of tangential wall and breast irradiation for carcinoma of the breast. Radiotherapy and Oncology 23: 118–126

Siddon R L, Tonnesen G L, Svensson G K 1981 Three field technique for breast treatment using a rotatable half beam block. International Journal of Radiation Oncology, Biology, Physics 7: 1473–1477

Valdagni R, Italia C 1990 Early breast cancer irradiation after conservative surgery: quality control by portal localisation films. Radiotherapy and Oncology 22: 311–313

Van Dongen J A, Bartelink H, Fentiman I S et al 1992 Factors influencing local relapse and results of salvage treatment after breast conserving therapy in operable breast cancer. EORTC trial 10801, comparing breast conservation with mastectomy in TNM stage I and II breast cancer. European Journal of Cancer, in press

Van Tienhoven G, van Bree N A M, Mijnheer B J, Bartelink H 1991a Quality assurance of the EORTC trial 22881/10882: 'assessment of the role of the booster dose in breast conserving therapy': the dummy run. Radiotherapy and Oncology 22: 290–298

Van Tienhoven G, Lanson J H, Crabeels D, Heukelom S, Mijnheer B J 1991b Accuracy in tangential breast treatment set-up: a portal imaging study. Radiotherapy and Oncology 22: 317–322

Westbrook C, Gildersleve J, Yarnold J 1991 Quality assurance in daily treatment procedure: patient movement during tangential fields treatment. Radiotherapy and Oncology 22: 299–303

17

Head and neck techniques

PRINCIPLES OF BEAM DIRECTION USING SHELLS

Beam direction shells (Fig. 17.1) are used to assist treatment delivery to any site where immobilisation plus complex field direction marks are needed. Although this chapter primarily relates to treatment of head and neck sites, using beam direction shells, similar principles apply when using shells for treatment of other sites such as limbs.

The first treatment planning procedure is the selection of an appropriate patient position, followed by manufacture of a shell (Chandler 1988) which is appropriate to need.

Field and shielding marks and beam direction

It is impractical to use skin marks for high precision treatments (Griffiths et al 1987), and especially unacceptable to the patient for treatment of the head and neck region. Where a head support system is used without a shell, although simple fields may be applied for palliation purposes, it is difficult to apply fields of more complex shape using marks on the patient's surface, unless tattoos are used, which is not allowed on the head and neck in the UK.

Even where immobilisation is achieved by means of a bite block system (Fig. 17.2), it is appropriate to mark field and shielding limits on a shell, together with beam entry and exit points. It is important to have field marks on the shell, even with isocentric techniques, so that all visible field entry positions can be checked with the marks.

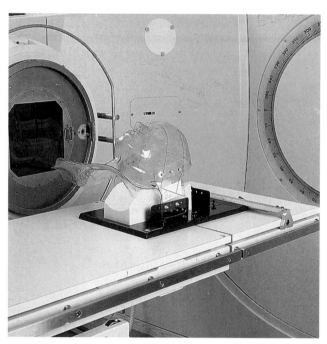

Figure 17.1 Shell attached at two lateral points and a superior point to a low attenuation carbon fibre headrest system with possible field entry from any angle. (Courtesy of Sinmed bv.)

Treatment accuracy is then dependent on the quality of construction and fit of the shell, since fields are primarily set up to marks on the shell. Marks on a high quality shell giving good patient reproducibility will relate reasonably accurately to the patient anatomy. Where the day-to-day accuracy of the treatment is not known, i.e. proven by extensive analysis (see Ch. 12), it is

useful to mark anatomical points which can be seen beneath the shell, in order to check that these coincide each day with the anatomy. Where field or shielding marks on the shell appear not to fulfil their intended purpose, e.g. the eye shielding appears to be inadequate, this should be investigated before treatment proceeds. If any alteration to the shell fit occurs, repeat planning checks or simulator verification should be performed before treatment continues.

Shell construction and fit

Shells used alone for immobilisation are usually constructed from a rigid clear plastic material moulded on a plaster cast of the patient. Increasingly, an opaque, meshed plastic material, which can be moulded directly on the patient, is used.

To be effective, shells must be close-fitting and rigidly constructed and/or rigidly fixed, so that the patient is immobilised in a reproducible position for each planning and treatment procedure. The shell construction should include suitable devices for attachment to a treatment couch

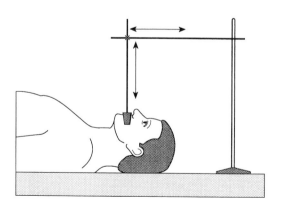

Figure 17.2 Bite block system to provide immobilisation of the head in all directions.

accessory system, so that the patient is immobilised on the relevant couch section but can be quickly released if necessary. Patient movement should not be possible once the shell is fitted. However, the larger the region enclosed by the shell, the more potential problems there are related to shell distortion, which may allow some patient movement.

The shell is attached at a minimum of two lateral points, with a superior point optionally, or a bite block arrangement (Figs 17.1 and 17.2). Ideally, a head shell should also attach at shoulder level so that shoulder position is reproduced, giving better reproducibility of the angle of the neck to the horizontal. Planning processes using the shell should be performed with the patient in the shell, as distortion may occur with an empty shell. Weight or contour change during treatment, which may affect fit, should be monitored.

Suitability of the shell for the treatment type envisaged

There is a need for detailed instructions, or standard protocols (such as supine or prone, head raised or flat) regarding patient positioning for treatment to be applied to a particular site. The likely field entry sites should be considered so that the patient position and shell construction is

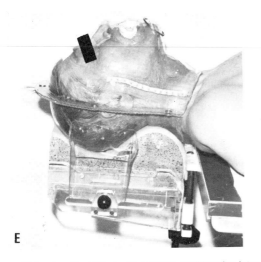

E

Figure 17.3 A patient fitted with a flange shell bearing lateral marker ladders and an anterior magnification ring. The patient has a bite block. (Reproduced from Walter et al 1982.)

suitable. Parts of the shell may be cut away to improve the acceptability to the patient.

The area of the face may be largely cut away for lateral neck fields. Once fields are defined, parts of the field area may also be cut away to retain full skin-sparing, leaving points carrying marks and retaining the strength and shape of the shell. Where shells are made in two halves, the joining zone, usually flanged (Fig. 17.3), must not coincide with crucial setting-up points. Similarly, flanges should be situated away from the entry ports for electron fields, to allow access for the electron applicator at the shell surface.

Similarly, for any other site, positioning and shell construction should be appropriate for field access.

PLANNING AND TREATMENT PRINCIPLES

Patient positioning

The patient position is set at the time of the impression or moulding. It is important that the required neck curvature is achieved via a suitable neck rest shape, which also contributes to head and neck immobilisation by preventing chin movement up and down and head roll from side to side, once the shell is fitted. Therefore several different shapes of headrest are required, so that a good fit can be achieved for each patient. Identical headrests and attachment systems should be available in each planning and treatment unit (Fig. 17.1).

The head should normally be straight. This is achieved by the use of sagittal and lateral lasers in the mould room (prior to and during plaster bandaging), with laser alignment marks being drawn on the shell later for use on each set-up. Where a shell is under manufacture for a child, sedation or anaesthetic procedures may be required.

Headrest systems

Ideally, a headrest system is required which attaches to any couch, but allows movement of the head support base both laterally and longitudinally before locking into position (Fig. 17.1).

An extension to the couch top may be useful where the longitudinal couch movement allows sufficient clearance from the isocentre (see Fig. 9.4).

Any system must allow access for the application of posterior oblique or vertical fields, without physical obstruction of the beams by high density couch or headrest components. Low attenuation headrest components are essential if this unobstructed field access from any direction is required. (Visual obstruction is not problematical for isocentric set-ups.) The system should also be compatible with use on a CT or MRI planning unit.

Localisation and simulation

Localisation may be undertaken on a CT or MRI unit, when three-dimensional digital data may be directly transferred into the treatment planning system, or on a treatment simulator (which may have an integral CT facility).

Using a simulator without CT facility, a pair of orthogonal films are required, on which target volumes are delineated. Marker ladders attached to the surface of the shell, one sagittal and two laterally (Fig. 17.3), serve to identify the shell surfaces (Fig. 17.4) and allow film magnification to be calculated. The films provide information, which is limited, but in three axes, for use in treatment planning.

As an alternative to planning from orthogonal films, the patient may be screened to allow inclusion of the target tissue within proposed treatment fields, and films of each field taken.

Following one of these procedures, a treatment plan is devised. A simulator portal check of some or all treatment fields is then undertaken.

Contour accuracy and dosimetry

Contours may be available from CT or MRI images, but otherwise may be taken directly from inside or outside the shell. The dose distribution actually obtained in tissue will then depend on shell fit. Also, if the contour is taken from a badly fitting shell, or from an empty shell with distortion, the plan may be invalid and the target tissue

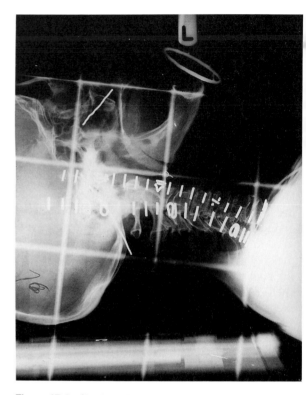

Figure 17.4 Simulator film with markers.

may be partially missed on each treatment. Where electron fields are applied, using an energy chosen to cut-off short of the spinal cord (see below: 'Two-phase treatments'), tissue contour accuracy becomes crucial to avoid an overdose to the cord.

Portal verification

It is recommended (Bleehen et al 1991) that for head and neck treatments, portal films of each field should be taken at least on the first set-up (Fig. 17.5). These should be repeated if there is doubt about the efficacy of the set-up, especially where critical organs are near to the treatment region. It is not physically possible for certain fields to be simulated because of the bulk of the image intensifier. The anatomy is not totally symmetrical, equipment is not perfect and beam divergence is in opposite directions, and as a result right and left lateral opposed fields may not appear to cover the same anatomy. Portal films should be directly comparable with a simulator

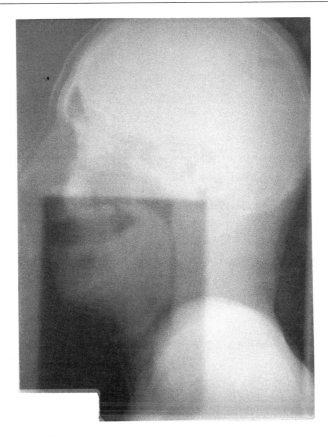

Figure 17.5 Double-exposed portal film.

field verification film where possible. Therefore a left lateral portal film should be compared with a left lateral simulator film.

Field arrangements

Many head and neck sites utilise a parallel, or near-parallel, pair of laterally directed fields, usually to a patient lying supine (the prone position being used for patients with posterior brain tumours). Other commonly used arrangements are:

- An anterior field with one or more lateral fields, for sites such as the maxillary antrum, where the anterior field goes through one eye. With a megavoltage beam the lens may be spared, but not the retina, so that depending on the dose given, the eye may have to be sacrificed. The other eye should be protected.
- Two fields, wedged in different axes (Fig.

17.7A), or a wedged and unwedged field applied via one portal, where a dose distribution improved over that from a single field is achievable and desirable.
- A combination of three or four angled fields, particularly to sites in the brain (see Ch. 23). It has been shown that reducing the dose through one portal by increasing the number of fields, minimises the chance of permanent alopecia or uneven hair growth following treatment (Vandevelde 1992).

Protection of critical organs

Field shaping and orientation

Any field may be shaped to protect normal tissue such as the brain, or critical organs such as the eye, optic chiasma and spinal cord. It is also important to avoid treating the whole of both lips, where possible. Shielding may be used.

Alternatively, the fields or patient may be orientated so as to avoid critical tissue being included in the treatment beams (see Ch. 23) which simplifies treatment delivery by reducing the need for shielding. Shielding systems placed relatively close to the patient result in a scatter dose at the patient surface which may be unacceptably high as an eye dose. A mouth bite block, incorporating an air passage, may be used to push the upper jaw and/or tongue out of the treatment volume. Often the collimator angle and patient position are carefully selected so that the spinal cord runs parallel with a field border (Fig. 17.6), which brings various advantages, particularly for two-phase treatments.

Dose monitoring. The eye dose may be estimated from strategically placed thermoluminescent dose (TLD) sachets, or by direct reading dosemeters. The relationship of the measuring device to the eye, and to the treatment beam edge and central axes, is important. The dose estimated may be superficial scatter if the device is outside the beam, i.e. an estimated lens dose, which may be a relevant indicator where the lens is also outside the beam. A measurement made at the outer canthus is more relevant to the estimation of dose to the retina, for example as a check near a divergent beam exit path running close to the eye.

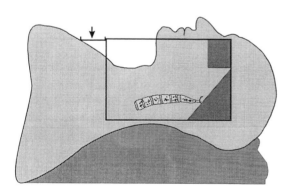

Figure 17.6 Large left lateral shaped field with 0° collimator angle, running parallel with spinal cord, for phase one treatment. The gantry angle for the anterior SCF field is 0° plus 1–2° so that the superior edge is vertical for matching to the inferior edges of both lateral fields.

Two-phase treatments

Sites requiring treatment to a relatively large risk area often require a boost dose to a smaller high risk site within the field area, or a replanned treatment after a certain dose, to prevent overdosage of critical tissues within the treatment volume. Treatment of these sites in the head and neck may necessitate an irradiation of the spinal cord which approaches the tolerance limit in the first phase. In the second phase, reduced size fields are planned to exclude the cord. A matched electron field may then be added to boost the dose to the remaining tissue lying lateral to the cord (Figs. 17.7A, B, C).

Use of asymmetric fields. Asymmetric fields may be used either to achieve a reduced field size, using the original setting-up points, and/or to reduce the need for shielding. Asymmetric fields may be planned so that the central axis passes through critical zones, for example close to the eye (see Ch. 19), in order to avoid divergence into critical structures.

Matched field techniques

Various head and neck sites require the use of adjacent fields matched to a line where they meet. The matched fields may be orthogonal or parallel to each other.

Orthogonal matched fields

Orthogonal matched fields are used to treat the nasopharynx and sites having high risk of spread down the lymphatics of the neck to the SCF nodes. Parallel opposed lateral fields are used to treat down to the root of the neck where they match to an orthogonal field to the SCF area (Figs 17.7 and 17.8).

Collimator and gantry angles. The collimator angle for the lateral fields is used for the gantry angle for the anterior field, with a 1° or 2° correction for the divergent angle of the 50% isodose curve, represented by the light beam edge, of the anterior field (Fig. 17.8). The edges of the fields (light beams) are set to the matchline and the lateral collimator angles checked to be within 2° of the anterior gantry angle.

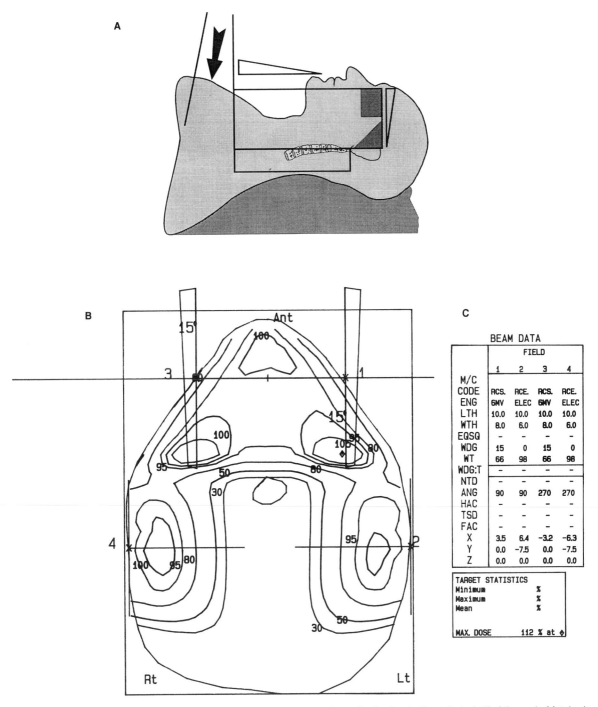

Figure 17.7 **A** Smaller photon field, wedged in two axes to improve the dose distribution, to the anterior half of the neck. Matched electron field to the posterior half of the neck, for a phase two treatment. **B** Cross-section showing field arrangement for A, with cord spared from the electron fields by virtue of the selected energy and cut-off depth. The central axes of both the photon and electron fields on each side of the neck are parallel. **C** Beam data for B.

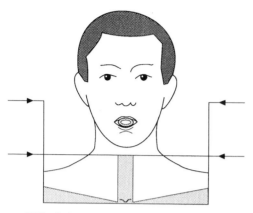

Figure 17.8 Orthogonally matched field arrangement.

The collimator angle must be zero for the anterior field (Fig. 17.9A) as any twist will disturb the horizontal geometry of the beam match (Fig. 17.9B). The couch has to be turned through 90° for the anterior field and often the match is uneven from one side of the neck to the other. Any adjustment necessary to achieve a good match at both sides of the neck must be achieved by a small couch twist, which does not disturb the geometry in the same way as a collimator twist. A small couch twist may be inevitable because of the limitations in equipment accuracy which are manifest when using orthogonal table angles.

Matching light edges on the sloping patient surface. A method of matching the orthogonal fields at the matchline is required, and this involves using the light beam/field edges. This type of surface match requires divergence in all matched edges or in none. It is possible to match two orthogonal field edges along a 45° plane, if they have similar angles of divergence. The anterior contour of the neck at the match level approximates to two 45° slopes in the orientation required for this match. If an attempt is made to match one nondivergent edge with one divergent edge, the visual match is difficult to achieve and edge angles will differ by 6° or so, in a direction tending to overlap of the beams at a depth. Asymmetry may be used to give nondivergent edges at the matchplane, but the narrower penumbra effect presents an increased potential for overdosage at the junction.

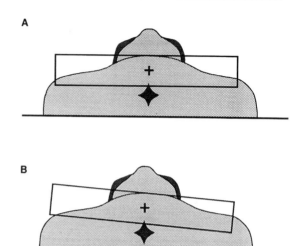

Figure 17.9 **A** Anterior SCF field from an exaggerated off-vertical beam's eye view aspect to demonstrate that with a 0° collimator angle the beam axis is horizontal. **B** Anterior SCF field viewed as in A, but with small collimator twist so that the axis is not horizontal and therefore incorrect for a geometrical match at either side of the patient.

Parallel matched fields

Head and neck regimes often require a boost phase with lateral photon fields matched to parallel electron fields over the cord (Fig. 17.7A, B). The match is critical because of the divergence of the isodose curves from the electron fields below the surface (see Ch. 5), into the adjacent photon field. There may need to be a small surface gap between the fields. It is particularly important to ensure that gantry, collimator and floor angles are constant (within 1–2°) for both the electron and photon field. It is desirable, for accuracy, not to move the patient between the application of one matched field and another. However, with older linacs there is a safety requirement to check that the swtich from one mode to the other is properly effected. This is checked by calibration or by running and monitoring a beam, so that the patient has to be removed from the room between fields.

Isocentric versus f.s.d. techniques

Set-ups using beam direction shells may be either fixed f.s.d. or isocentric. Set-up time is minimised with an isocentric technique, and more flexibility for using posteriorly directed fields is obtained, since set-up may be achieved via gantry, couch and collimator rotations. Any centring inaccuracy arising during couch rotations (owing to equipment accuracy limitations) must, however, be corrected for by using couch movements. It may not be possible to see the centring point of any through-couch field, therefore some means of visual check using the lasers must be incorporated into the method.

A potential advantage of an f.s.d. set-up is that fields are necessarily always visually checked on the shell. Also, increased clearance between the patient and the machine allows better visibility during set-up, and reduces the scatter dose from the shielding and from machine hardware (see Ch. 8).

REFERENCES AND FURTHER READING

Bleehen N M et al 1991 Quality Assurance in radiotherapy. Report of a Working Party. Standing Subcommittee on Cancer of the Standing Medical Advisory Committee

Chandler M 1988 Behind the mask. Change, Stoke-on-Trent

Dobbs J, Barrett A, Ash D 1992 Practical radiotherapy planning, 2nd edn. Arnold, London

Griffiths S E, Pearcey R G, Thorogood J 1987 Quality control in radiotherapy: The reduction of field placement errors. International Journal of Radiation Oncology, Biology, Physics 13: 1583–1588

Huizenga H, Levendag P C, De Porre P M Z R, Visser A G 1988 Accuracy in radiation field alignment in head and neck cancer: A prospective study. Radiotherapy and Oncology 11: 181–187

Mould R F 1985 Radiotherapy treatment planning, 2nd edn. Adam Hilger, Bristol

Vandevelde G 1992 Presentation at postgraduate teaching course for radiographers. ESTRO (European Society for Therapy, Radiology and Oncology

Verhey L V, Goitein M, McNulty P, Munzenrider J E, Suit H D 1982 Precise positioning of patients for radiation therapy. International Journal of Radiation Oncology, Biology, Physics 8: 289–294

Walter J, Miller H, Bomford C K 1982 A short textbook of radiotherapy, 4th edn. Churchill Livingstone, Edinburgh

18

Treatment principles for large, complex shaped fields

For certain diseases such as lymphoma and seminoma, a relatively large region of the body requires the application of large, parallel opposed, treatment fields. Tissue not requiring treatment is shielded within the large area so that a complex field shape is created. The nature of these fields and the accuracy required demands special methods to achieve a high level of precision.

These diseases are radiosensitive and therefore eradicated by a relatively low radiation dose, so the patient has a high chance of cure following well executed radiotherapy. There is evidence that inadequate technical methods cause large differences in both marginal and in field relapse rates for Hodgkin's disease (Kinzie et al 1983). A study of Grant et al (1973) into the reasons for recurrence following the mantle technique also suggested that recurrence may be due to technical failure rather than radioresistance. This chapter describes the principles used and ways to avoid the pitfalls. Many of the principles apply to any field with a complex shape.

For diseases commonly treated by these techniques it is particularly relevant to describe the sites included in the fields, as these determine the field shape and accuracy criteria. A check of the light beam cover on the anatomy against the expected or prescribed cover is carried out as part of the setting-up process.

FIELD SHAPES FOR SPECIFIC DISEASES

Above the diaphragm

In a 'full mantle' technique, the mediastinal, supra- and infraclavicular, axillary and cervical lymph node chains are treated, using fields extending from the angle of the mandible to the xiphisternum (Fig. 18.1), usually for Hodgkin's disease. For this condition, a tumour dose of 35–40 Gy in 4 weeks is used. The lungs are shielded, also the larynx anteriorly and cervical cord posteriorly, if there is no central disease in the neck. The whole length of spinal cord is shielded on the posterior field after 20–25 Gy tumour dose. Depending on the stage of the disease, smaller portions of the mantle fields may be used. However, in the case of a smaller field, the same precise technical methods are required as the possibility of the patient having treatment, to an adjacent node chain, 'matched' to the original treated area at a later date has to be considered. For disease presenting in the mediastinum, the mediastinal field is extended down to the level of the second lumbar vertebra to include upper paraaortic nodes.

Occasionally, for example in non-Hodgkin's lymphoma, the upper border will be extended to cover the preauricular nodes and Waldeyer's ring. Alternatively, lateral fields, matched to the superior mantle border at the level of the angle of the mandible, may be used for these nodes.

Below the diaphragm

A field shape called a 'dogleg' (Fig. 18.2) is used for treating paraaortic node chains in continuity with ipsilateral iliac nodes for patients with seminoma (or a long paraaortic field alone may be used, as in a current trial). An 'inverted Y' field shape (see below: 'Total nodal irradiation') is sometimes used for treating paraaortic node chains in continuity with bilateral iliac nodes, usually for lymphoma. In either case the kidneys are shielded.

Other diseases may be treated using similar methods, for example, whole abdominal fields

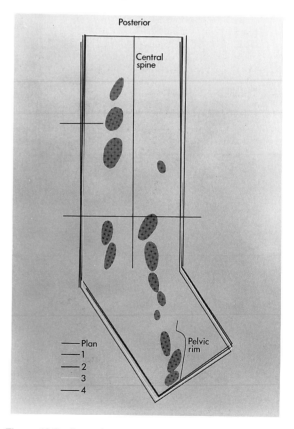

Figure 18.2 Several posterior field treatments of a dogleg field, using a reproducible (supine-and-prone) technique. Node positions are shown within the field.

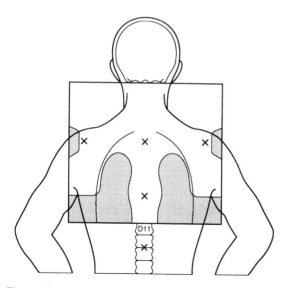

Figure 18.1 Mantle field with tattoo points (shown as crosses).

with kidney shielding, or gynaecological fields extended to include the paraaortic nodes.

CHALLENGES OF LARGE, COMPLEX SHAPED FIELDS

The large size of the fields, together with complex shielding, present a need for high precision to overcome a number of problems, of which both planning and treatment staff need to be aware. Complex shaped fields are prone to significant placement errors, identifiable only with portal imaging, arising from the magnification of small variations in equipment setting or patient positioning. Specialist, well researched techniques are required.

The two main challenges are:

• to ensure that the shielding blocks are always aligned with submillimetre accuracy in relation to the field axes
• to ensure that the shaped field is always applied correctly to all the target anatomy.

Template technique: the basis of an accurate method

The template technique is the basis of any accurate method for treating large, complex shaped fields. A template, carrying field and shielding alignment marks, is used as a fixation point for shielding blocks, at tray level. This sets the field shape and is used for projecting alignment marks on to the patient.

The processes used may vary and the overall effectiveness will depend on the accuracy of each of the constituent processes. There are several key factors influencing the accuracy achievable:

• compatibility between the simulator and treatment tables
• the method of positioning the patient, and support devices used
• the body position/s used
• limitations in machine accuracy and the way equipment is used
• the f.s.d. used
• the type of skin reference marking system used

• the shielding system used
• the treatment field verification methods and protocols for assessing and correcting.

The effects of these factors interlink, so they must be considered together.

Patient positioning and supports used

Any support or accessory used in positioning the patient must be identical on planning and for each treatment. Special patient positioning methods are required to ensure that the anatomy of the patient is 'arranged' each day so that the spatial configuration of a series of reference tattoos around the target region conforms exactly to that when tattooing took place.

The patient is usually required to lie flat, supine or supine-and-prone, and as straight as possible. Those who have difficulty with this should not be manipulated into a position which is too unnatural or uncomfortable, since this will lead to an unreproducible treatment set-up and/ or movement during treatment delivery.

Lateral laser points should be used to correct lateral rotation (see Figs 13.5 and 13.6) and well spaced midline tattoos (see Fig. 13.3) are used to align the patient with the sagittal laser or field axis line. Additional tattoos on the shoulder area (Fig. 18.1) should be used for aligning mantle patients. Reproducible positions for the head, arm and shoulder are crucial.

Abdominopelvic fields

The patient's head should be on a firm support so that the relationship of the spine to the couch top is reproduced. This assists in preventing a shift of the tattoos along the longitudinal body axis. The hand and arm position relative to the trunk and the couch top should also be reproduced to ensure a consistent relationship of the tattoos to the internal anatomy.

Mantle technique

Head position. For a patient lying supine, the head should be held straight with the chin extended so that the mandible is aligned with the angle of divergence of the superior border of the anterior field. This border usually extends to the level of the angle of the mandible (Fig. 18.3A) and to just below the external auditory meatus (EAM) bilaterally.

A measurement from the chin to the SSN should be used at each set-up to check the chin position. A head support is required to ensure that the position is held and reproduced on each treatment. Such a support should encompass a

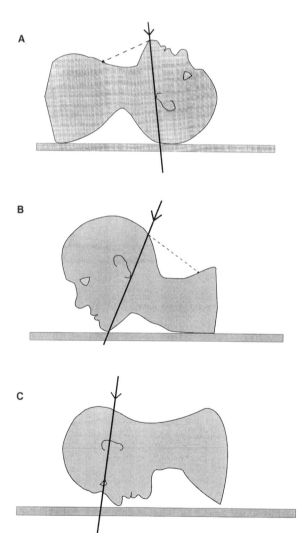

Figure 18.3 Alignment of upper field border through the head. **A** Anterior field. **B** Posterior field. **C** Posterior field misaligned owing to incorrect chin/head angle.

bite block or support which fits under the nose. If the chin drops during treatment, the teeth and gums will be irradiated, causing dental problems later.

For a patient lying prone, the chin position should also allow the superior posterior field border to run approximately along the angle of the mandible (Fig 18.3B), just below the EAM. If the chin drops, the eyes may be irradiated (Fig. 18.3C) to up to 25% of the prescribed dose (Grant et al 1973) and the suboccipital nodes may be above the field edge. A measurement from the occiput to a tattoo over the dorsal spine should be used at each set-up to adjust the head position.

Arm position. Variations in arm position are in use, each having advantages and disadvantages:

1. When the arms are allowed to rest on the couch top next to the trunk, the shoulder position can be easily reproduced by means of appropriate tattoo points. The tissue contours are thus simplified and the axilla is enclosed within a thickness of tissue so that it receives a high dose. However, the skin of the axilla may suffer severe reaction, since the skin-sparing effect is lost.

2. The hands may be placed on the hips, which allows some skin-sparing of the axilla. This position can be well reproduced but can be difficult to sustain unless the weight of the arms is supported on the couch. The use of supports under the shoulder has been advocated (Grant et al 1973) to alter the position of certain lymph nodes, but we have found reproducibility to be poor when using such pads.

3. An additional couch section with lateral extensions for the arms to rest on (crucifix technique) may be used. The authors have no experience with this technique.

4. The arms may be raised above the head; however, reproducibility will be poor unless a well designed support with handgrips is available. The angle at which the arms are held may be very variable leading to an inconsistent relationship of the skin and marks to the target anatomy, giving rise to variations, particularly in the longitudinal axis (Fig. 18.4). Also, this position tends to pull certain lymph nodes over the humeral head so that joint shielding is not possible (Weisenburger & Juillard 1977). The skin

Example of 1cm Caudo-Cephalic Shift
Causing Node Shielding

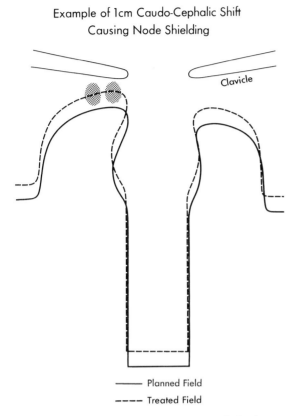

—— Planned Field

---- Treated Field

Figure 18.4 Effect of field shift in the longitudinal axis.

around the shoulder region is stretched and creased, and so unsuitable for bearing tattoos.

Treatment planning and simulation

Following accurate staging confirmed from diagnostic CT scanning, the patient may have the target tissue defined from planning CT images. The feasibility of this depends on both the availability of CT planning facilities, and on whether the patient can be scanned in the treatment position. More usually, the patient is planned from anteroposterior (AP) and posteroanterior (PA) simulator films which cover the entire body region at risk.

Simulation

Compatibility between the simulator and treatment tables. Simulation must be carried out on a table surface with the same degree of rigidity as the treatment couch, otherwise there is little chance of a consistent relationship of anatomy and reference marks throughout planning and treatment (see Ch. 13).

Patient position. The patient is positioned as required for treatment, for each set of films to be taken. Even where only one patient position is used for both fields (see discussion later in this chapter), fields should be planned and verified individually.

f.s.d. setting. The patient is set at the f.s.d. required for treatment, at one of the marked points. If the f.s.d. is set at differing points on the patient at simulation and treatment, inaccuracies in the field cover will arise.

Treatment reference marks. Selected reference points along the patient's central axis, as defined by the sagittal laser or machine centre cross-wire, together with other key points, are marked on the skin. These reference points are subsequently used to realign the patient's anatomy correctly on each treatment. They should be tattooed at simulation so that they are not lost and can be relied on both during treatment and subsequently. All tattoos should be well spaced out, so that they are effective for alignment with the straight field axes (Fig. 18.1).

Planning films

The reference points are marked by radio-opaque crosses placed on the skin. These represent the reference points and their relationship to the simulator centre cross, on the films.

Field planning

A film is taken of the area of interest, with the patient in the selected treatment position. Overlapped films, with markers for use in joining them together, may be required if the area of interest, magnified by the patient-to-film distance, is larger than the largest film available. The clinician marks the planning volume and shielding, with appropriate margins, on the image (Fig. 18.5). Safety margins should be as small as

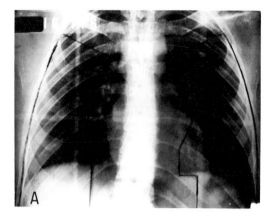

Figure 18.5 Simulator film outlined with shielding. (Reproduced from Walter et al 1982.)

possible, to minimise the irradiated volume, but appropriate for the accuracy achievable (see Ch. 12).

The field size is determined by the peripheral limits of the target tissue in the longitudinal and lateral axes. The simulator centre will thus not be the exact treatment field centre. The reference points, rather than the field centre, are subsequently used to align the patient with the treatment beam.

Dosimetry

The dose received at various points within a mantle field may differ with body contours and field shape, by around ±10% of the prescribed target dose. The dosimetry within mantle fields varies with the size of the field portion, since the penumbra effect of the shielding, combined with small effective field sizes within the area, causes a marked decrease in dose levels (Fig. 18.6A). Thus it is likely that very few areas actually receive the full prescribed dose. Some shielded areas receive up to 20% of the central axis dose (Fig. 18.6B). The reasons for this are described in detail by Marrs et al (1993).

Conventional dose calculation provides dose estimates only at specific points and planes. Accurate dose determination for specific areas or critical tissues is not possible. A more accurate and detailed dose distribution can be achieved by transferring anatomical information from CT images to the planning system (Rathmell et al 1992),

in order to compute the combined effects of shielding blocks and body contours. Tissue compensators may be required.

Template and shielding block production

A template of the treatment field, with shielding block positions marked, is produced, with dimensions which are correct at the shielding tray height for the treatment machine to be used. Beam-shaped shielding blocks of the required shapes are produced from low melting point alloy. A block fixation system is required.

Field verification

Verification of the treatment field and shielding accuracy may be achieved on the treatment machine or the simulator by setting up the patient as if for treatment, using the actual blocks (see Ch. 8). A film for each field is taken and must be accepted, or a second set accepted after any adjustments, before a treatment dose is delivered. Portal films (Fig. 18.7) are then used to check the set-up on at least the first treatment (see Ch. 12), since one piece of equipment always differs slightly from another (Fig. 18.8). If the reproducibility is good (see Ch. 12) then further films are only required if there is a change in set-up, such as the addition of spinal shielding, or if a long break in treatment or excessive weight loss occurs.

TREATMENT DELIVERY AND QUALITY

Quality of information and staff continuity

The information relating to the patient position and set-up must be clearly and fully recorded for use by the treatment staff, who start the treatment without the advantage of a simulator for a visual field check, and without having seen the patient or the set-up before. There should be some information available for checking field borders against anatomical landmarks, and to give an indication if the patient position is unusual, e.g. twisted due to scoliosis. It is difficult to verify the block shadows on the patient are

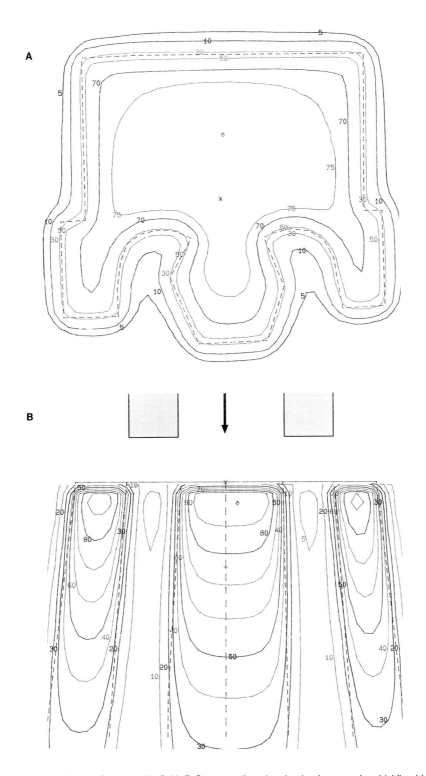

Figure 18.6 **A** Isodose distribution for a mantle field. **B** Cross-section showing isodoses under shielding blocks.

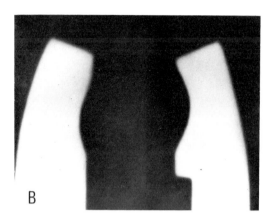

Figure 18.7 Mantle verification film. (Reproduced from Walter et al 1982.)

FIELD SHIFT BETWEEN SIMULATION AND TREATMENT

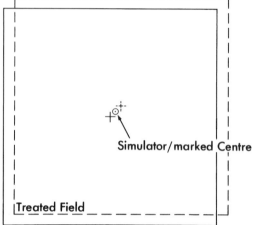

Simulator/marked Centre

Treated Field

Simulator Planned Field

Both machines working at limits of accepted accuracy specification.
Worst case = 8mm shift

Figure 18.8 Differences in the accuracy characteristics of equipment may lead to a shift of the field in any direction, necessitating a portal check on any machine used for high precision work.

correct, but if a member of the planning team attends the first treatment set-up, a visual check of consistency can be made.

Gantry angle

The gantry must be set exactly vertically, as a discrepancy of 0.5° produces an error of 2.5 mm or more at the distal surface of the patient (Fig. 18.9). Equipment setting scales are accurate only to ±0.5° and additional 'true vertical' setting indicators are required.

If the sagittal laser runs to one side of the central axis, it is likely that the gantry is not set vertically.

Diaphragm angle

The diaphragms must be set on the same quarter-circle angle throughout treatment, to prevent changes such as a longitudinal or lateral shift of the field resulting from the use of different diaphragm orientation. Diaphragm angle scales are accurate only to ±0.5° and 0.5° diaphragm rotation leads to a 3.5 mm inaccuracy at the end of a 40 cm long field at 100 cm f.s.d. (greater at longer f.s.d.) (Figs 13.1 and 13.2).

The f.s.d.

Any inaccuracy in machine or block positioning is magnified by increased f.s.d., and most linacs

provide a field size of 40 cm × 40 cm at the isocentre, which is large enough for most fields. Thus the technique is more accurate at shorter f.s.d. However, shielding blocks are larger and heavier, which increases safety hazards.

Shielding

Individually moulded beam-shaped shielding blocks, the positions of which are fixed in relation to the field centre (see Ch. 8), are required. Blocks may be placed individually on the template during set-up, each block pegging into the template in a unique manner (Pearcey & Griffiths 1986), reducing the lifting hazards. Often, the shielding blocks cover one or more of the reference points, so that set-up is completed before one or more blocks are inserted (particularly spinal lead). It is important to ensure that the patient does not move once the reference points are obscured.

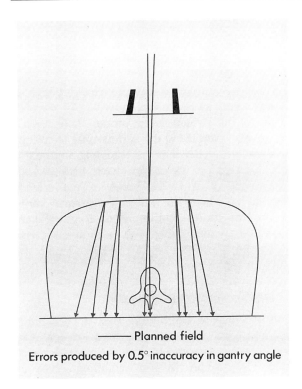

———— Planned field

Errors produced by 0.5° inaccuracy in gantry angle

Figure 18.9 Effect of slight gantry angle inaccuracy.

Template identification and orientation

The template is aligned along the longitudinal axis of the machine centre cross or sagittal laser. A checking procedure is required to ensure that the correct template is used and that it is accurately located in the shielding tray.

Potential pitfalls and their origins

Field rotation

Rotation of the field will be seen (see Figs 13.1 and 13.2) if the patient is lying slightly skew. This rotation is likely to occur where the midline tattoos, used to set the straight field axis or sagittal laser, are close together, e.g. all within 10–12 cm length. The potential for inaccuracies, even when the field centre is well aligned, increases with distance from the field centre especially at points where shielding is used, and

can be significant at the upper paraaortic and lower mediastinal areas (see Fig. 13.2 and see below: 'Limitations in machine accuracy'). The more widely spaced are the tattoos (Fig. 18.1), the more effective they are in preventing rotation.

Field rotation may arise where the relationship between the field centre cross and the sagittal laser are different on the simulator and treatment machine. Where the machine centre cross is slightly skew (see Fig. 9.13), it will not coincide with the sagittal laser.

Shielding system

Differences between machines. Where a tray with fixed blocks is interchanged between the simulator and the treatment machine, problems may occur with field symmetry about the blocks. Variations will also occur if the patient is transferred to a different machine.

Manually placed blocks. If unmounted blocks are used without a fixation system, shielding is not accurate and relies on subjective judgement in aligning blocks with lines. Small discrepancies at tray level are magnified by a long tray-to-patient distance. This usually leads to overshielding (Fig. 18.10), which, in a mediastinal field portion bounded by shielding on both borders, can result in field narrowing of up to 2 cm (Griffiths & Pearcey 1986).

It is particularly important that shoulder shielding is accurately placed, using shoulder alignment tattoos and fixed blocks, since the gap between this and the lung blocks is narrow, already reducing the dose by 6–10% (Grant et al 1973). Also the axilla is at risk of being shielded by laterally misplaced lung blocks, or by shoulder blocks, especially where the shoulder position is not well reproduced.

Skin marks

Skin-marked field or shielding outlines should not be used where accuracy is required (Griffiths & Pearcey 1985). Where blocks are lined up with shielding outlines on the skin, shielding misplacement occurs since the shape and position of marks varies with patient position.

'Field' Width Altered by Shielding Block

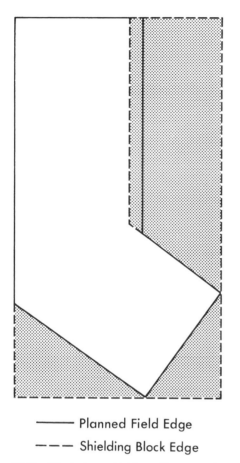

——— Planned Field Edge

– – – Shielding Block Edge

Figure 18.10 Effect of overshielding, with a manual system, on a dogleg field.

Through-couch fields

There are additional problems for these fields, discussed below.

Supine-only versus supine-and-prone technique

There is a continuing debate as to how complex fields such as mantles should be treated. When using the supine-only position, with the posterior field treated through the couch, it is assumed that the patient position and anatomy remains constant, and thus is treated by truly parallel opposed fields. These fields may then be planned from above the couch only and a mirror image of the field and shielding blocks used for the under-couch field.

There are anatomical changes when a patient is turned over, necessitating individually planned fields to the patient lying prone, then supine. However, when using the supine-only technique it is acknowledged that the shielding accuracy is less accurate on the under-couch field (Sebag-Montefiore et al 1992). Some of the reasons for this have been identified by means of verification film studies, and improved accuracy demonstrated when using the supine-and-prone technique (Griffiths et al 1987). These are summarised below.

Limitations in machine accuracy

The accuracy of equipment used is particularly significant for large complex field set-ups. Any small inaccuracy is doubled on the through-couch field (Fig. 18.11A, B) and magnified where an increased f.s.d. is used (Griffiths & Pearcey 1985).

• A droop of the gantry leads to a longitudinal shift of the field between the over-couch and under-couch field. The two fields will not be coincident in the patient because the over-couch field points back towards the gantry and the under-couch field points away from the gantry.
• A small discrepancy in the gantry scale will lead to a lateral shift of the field which is doubled on the under-couch field.
• A slight diaphragm rotation may be doubled on the under-couch field.
• With an extended f.s.d. set-up, there is considerable couch travel between fields, for example 60 cm for 120 cm f.s.d.. During 10 cm of vertical travel there can be 1 mm of couch top movement, e.g. laterally. Thus for 60 cm travel, there could be 6 mm movement.

In the authors' experience, most of the errors are random. The effect can be demonstrated on any machine used for the technique, by setting up the over-couch field on to paper stuck to the couch top, tracing the field and shielding, then setting up the under-couch field to compare their co-incidence. The couch heights must be set so that

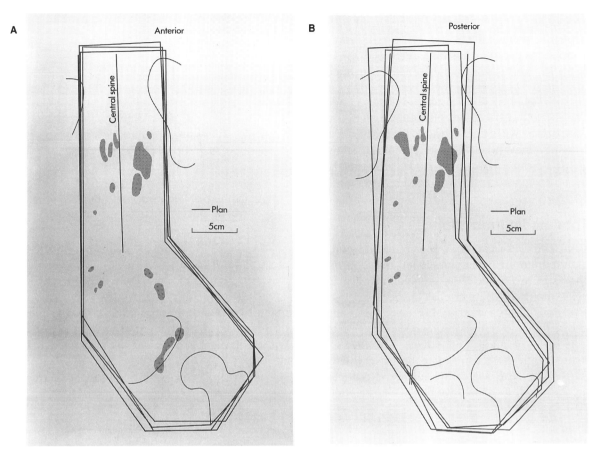

Figure 18.11 Three treatments (supine-only technique) of a dogleg field, related to the plan. **A** Anterior fields. **B** Posterior fields, treated through the couch, on the same three treatment occasions as shown in A. This demonstrates large and random field rotation and lateral shift inaccuracies on the under-couch field.

the vertical travel of the couch used simulates the patient set-up. The process should be repeated several times, changing the variables, such as having a different person setting up.

Beam divergence

The divergence of the two opposed beams differs, so that planning from the over-couch field only is inadequate for any target tissue lying below the midplane (see Fig. 15.5), especially that which is near to shielding blocks or field edges. Tissue which is encompassed in the over-couch beam may be inadequately treated by the under-couch beam, even if the patient remains still, unless fields are planned individually.

Procedure time and patient movement or shape changes

Treating both fields may take 20 minutes or more, so with a supine-only technique these points should be taken into consideration:

• The patient has to lie still while both fields are applied, an ordeal for any patient, who may move a little.

• There is a need to verify that the patient has not physically moved during the setting-up of the under-couch field, or gradually moved during the treatment process (all reference marks being on the uppermost patient surface).

• The authors have observed that when a patient has been lying on the table for 10–20 minutes, a longitudinal table movement becomes necessary to realign the field centre. During this time, the patient tissue has relaxed so that the interfield separation has also decreased by 1 cm or more, indicating a change in the body shape so that the position of a marked reference point may have changed in relation to the target anatomy. Therefore, if a treatment procedure is lengthy in comparison with the planning procedure, a discrepancy may arise. The length of duration of any CT scan from which node positions have been determined, may also be relevant.

Total nodal irradiation

Total nodal irradiation is now only occasionally required, to treat the whole of the lymphatic chains in the trunk. This involves using mantle fields matched to 'inverted-Y' fields (Fig. 18.12). The principles used for either field alone apply, with additional complications related to the junction zone. Mantle and inverted-Y fields are treated with a calculated gap between them on the surface. The size of the surface gap depends on the depth at which the fields are intended to

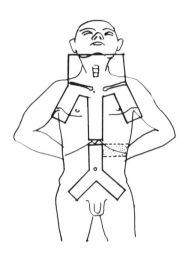

Figure 18.12   Mantle and inverted-Y fields for total nodal irradiation. (Reproduced from Walter et al 1982.)

meet. The mantle and inverted-Y field sequence on one side of the patient should be completed without patient movement, as for any matched fields.

The principles of moving the junctions are the same as for total neuraxis irradiation (see Ch. 19).

REFERENCES AND FURTHER READING

Creutzberg C L, Visser A G, De Porre P M Z R, Meerwaldt J H, Althof V G M, Levendag P C 1992 Accuracy of patient positioning in mantle irradiation. Radiotherapy and Oncology 23: 257–264
Dobbs J, Barrett A, Ash D 1992 Practical radiotherapy planning, 2nd edn. Arnold, London
Grant L, Jackson W, Isitt J 1973 An investigation of the mantle technique. Clinical Radiology 24: 254–262 .
Griffiths S E 1986 Reproducibility in radiotherapy. Radiography 52: 167–169
Griffiths S E 1989 Hit or miss – is perfection achievable in radiotherapy? Radiography Today 55: 24–26
Griffiths S E, Pearcey R G 1985 The reproducibility of large lead protected fields to the abdomen and pelvis. Radiography 51: 247–250
Griffiths S E, Pearcey R G 1986 The daily reproducibility of large, complex shaped radiotherapy fields to the thorax and neck. Clinical Radiology 37: 39–41
Griffiths S E, Pearcey R G, Thorogood J 1987 Quality control in radiotherapy: the reduction of field placement errors. International Journal of Radiation Oncology, Biology, Physics 13: 1583–1588
Griffiths S E, Khoury G G, Eddy A 1991 Quality control of radiotherapy during pelvic irradiation. Radiotherapy and Oncology 20: 203–206
Hulshof M, Vanuytsel L, Van den Bogaert W, Van der

Schueren E 1989 Localization errors in mantle field irradiation for Hodgkin's disease. International Journal of Radiation Oncology, Biology, Physics 17: 679–683
Kinzie J J, Hanks G E, Maclean C J, Kramer S 1983 Patterns of care study: Hodgkin's disease relapse rates and the adequacy of portals. Cancer 52: 2223–2226
Marks J E, Haus A G, Sutton H G, Griem M L 1976 Localisation error in the radiotherapy of Hodgkin's disease and malignant lymphoma with extended mantle fields. Cancer 34: 83–90
Marks J E, Haus A G, Sutton H G, Griem M L 1976 The value of frequent treatment verification films in reducing localisation error in the irradiation of complex fields. Cancer 37: 2755–2761
Marrs J E, Hounsell A R, Wilkinson J M 1993 The efficacy of lead shielding in megavoltage radiotherapy. British Journal of Radiology 66: 140–144
Pearcey R G, Griffiths S E 1985 The impact of treatment errors on post-operative radiotherapy for testicular tumours. British Journal of Radiology 58: 1003–1005
Pearcey R G, Griffiths S E 1986 An investigation into the daily reproducibility of patient positioning for mantle treatments. Clinical Radiology 37: 43–45
Rathmell A J, Workman G M, Clinkard J E, Taylor R E, Carey B 1992 Use of CT planning to improve mantle radiotherapy dosimetry. British Journal of Radiology 65 (Suppl): 17

Richards M J S, Buchler D A 1977 Errors in reproducing pelvic radiation portals. International Journal of Radiation Oncology, Biology, Physics 2: 1017–1019

Sebag-Montefiore D J, Maher E J, Young J, Hudson G V, Hanks G 1992 Variation in mantle technique: implications for establishing priorities for quality assurance in clinical trials. Radiotherapy and Oncology 23: 144–149

Walter J, Miller H, Bomford CK 1982 A short textbook of radiotherapy, 4th edn. Churchill Livingstone, Edinburgh

Weisenburger T H, Juillard J F 1977 Upper extremity lymphangiography in the radiation therapy of lymphomas and carcinoma of the breast. Therapeutic Radiology 122: 227–230

19

Craniospinal irradiation

Introduction

Craniospinal irradiation (CSI) is used to treat those brain tumours which are associated with a high risk of spread via the cerebrospinal fluid (CSF), such as medulloblastoma, primitive neuro-ectodermal tumour (PNET), and germ cell tumours. CSI is also used to treat the neuraxis in patients with acute lymphoblastic leukaemia (ALL), who present with leukaemic cells in the CSF or who relapse with spread to the central nervous system (CNS). (Cranial irradiation alone is generally used for ALL.) A high precision technique with a beam direction shell is normally used. There is evidence to link recurrence to dose received, so the quality of radiotherapy delivery can influence survival (UKCCSG 1992).

Cytotoxic drug treatment such as intrathecal methotrexate may be given prior to, or concurrently with radiotherapy to control leukaemic deposits in the spinal region. Twice-weekly blood counts are necessary. Dexamethasone treatment may be necessary to prevent increased intracranial pressure during radiotherapy. The majority of patients undergoing craniospinal radiotherapy are children so it is appropriate to consider the special problems of children and radiotherapy at this point.

CHILDREN AND RADIOTHERAPY

Children are naturally nervous of unfamiliar procedures and may expect to be hurt by the radiotherapy process. Thus it is extremely important that the paediatric oncologist communicates well with the family, and that time is made available on the first visit to the department to help to put the child at ease. A pretreatment video may help (available from the Radiotherapy Department, Nottingham).

The use of 'play' activities can help the child to adjust to treatment procedures, and to be cooperative (Barrow 1992). Radiographers can help by allowing a child to raise or lower the couch with a favourite toy to view on the TV monitor. A few minutes spent in this way can cajole a child into participating in the 'game' by lying still on the couch as required. The use of a personal cassette recorder with a suitable tape can help the child to cooperate for the duration of each treatment. A blanket and restraining ties can be used to secure the child on the couch top if necessary for safety.

Babies and very young children, e.g. aged less than 3 years, may need a fast-acting narcotic to provide sleep conditions for shell preparation, planning and treatment sessions. This adds complications to the process but aids accuracy where the child cannot cooperate. A short acting narcotic such as Diprivan, a barbiturate or ketamine can be used and is given by injection just before treatment. After a few minutes the child is asleep but does not require assistance to breathe, and can be left alone in the treatment room for each exposure. The pulse and arterial oxygen saturation can be monitored using a pulse oximeter with a closed-circuit TV system. The child 'sleeps' only for few minutes, so top-up doses of drug are given via a butterfly needle if movement occurs before treatment is complete. Care should be taken to ensure that nutrition is adequate, since there is a likelihood that children who are drugged miss their meals (Dobbs et al 1991).

Most radiotherapy centres treating children are specialist paediatric oncology centres, since considerable expertise is required for the optimal treatment of what is still a small number of patients, even in a centralised facility. There is a 60–70% cure rate for children and often a good rapport is built up between staff and children, so that treatment can be rewarding for staff because of positive outcomes. Ideally there should be a paediatric ward where the arrangements for children can be coordinated. Pre- and post-anaesthetic activities can then be carried out in the ward, and there also the family can spend time waiting for transport or treatment. It is essential that good communication with the childcare team is maintained. Often radiogra-

phers reward children with sweets for being cooperative, so they need to know on which days the child is having other procedures after radiotherapy, such as lumbar punctures, which require starving.

Special policies should be adopted for children undergoing radiotherapy. A specialist team of paediatric radiographers should be available in a centre of excellence.

PRINCIPLES OF CRANIOSPINAL IRRADIATION

Treatment of the cranium plus spine requires a complex treatment technique to deliver 35 Gy in 4 weeks to the whole neuraxis. A pair of lateral opposed fields are applied to the cranium, down to the level of C2 for ALL, or to C5 for medulloblastoma which tends to local extension into the cord. A single vertical field, or two abutting fields, depending on the total length of spine to be treated and the maximum field length available, is/are applied to the spine (Fig. 19.1). The upper border of the spinal field is matched to the edges of the cranial fields in the neck.

For PNET a smaller boost field parallel pair is used, usually to the posterior fossa (Fig. 19.2) but possibly elsewhere depending on the tumour site, and applied after completion of the neuraxis treatment. However, it may be begun in midcourse if the blood count falls and necessitates suspension of the spinal fields for several days. The boost fields give an extra 20 Gy in 12 fractions to the tumour bed or highest risk site and are not critically matched to other fields. Several important factors contribute to the successful achievement of the prescription for CSI:

- geometrical arrangement of fields and beam divergence
- centring and symmetry of fields, shielding system and field shape
- junction planning
- junctions
- compensation for spinal cord depths
- patient position, shell fit, patient cooperation and immobilisation
- setting-up procedure
- portal and parameter verification.

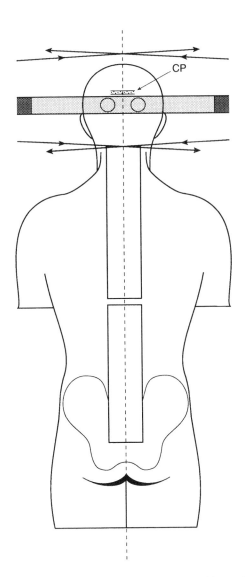

Figure 19.1 Lateral opposed cranial fields with matched spinal fields to treat the whole neuraxis. Note the nondivergent axis at eye level to avoid shielding the cribriform plate (CP).

A

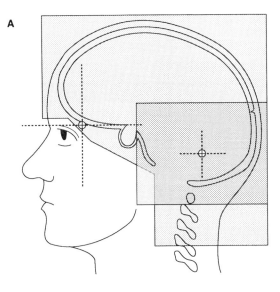

B

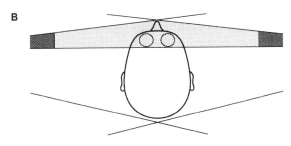

Figure 19.2 **A** Asymmetrical lateral cranial field centred at outer canthus, with inset posterior fossa boost area marked. **B** Nondivergent axis with eye shielding.

Simulation principles

Simulation is performed in two stages with the patient in a shell in the treatment position. Firstly the spinal length is determined by screening, so that the diaphragm angle of the head fields can be calculated, and the head fields are then screened, centred on the outer canthus, and marked. Lateral films with magnification markers and reference markers on the skin over the spine, are taken to cover the whole neuraxis.

Eye shielding, junction levels and the diaphragm angle for the head field are marked on the films. Junction planning and shielding and compensator construction are performed. At the second simulation session the eye shielding is checked and finalised, junctions and field centring points are marked and the fields verified.

Geometrical arrangement of fields and beam divergence

Matching field from two orthogonal directions principally requires certain diaphragm and gantry angle settings to be correct. The radiation beams will only relate to each other in the planned way within the patient if the patient is correctly aligned in the beam for each field, without moving or being moved between fields (apart from the required table movements).

The approximate length of the upper spinal field determines the divergent angle, for example for a symmetric field approximately 20 cm long, the angle of divergence of one edge is 6°. Thus to match lateral head fields to this at a neck junction, the diaphragm rotation angle for the head fields will also be 6° (Fig. 19.3).

At some centres the couch is angled for each head field, by the divergent angle of the head fields, to eliminate divergence in the lateral direction across the junction (Fig. 19.4). However, this is not a recommended practice for reasons described below. The effect of beam divergence will be further considered with junction planning.

Centring, symmetry of fields, shielding system and field shape

Beam divergence is also an important consideration in protecting the eye. The head fields should be centred just behind the eye so that there is minimal divergence in the region of the

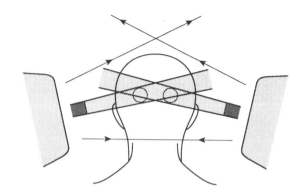

Figure 19.4 Effect of angling couch (for achieving straight light field edge across neck) on eye shielding.

eye and the cribriform plate which lies just above the eye, and the coincident straight beam axis for the fields passes evenly behind both eyes. As much of the eye as possible is shielded (Figs 19.1 and 19.2), while treating the whole of the cribriform plate, a high risk site for recurrence of disease (Carrie et al 1992). Recurrence here may be due in part to inadequate dose, owing to overshielding the eye, and is not easily treatable so the outlook for the patient is then poor. Thus

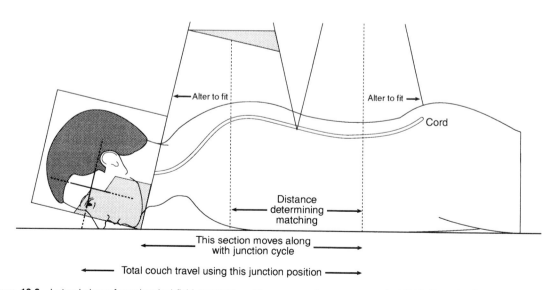

Figure 19.3 Lateral view of craniospinal field geometry, with compensator on upper spinal field. Note the field edges where alteration of size (asymmetric, keeping centre position) may be used on a daily basis if necessary for matching. Note also the edge geometry of two divergent edges matched at the anterior surface of the dorsolumbar spine.

adequate treatment of the cribriform plate is more important than fully protecting the eye. If a cataract arises later owing to eye dosage, it can be treated successfully by surgery. The advantages and disadvantages of various shielding methods have already been discussed in Chapter 8. In cranial irradiation it is essential for accuracy that beam-shaped shielding is used, and that its adequacy is checked by portal films or images.

Centring the fields near the eye requires the use of a very large overall field size, or the use of asymmetric fields (Fig. 19.2). The required facial shielding can be achieved by a single block incorporating the eye shielding, or by a multileaf collimator system. A multileaf collimator system is preferable as it reduces planning time, daily set-up time and the scatter dose to the eye since there is no lead or shielding tray close to the eye. Also, in conjunction with an MVI device multileaf collimators could be adjusted on the treatment machine to achieve the best fit.

The above principles apply equally when head fields are used alone.

Junction planning

Often, there is a surface gap between field edges at junctions. Whether there is a gap, and the size of the gap, depends on the depth of the spinal cord or the critical zone beneath the surface, and on the divergence of fields to be matched. The principle used with symmetric fields for a spinal–spinal junction is shown in Figure 19.3, where the edges of the two fields meet at the critical depth, which determines the gap on the surface. The use of asymmetry to change the divergent angle of one or both fields can improve the gap dosimetry and alters the surface gap. An example of junction dosimetry is given in Figure 19.5A, B.

The neck gap is complicated by the divergence of the head fields across the junction. However, the high value isodose lines for parallel opposed fields do not diverge (see Ch. 6), therefore the lateral pair effectively produce a 'beam edge' plane parallel with the collimator angle, which is matched with the spinal field edge as described above (Figs 19.1 and 19.3). Only the low value isodose lines follow the divergence of the field

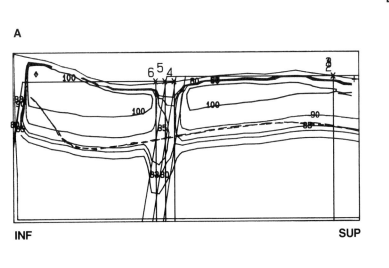

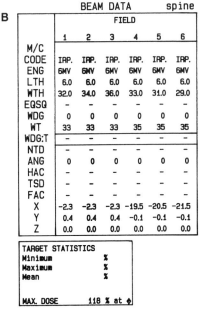

BEAM DATA						spine
	FIELD					
	1	2	3	4	5	6
M/C CODE	IRP.	IRP.	IRP.	IRP.	IRP.	IRP.
ENG	6MV	6MV	6MV	6MV	6MV	6MV
LTH	6.0	6.0	6.0	6.0	6.0	6.0
WTH	32.0	34.0	36.0	33.0	31.0	29.0
EQSQ	–	–	–	–	–	–
WDG	0	0	0	0	0	0
WT	33	33	33	35	35	35
WDG:T	–	–	–	–	–	–
NTD	–	–	–	–	–	–
ANG	0	0	0	0	0	0
HAC	–	–	–	–	–	–
TSD	–	–	–	–	–	–
FAC	–	–	–	–	–	–
X	-2.3	-2.3	-2.3	-19.5	-20.5	-21.5
Y	0.4	0.4	0.4	-0.1	-0.1	-0.1
Z	0.0	0.0	0.0	0.0	0.0	0.0

TARGET STATISTICS	
Minimum	%
Maximum	%
Mean	%

MAX. DOSE	118 % at ◆

Figure 19.5 **A** Overall isodose distribution at gap for three-phase junction cycle, using one nondivergent (sacral) edge and one divergent edge. The isodose value at cord level is 75%, planned to be low to allow for a small discrepancy in matching without risk of overdosing the cord. Modal dose prescribed at 79% isodose. **B** Beam data.

edges. Rotating the couch for the head fields has doubtful value and may lead to underdosage in the junction. It has the further disadvantage of angling the fields towards the eyes, so that eye protection is poor (Fig. 19.4).

Junctions

Matching adjacent fields is a critical process, especially where the spinal cord is included in the junction zone. Radiotherapy is not a precise procedure, for once the patient is introduced into the beam, any slight movement can disrupt junction dosimetry in the patient. If the dose at the junction is too high, late complications such as spinal cord damage and paralysis may occur. If part of the junction zone is underdosed, there is a risk of recurrence.

Moving junctions are often used, so that the uncertainty in dosimetry is spread across a longer tissue volume. For example, three different junction lines 1 cm apart are used on a daily or weekly cyclical basis (Fig. 19.6). This requires three sets of field sizes and setting-up information, so a fail-safe system of coding the sequence is required. Colour coding the junction points and the corresponding setting-up details works well.

Setting-up may be achieved by marking the gap on the shell or skin to check the light field match, but a complication arises when the junction is situated on a sloping area such as the neck or lower back. The gap required is a horizontal distance. A slope, which may vary from day to day, distorts the field edge on the surface so that measurement of a horizontal distance at the surface is variable. A method should therefore be used which allows the distance between the two field centres to be measured in order to reproduce the required horizontal gap (Fig. 19.3).

A single, long field may eliminate the need for a midspine junction. However, the spinal contour may result in a dose variation down the spine, and compensation may be required.

Dose prescription

The aim is to avoid a variation of more than 5%

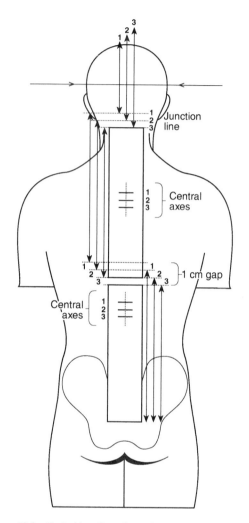

Figure 19.6 Coded junctions for a three-phase cycle. Note asymmetric sacral field. There is an equal distance between spinal field centres on each phase so that gap geometry remains constant.

from the modal dose and the following criteria are used in dose specification:

• The modal dose is generally prescribed to the anterior surface of the spinal cord (posterior surface of vertebral bodies).

• The cranial dose is prescribed at the midplane (central axis dose) of the opposed fields.

• The posterior fossa dose is prescribed at the midplane of the widest diameter of the posterior fossa, and wedging or compensators applied if necessary.

Compensation for spinal cord depths

Taken as a whole, the spinal cord varies in its depth below the surface. The position of the patient can even out the depth to some extent, but the cord will always be deeper at neck level than at sacral level. Depending also on the field/s positioning, patient contour along the spinal length and the consequent variation in f.s.d., a compensator or wedge may be required to achieve even dosimetry. For example, where the cord is deeper in the neck than it is at upper dorsal level (Fig. 19.3), the dorsal cord would receive a higher dose by virtue of being nearer the surface, and also because the f.s.d. is shorter. A compensator is required if the dose variation is greater than 5%. A similar situation may occur in the lumbosacral region.

Patient position, shell fit, patient cooperation and immobilisation

The prone position is used for craniospinal techniques, with the head supported at a particular angle by an appropriate face rest. The degree of curvature of the spine, and to some extent the cord depths, is determined by the exact position of the patient. The spinal curvature at the lumbar level may be reduced by introducing a thin wedge under pelvis. The neck curvature may be reduced by arranging for the forehead to be lower than the rest of the body. This evens out the f.s.d. over the neck and upper back, as well as facilitating easier junction planning and marking but spinal fields may irradiate the mouth.

The technique requires precision in set-up, and good immobilisation of the patient. A beam direction shell which fits the head well and gives precise reproducibility of patient position each day is essential, as is the cooperation of the patient in keeping still for 20 minutes or so while all fields are set up and treated. The shell should extend over most of the dorsal spine so it can carry the marks for the upper junction and centring points for the upper spinal fields. The shell should be checked, at each planning session or treatment, for straightness over the length of spine covered, since most shells will not necessarily ensure that the patient is straight but are used to carry treatment marks.

Acceptable reproducibility of the spinal fields, especially in the pelvic and lumbar region where the cord lies up to 8 cm deep in the body, may require the use of special positioning aids. Lateral tattoos at pelvic level have been shown to give a random error within 2 mm for the pelvis (Griffiths et al 1991). At present a quality assurance study is being set up by the UKCCSG/SIOP group for CSI. The study will assess accuracy using body casts or moulded patient supports. A study by Hulshof et al (1989) reported that body casts did not increase accuracy for the trunk owing to distortion of the casts.

Unless a whole body shell or alpha cradle (Soffen et al 1991) is used, lateral laser points should be marked on the patient so that excessive lateral rotation can be avoided.

If swelling of the face due to dexamethasone treatment compromises shell fit in midcourse, it is essential to make adjustments or a new shell so that the accuracy of marks on the shell in relation to the anatomy is maintained.

Setting-up procedure

The sequence in which fields are set up may vary, as may the technique and junction symmetry. The process for setting up a patient with two spinal fields will illustrate the type of choice made during set-up when field sizes do not exactly match markings on the shell. The reasons why lengths etc. may not fit exactly, include limits in the accuracy of equipment, with resulting slight differences from day to day and from machine to machine, and differences in the length of the spine with patient position and possibly with the time of day. With a well planned and carried out treatment sequence, administered at a broadly similar time each day, field lengths may vary slightly (e.g. 5 mm in 25 cm) on the first treatment from the planned length, but should be reasonably consistent on each treatment. Where there is an adjustment to make, it is most important to ensure that the geometry at the junctions is still correct.

Example of a set-up process. It is important to establish a routine which allows all fields to be treated consecutively, without disturbing the patient's position between fields. For an adult or tall child, this may involve measuring the total distance between the cranial and sacral field centres (Fig. 19.3) and establishing where the patient must be positioned on the couch to achieve the required longitudinal couch travel. The patient should be central on the couch to allow treatment of both lateral head fields.

The patient is positioned in the shell and straightened using the lasers, especially down the spinal length. The patient is checked for comfort and encouraged to keep still. The fit of the shell is checked, ensuring that anatomical landmarks, particularly near the eye, correspond to appropriate points on the shell. If dosimetry checks for the eyes are required, capsules or detectors are placed at specified points, such as just anterior to the outer canthus.

Head fields. The first head field is set up and checked for beam cover, using independent or asymmetric collimators to optimise cover. A minimum clearance of 5 mm is required to ensure that the skin surface is well within the beam (Fig. 19.2) and not in the penumbra (the dermal lymphatics are often considered to be at risk, and also hair regrows more evenly following even loss). If necessary, any adjustments required should be made to the field size, but keeping the junction match correct, rather than adjusting centring which would alter the position of the shielding. The position of eye and facial shielding is checked against anatomy and landmarks on the shell. After exposure, the opposing field is treated in the same way.

Spinal fields. The cervicodorsal spine field is centred on the appropriate centre point and matched to the corresponding junction at the neck, adjusting the length of the superior half of the field, if this is needed to achieve the match. The fit along the spine is checked, if necessary adjusting the patient gently from the hip region rather than the neck to preserve the upper junction geometry. The inferior field limit is marked, and any wedge or compensator inserted, then the field is irradiated. Finally the lumbosacral field is set up, moving the couch longitudinally for the measured horizontal distance between the two spinal field centres (Fig. 19.3), and checking the superior border against the lower limit of the upper spinal field, to ensure that there is no overlap and that the geometry is approximately as expected. The length of the sacral half of the field is adjusted, to ensure fit to the lower sacral border marked on the patient or shell. Any compensator or wedge is positioned and the field treated.

If patient-generated movement has occurred during treatment, the junction geometry and dosimetry is compromised. The advice of the oncologist should be sought for subsequent treatments.

Portal and parameter verification

Portal films of all fields are performed on the first treatment, particularly to check the cover in the cribriform plate area. Parameters used on each treatment should be recorded and a careful check kept that the required junction movement sequence is performed.

REFERENCES AND FURTHER READING

Barrow S 1992 Play therapy in the radiology department. Radiography 58: 12–16
Carrie C, Alapetite C, Mere P et al 1992 Quality control of radiotherapuetic treatment of medulloblastoma in a multicentric study: the contribution of radiotherapy technique to tumour relapse. Radiotherapy and Oncology 24: 77–81
Dobbs J, Barrett A, Ash D 1992 Practical radiotherapy planning, 2nd edn. Arnold, London, Chs 18, 33
Griffiths S E, Khoury G G, Eddy A 1991 Quality control of radiotherapy during pelvic irradiation. Radiotherapy and Oncology 20: 203–206

Hulshof M, Vanuytsel L, Van den Bogaert W, Van der Schueren E 1989 Localization errors in mantle field irradiation for Hodgkin's disease. International Journal of Radiation Oncology, Biology, Physics 17: 679–683
Lanzkowsky P 1989 Manual of paediatric haematology and oncology. Churchill Livingstone, Edinburgh
Plowman P N 1986 Tumours in children. In: Hope-Stone H F (ed) Radiotherapy in clinical practice. Butterworths, London
Soffen E M, Hanks G E, Hwang C C, Chu J C H 1991 Conformal static field therapy for low volume, low grade prostate cancer with rigid immobilisation. International

Journal of Radiation Oncology, Biology, Physics 20: 141–146

Thatcher M, Glicksman A 1989 Field matching considerations in craniospinal irradiation. International Journal of Radiation Oncology, Biology, Physics 17: 865–869

UKCCSG Radiotherapy Group 1992 Quality assurance for cranio-spinal axis irradiation in UKCCSG/SIOP PNET 111 (UKCCSG 9102), UK Children's Cancer Study Group, Leicester

20

Brachytherapy techniques and practice

BASIC PRINCIPLES FOR AFTERLOADING PRACTICE

The use of brachytherapy is developing to include many sites. Although the regimes and source arrangements vary according to the size and site of the tumour, similar principles apply to all applications where afterloading machines are used. The following procedures are common for most sites:

- applicator insertion
- positional assessment of applicator(s) radiographically (CT), or using MRI
- adjustment of applicator positions if required
- computation of dose distribution and determination of source configurations needed
- programming of afterloading machine, checking program
- treatment administered
- treatment details including applicator types recorded and filed with patient records.

Safety and operator training

The practice and equipment for afterloading techniques are totally different from those of external beam treatments. The potential exists for large dosimetry errors or a geographical miss even within one treatment fraction, if the source program used is in any way incorrect for fulfilment of the prescription. Safety and quality assurance in practice requires the use of well trained operators, usually radiographers or physicists, to carry out daily machine checks, exposure programming and dose delivery. These staff must also be trained in emergency procedures in case of a source staying in the exposed position.

Checks required

For each treatment or exposure given, there are a number of checks which must be carried out and checked by two operators before the sources are moved from the safe position. These are partly technique- and site-dependent and include:

- Every detail of the prescription (a third independent check is advisable).
- That the applicators programmed correspond with those actually in the patient, and where there are multiple channels with different programs, that each one is correctly placed.
- Any settings which are variable and which affect the program.
- That connections to the machine are correct and secure (although fail-safe interlocks prevent source movement if connections are defective).
- That the programmed source arrangement shown on the machine display or printout corresponds to the configuration required to fulfil the prescription.
- That the source configuration is programmed for the correct part of the catheter (many applications require the exposure to start at some distance from the end of the catheter, a potential geographical miss factor).
- That source dwell times are correct, checked by using a decay factor. (The factor changes each day for iridium sources, each month for cobalt sources.)

Intracavitary and intraluminal therapy

Intracavitary work has long been undertaken in gynaecological sites, using manually (i.e. forceps) handled radium or caesium sources, prior to afterloading systems being available. Intraluminal applications in palliative sites, particularly the oesophagus and bronchus are of increasing importance. A high radiation dose is delivered to a restricted volume to achieve maximum tumour growth restraint. The use of brachytherapy to boost the dose in the high risk

zone of the target volume, combined with external beam treatment to a larger volume, is developing for many radical treatments, for example in head and neck sites.

Gynaecological treatments

Cervix

Cancer of the cervix is the commonest condition treated using brachytherapy.

Source insertion. The insertion of sources or source carriers is usually carried out under general anaesthetic, since one long source is required within the uterus and its insertion requires dilatation of the cervical canal. Two further short sources are positioned in the fornices of the vaginal vault (Fig. 20.1A). The three sources are placed in an orientation which gives rise to a pear-shaped high dose volume containing the uterus and cervix (Fig. 20.1B, C). The number of applicators used may be dictated during the insertion depending on whether it proves possible to insert three applicators.

Planning films. Lateral and anteroposterior orthogonal radiographs (Fig. 20.1D), or CT scans are performed to establish reference points for dose computation. Alternatively, sagittal and axial MR images, showing applicators marked with gadolinium-DTPA may be used (Potter et al 1991).

Rectal dose and its assessment. In addition, the developing use of endovaginal and endorectal ultrasound probes (Mak et al 1989), with or without surface ultrasound application, allows accurate measurement of tissue thicknesses and thus more precise calculation of organ doses, e.g. rectal dose. Applicator systems incorporating strategically placed shielding may be used to protect the rectum. An innovative approach is the use of silk bags (Lei et al 1989) packed with pulverised tungsten, placed anteriorly and posteriorly of the implant to protect the rectum and bladder. The rectal dose is calculated by inserting a rectal tube containing barium, and measuring the distance between it and the applicators on the radiograph.

Alternatively the dose rate in the rectum may be measured from a calibrated source placed in one applicator. The positioning of the applicators may be adjusted if the rectal dose is too high. Applicators are held in place by vaginal packing, or by a rigid applicator fixation system.

Regimes and stage. Whether brachytherapy is used at all, alone, or in combination with external beam therapy, depends on the staging of the disease.

Early disease. For early stages, brachytherapy is used as the primary treatment (Joslin 1990), with external beam to boost the dose to pelvic nodes. High dose rate treatment may be 5 once-weekly insertions to a total dose of 37.5 Gy to point A (which is approximately 2 cm superior to the top of the vaginal fornices and 2 cm lateral to the central sagittal plane of the uterus), given concurrently with 4 fractions of external beam per week, to add 24 Gy at point A. Some central wedging or compensation must be used with the external fields to reduce the dose to the zone receiving the highest dose from the intracavitary treatment. The external treatment is planned multifield or uses parallel opposed fields (see Ch. 15).

Advanced disease. For advanced disease, brachytherapy is used as a boost to the higher risk site. External beam is given first, e.g. 50.4 Gy in 28 fractions, and brachytherapy follows, to add 15 Gy in 2 fractions.

Treatment routines for anaesthetised patients

Treating anaesthetised patients using high dose rate afterloading machines has disadvantages, apart from a lack of personal communication with the patient. The main drawback is that any time wasted means a higher anaesthetic dose, so there is some urgency about the procedure (and some impatience on the part of the anaesthetist when delays occur!). The time taken to achieve the insertion, imaging and dosimetry calculations is variable, which affects the working schedules of staff operating the afterloading unit and ultimately influences the patient throughput capacity. Often the machine cannot be programmed until the radiotherapist is ready to start the treatment and he/she plus the anaesthetist leave the treatment room and appear at the control panel and give a written prescription. The uncertainties for each insertion result in prescribing following completion of the insertion.

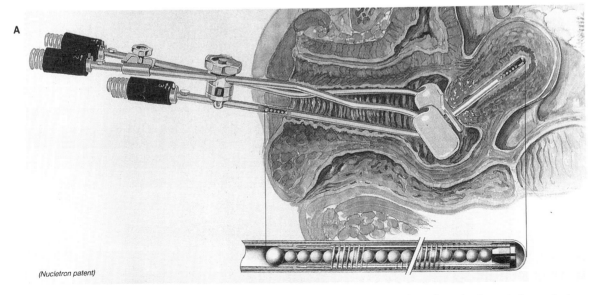

(Nucletron patent)

Figure 20.1   A Applicators for uterine cervix, lateral view, showing source train. **B** Isodose shape for three uterine applicators. **C** Cross-section through ovoids. **D** Anteroposterior view of applicators in situ. Some specific points are indicated, e.g. Manchester reference points A, B (Courtesy of Nucletron Trading Ltd.)

B

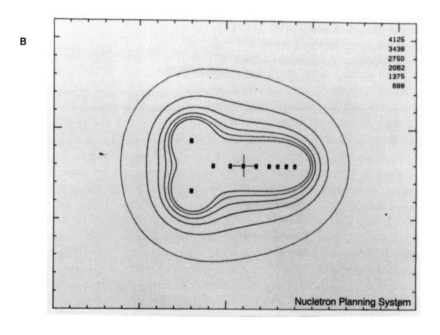

C

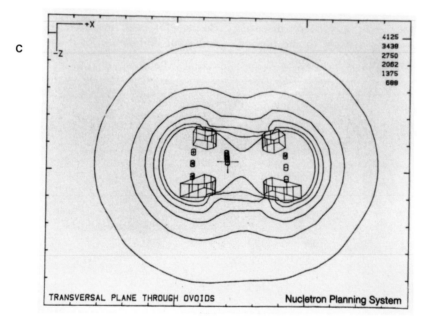

Figure 20.1 *(continued)*

D

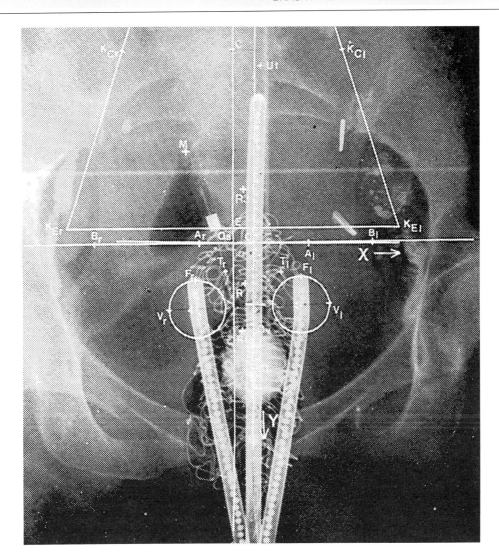

Figure 20.1 *(continued)*

Radiographer checks. Radiographers must check which applicators are in the patient, whether they are correctly connected, and note any setting used. Checking and communicating every detail prior to irradiating are extremely important as any incorrect factor can lead to a large dosimetry error, even within one fraction.

Programming. The unit is then programmed for the appropriate source configuration, times checked by using a decay factor, and the treatment administered.

Patient monitoring. The patient is viewed through closed-circuit TV as for other treatments, but additional viewing of anaesthetic systems and pulse monitors etc. is required. The desk therefore houses a number of patient-monitoring devices for the anaesthetist's use. Treatment is interrupted if the anaesthetist needs to check the patient's condition.

High, medium and low dose rate regimes. Treatment has been described above using a high dose rate machine, but the same dose distribution can be obtained by using a medium or low dose rate system, when treatment will take several hours or days. In these cases the patient has partially recovered from the anaesthetic before treatment begins, and so the urgency for completing procedures is lessened. Patients find the procedure more painful since the presence of the applicators, and their subsequent removal, must be endured while sedated but conscious.

Fractionation schedules differ. A complete course of external beam treatment may be given between two fractions of medium/low dose rate brachytherapy.

Manual insertions. Where afterloading systems are not available, similar treatments are given, now less and less frequently, using manually handled radium or caesium sources. Manual insertions tend not to involve radiographers except for imaging the source geometry.

Reproducibility. In insertions for the cervix there is some variation in source positioning, with regard to the relationship of sources to each other and to the anatomy. Treatment-to-treatment, and patient-to-patient variations can lead to altered doses to adjacent organs, and imprecision in dose distribution when combined with external beam wedged fields (see Ch. 23).

Fixation systems. Various devices have been developed to help to fix applicator positions. A special multiapplicator device designed to hold the sources at a fixed geometry, such as a ring applicator with built-in rectal retractor, may be used to improve the reproducibility of treatments (Abitbol et al 1990). The device is used without vaginal packing, which in itself reduces patient discomfort and prevents vaginal mucosal pressure necrosis. It also results in a lower dose to the small bowel, rectum and bladder owing to optimum positioning of the source carriers.

Uterus body

To treat cancer of the body of the uterus, brachytherapy may be used alone (following surgery) but is more often combined with external beam therapy.

Combined with external beam. As an example, 40 Gy in 20 fractions external beam may be followed by two to three intraluminal insertions to give a further 8 Gy to the vaginal lymphatics.

Brachytherapy alone. When brachytherapy is used alone, the uterus is packed with several small sources of equal activity, or specially designed afterloading source carriers such as

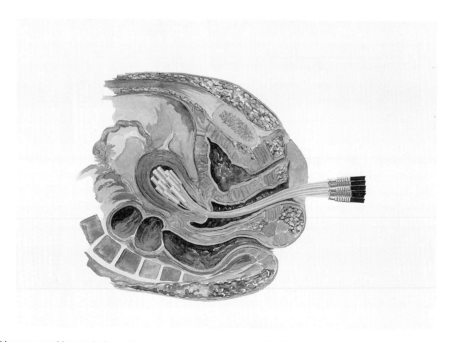

Figure 20.2 Heyman packing technique. Uterus body treatment using the Heyman packing method with Norman Simon applicators for connection to the microSelectron. (Courtesy of Nucletron Trading Ltd.)

Heyman, Norman Simon or similar applicators (Fig. 20.2). A CT-assisted dose planning package is used.

The applicators have flexible catheter connections for attachment to the Selectron or micro-Selectron and remain in place for a few days to allow fractionated high dose rate treatment to be given. A hyperfractionated regime may be used, giving an AIR Kerma of 27.5 mGy.m^2 (approximates to 4000 mg.hrs) in three fractions over approximately 24 hours, with a minimum treatment interval of 6 hours. Low dose rate treatment may be given as a single fraction using the same technique.

Early tumours: vaginal vault treatment only. Alternatively, for early tumours, following healing from radical surgery, a single vaginal source is used to treat the upper vagina, for example, five or six daily fractions to give 27–30 Gy in total.

These treatments are usually given on an outpatient basis, since no anaesthetic is required. The source is inserted via a cylindrical perspex applicator with a central lumen which carries an afterloading catheter. Various diameters, e.g. 2 cm, 2.5 cm, 3 cm, up to 4.5cm may be used. Doses are specified at 5 mm or 10 mm from the applicator surface. Treatment is best given using the widest applicator that the patient can tolerate so that the steepest dose fall-off occurs within the applicator and a more even dose gradient is obtained throughout the adjacent tissue envelope.

The length of the source (typically 3.5 cm), is chosen to treat only the upper two-thirds of the vaginal lymphatics, so as to avoid lower vaginal stenosis. It is important that the applicator is inserted to the same point on each treatment in order to achieve this sparing; a centimetre scale is etched onto the tube. The patient should be in a similar position to that used for any external beam treatment, so that the combined dosimetry can be estimated. The patient is subsequently asked to use a dilator regularly to keep the vagina open.

Bronchus

An advanced tumour in the bronchus may be treated in a sedated patient by passing a fine applicator through the tumour-bearing area, via a fibreoptic bronchoscope. The position of the applicator in the patient is radiographically checked in theatre and the source loading for the applicator determined. Sometimes more than one applicator is used (Fig. 20.3), when dose computation becomes more critical because of the larger volume.

The variable factors are the position of the active source positions relative to the distal end of the applicator, and the length to be irradiated, e.g. 6–10 cm. Single doses of 7.5 Gy to 15 Gy may be used. A dose of 15 Gy at 1 cm is common and may be given in about 10 minutes with the microSelectron. Sometimes treatment is given in two or three once-weekly fractions. Good symptomatic relief is obtained within days (Rowland et al 1989).

Oesophagus

The oesophagus may be treated with a single linear source, in a similar manner to treatment of the bronchus. The fine applicator is passed via a nasogastric tube. Brachytherapy is usually used in conjunction with external beam therapy for palliation at any oesophageal level, for radical treatment of the upper third or as preoperative treatment for lower oesophageal tumours. The dose used is similar to that for the bronchus, but is reduced if followed by five fractions of external beam. A second brachytherapy insertion may follow external beam if required.

For many of these new developments, the radiographer's role extends to the care of endoscopes and surgical equipment. The range of special applicators used are expensive and very easily damaged. For example, a 1 metre long 2 mm diameter plastic tube, used for endobronchial or oesophageal work, is easily kinked and thereafter needs replacing.

Skin moulds

Skin moulds may be constructed to fit closely to a surface bearing a tumour. The mould carries applicators (or holding points for these) for attachment to an afterloading machine, for

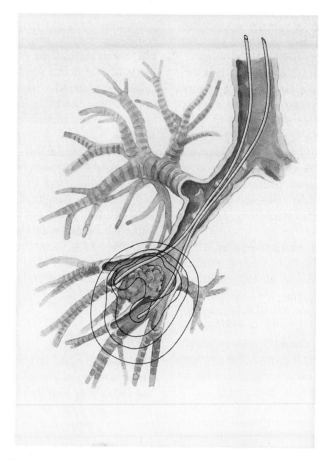

Figure 20.3 Two-applicator implant for bronchus. (Courtesy of Nucletron Trading Ltd.)

example the Selectron-LDR/MDR using caesium. Fractionated treatment at a high dose rate may then be applied on an outpatient basis, as described by Kitchen et al (1991) for the pinna. A single plane source arrangement using three applicator channels was used for eight fractions, each lasting about 90 minutes, to give a prescribed dose of 45 Gy at 7.5 mm from the source plane.

The use of moulds is a time-consuming process, both for mould preparation, planning and treatment, but produces less disfigurement than surgical excision. It is likely to be more cost-effective than an interstitial implant to produce a similar outcome. (Another treatment option is electron beam therapy, if a dual mode accelerator is available.)

Neutron brachytherapy

A future possibility is the development of afterloading machines for neutron-emitting sources such as californium-252 (neutrons plus gamma rays, modal energy 1.5 MeV, half-life 2.64 years), to utilise the radiobiological advantages of neutrons for radioresistant tumours. Intracavitary neutron treatment has been applied in various centres (in the USA, the former Soviet Union and Japan) and is thought to be advantageous for large bulky tumours, particularly in gynaecological sites, but also in the head and neck, if applied prior to external beam.

The use of californium in clinical trials has indicated that there may be faster tumour shrinkage than with conventional brachytherapy, with a lower incidence of normal tissue complications (Kal & Batterman 1989). The more widespread use of neutron brachytherapy is dependent on the development and provision of suitable equipment and of special treatment rooms to address the radiation protection problems.

INTERSTITIAL BRACHYTHERAPY

Exposing the centre of a tumour to radioactive sources by implanting applicators carrying them has many practical and theoretical advantages over fractionated external beam therapy. It may be considered to be a type of conformal therapy (see Ch. 23).

Features of interstitial brachytherapy

• High dose localised to the target volume with rapid fall-off, allowing the tumour volume to tolerate a higher dose.
• Continuous low dose rate, allowing recovery of normal tissue during treatment.

• Short overall treatment time, convenient to the patient.
• Radiation accurately applied to tumour: geographical miss factor removed, although inhomogeneity of dose distribution owing to higher doses nearer to sources may lead to failure if underdosage occurs in the target volume.

Treatment sites

This type of therapy may be used as the primary radical treatment in small, well localised tumours. Alternatively it may be used as a boost to the tumour site, occasionally before but usually following regression gained using external beam radiation, for example in the neck (Fig. 20.4). It may also be used as salvage therapy in recurrence sites. Intraoperative or perioperative therapy involves positioning the sources visually during surgery at sites of risk of recurrence. The techniques will increasingly be adapted for use with low dose rate and pulsed afterloading equipment to increase operator safety.

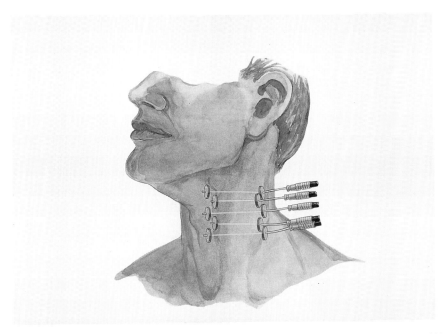

Figure 20.4   Head and neck implant, with flexible implant tubes connecting to the microSelectron. (Courtesy of Nucletron Trading Ltd.)

The tumours practically amenable to an interstitial approach are those which are small with accurately defined edges, without bone involvement and which are easily surgically accessible (Ash 1986). Typical sites treated include:

- tongue, floor of mouth, lip, cheek
- anal canal and rectum
- penis, prostate
- skin
- breast, vagina
- urethra, bladder
- brain

Dose planning

Similar general principles to those for intracavitary therapy apply. However, more source carriers tend to be used for most interstitial work, so that the implantation and checking procedures are more complex, as is the computation of dosimetry.

Source geometry and fixation devices

The arrangement of sources must be suitable for the application of established dosimetry systems. To assist the radiotherapist to achieve this, a number of devices have been developed which carry rigid source carriers with known geometry (Fig. 20.5). These devices, the simplest being a hairpin-type structure having two parallel needle source carriers, are implanted into tissue, leaving access to the sources from one end. The sources are fed into the carriers either manually (iridium wire), or from afterloading machine connections to the carriers. Example of use are given below.

Breast

Boost

A breast boost or top-up dose to the lumpectomy site may be given using a double plane implant to give 15–20 Gy, as salvage therapy for local recurrence, or as a boost to tumour residue after external beam treatment of inoperable disease.

Whole breast/chest wall

Interstitial brachytherapy may also be used alone following local excision (Rowland et al 1989). A

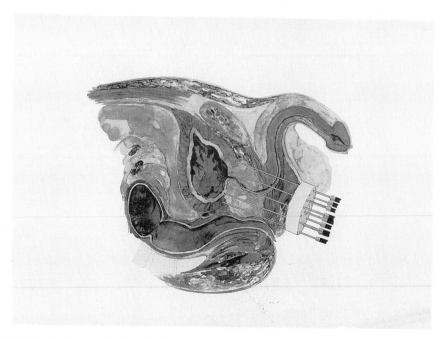

Figure 20.5 Prostate implant connecting the microSelectron to a template with rigid needles. (Courtesy of Nucletron Trading Ltd.)

larger implant may be used for total breast treatment, using either low or high dose rate. The implant may be carried out under local anaesthetic, and the breast squeezed into a two-plate template applicator through which the implant needles are passed to give an arrangement similar to that in Figures 20.6 and 20.7. Protective rubber caps are pushed onto the cutting ends of the needles.

The devices may be worn overnight between fractionated treatments, with protective end caps on both ends of the needles. Oedema following the implant cannot distort the geometry because of the containing effect of the template. The

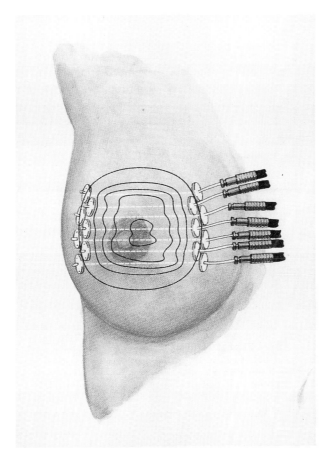

Figure 20.6 Breast implant showing isodose pattern. (Courtesy of Nucletron Trading Ltd.)

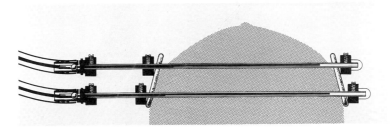

Figure 20.7 Breast implant fixation system. (Courtesy of Nucletron Trading Ltd.)

central plane cross-sectional dosimetry pattern is shown in Figure 20.8. Doses used for primary treatment of small (less than 3 cm) tumours include 28 Gy in four, or 20 Gy in two, high dose rate fractions. For a boost following external beam, 14 Gy in two fractions may be used (Rowland et al 1989). These high dose rate treatments are still developmental.

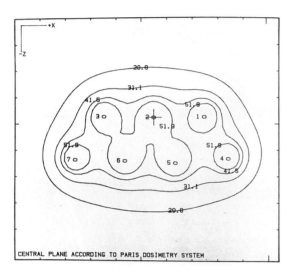

Figure 20.8 Cross-sectional isodose distribution of breast implant as in Figures 20.6 and 20.7. The seven wires are at the points of equilateral triangles. (Courtesy of Nucletron Trading Ltd.)

Childhood tumours

High dose rate afterloading interstitial implants may be used for some solid paediatric tumours, to achieve high local dose whilst sparing normal tissue to an extent not achievable with external beam treatment (Nag et al 1990). Lower dose rate treatment is not practical due to the need for sedation, immobilisation and parental or nursing care of the infant or child during the implant.

Brain

Fractionated high dose rate stereotactic treatments (see Ch. 23) may be applied to sites in the brain via interstitial catheters. Trials of this technique in combination with interstitial hyperthermia are in progress (Garcia et al 1992).

REFERENCES AND FURTHER READING

Abitbol A A, Houdek P, Schwade J G, Lewin A A, Serago C, Brandon A 1990 Ring applicator with rectal retractor: applicability to high dose rate brachytherapy of cervical cancer. Selectron Brachytherapy Journal 4(3): 68–69

Ash D V 1986 Interstitial therapy. In: Hope-Stone H F (ed) Radiotherapy in clinical practice. Butterworths, London

Garcia D M, Marchosky J A, Nussbaum G, Drzymala R 1992 Interstitial HDR brachytherapy and long duration interstitial hyperthermia in the treatment of newly diagnosed malignant gliomas. Selectron Brachytherapy Journal 6(2): 70–74

Hishkawa Y, Kirisu K, Taniguchi M, Kamikonya N, Miura T 1991 High dose-rate intraluminal brachytherapy for oesophageal cancer: 10 years experience in Hyogo. College of Medicine Radiotherapy and Oncology 21: 107–114

Joslin C A J 1990 Quality assurance in brachytherapy: clinical aspects. Selectron Brachytherapy Journal 5(2): 63–68

Kal H B, Battermann J J 1989 Brachytherapy with californium-252 neutrons. Brachytherapy 2. Nucletron, Leersum

Kitchen G, Dalton A E, Pope B P, Smith P D, Powner M 1991 Surface applicator for basal cell carcinoma of the right pinna: a case report. Selectron Brachytherapy Journal 5(3): 140

Lei Yan-Fan, Chen Di-Xia, Jun-Yuan, Wang Yi-Tao 1989 Brachytherapy of cervical carcinoma with the Selectron HDR. Brachytherapy 2, Nucletron, Leersum

Mak A C A, Kuipers Tj, van't Riet A 1989 Endovesical and endorectal ultrasound imaging applied for dosimetry of gynaecological intracavitary brachytherapy. Brachytherapy 2, Nucletron, Leersum

Martinez A A, Orton C G, Mould R F (eds) 1989 Remote afterloading: State-of-art, Brachytherapy HDR and LDR. Nucletron, Leersum

Mate T P, Gottesman J, Hatton J 1992 Remote afterloading conformal brachytherapy of the prostate: an update. Selectron Brachytherapy Journal 6(2): 51–54

Minsky B D, Cohen A M, Fass D, Enker W E, Sigurdson E, Harrison L 1991 Intraoperative brachytherapy alone for incomplete resected recurrent rectal cancer. Radiotherapy and Oncology 21: 115–120

Mould R F (ed) 1989 Brachytherapy 2. Nucletron, Leersum

Nag S, Ruymann F, Su Cheng Ming, Pieters R S, Gahbauer R A 1990 The use of high dose rate brachytherapy in paediatric tumours. Selectron Brachytherapy Journal 4(2): 22–23

Pierquin B, Wilson J-F, Chassagne D 1987 Modern brachytherapy. Masson, New York

Potter R, Kovacs G, Lenzen B, Prott F J, Knocke T H, Haverkamp U 1991 Technique of MRI assisted brachytherapy treatment planning. Selectron Brachytherapy Journal 5(3): 145–148

Rowland C, Ingham D, Cook S, Robins M 1989 Breast conservation: High dose rate breast implants. Selectron Brachytherapy Journal 2: 1–3

Sidorchenkov V O 1991 Intracavitary brachytherapy for rectal cancer. Selectron Brachytherapy Journal 5(3): 137–139

21

Treatment of tumours using particle radiations

A range of modalities employing particle radiations is used in the treatment of malignancies. The indications for use are limited to where a technical or clinical advantage over photon beams is gained (see Ch. 5). The most commonly used modality is electron beam therapy, since this facility is available in most radiotherapy departments.

There follows an overview of the use of each modality.

ELECTRON BEAM TREATMENTS

Treatments using electron beams are usually single-field techniques, the principles of which are discussed in Chapter 15. These may form part of a more complex treatment, such as for a head and neck tumour where electron fields are used in combination with and are matched to photon fields (see Ch. 17). Electron fields may also be used to give a boost dose to the breast (see Ch. 16); however, depending on the machine used and thus the skin dose, late damage to the skin in the form of brown pigmentation of the treated area may make this unacceptable for cosmetic reasons.

The overriding reason for using electron beams clinically is the sharp cut-off of dose at a depth corresponding to the beam energy (see Ch. 5). Shallow tissue volumes can be treated without high dose to the underlying structures, i.e. there is a depth sparing effect.

Matching the cut-off depth with the clinical site

Where an electron field is being planned, there may be a need to establish the exact tumour depth in order to choose an appropriate beam energy to treat the tumour or protect underlying structures. For example, if treating over lung, the thickness of the chest wall over the area may be determined by ultrasound or CT (see Ch. 11), in order to choose an energy which will not give high dosage to underlying lung.

Where electron fields are used to treat tissue overlying the spinal cord (Fig. 17.8B), particularly for a boost treatment where the cord has been treated to its tolerance dose, the tissue contour and spinal cord depth must be accurately known to avoid treating the cord.

f.s.d., applicators and setting-up implications

The standard f.s.d. for electron beams is 95 cm, so that set-ups are not isocentric and are therefore more tedious to perform. The applicator and end-frame obscure the view of the treatment marks once the required set-up is almost achieved. Also the bulk of the applicator end limits access to set-ups for irregularly shaped areas of the body such as the lower neck. Lateral fields to the root of the neck are impossible to set up using 95 cm f.s.d. Because of these limitations, many departments use f.s.d.s of 100 cm or more. However, this affects the beam flatness by altering the shape of the isodose curves, which become more pointed at the central axis with increasing f.s.d., thus compromising the useful features of the beam.

Shaping the treatment field

Cutomised end-frames either cut or shaped from low melting point alloy can be made for each field (see Ch. 5). The cut-out slots into the electron applicator, so that it is secured in the beam. Set-up of an irregularly shaped field is then as simple as for a rectangular field.

Verification of the field

Field placement can be verified by portal film as for a photon beam (Fig. 21.1).

Figure 21.1   A verification film of an electron field, showing the applicator and treated area against the background anatomy.

Use of bolus

When bolus is used to raise the skin dose, the bolus thickness must be carefully chosen and accurately applied as it influences the volume of tissue treated by altering the cut-off depth. Where bolus is used to provide a particular effect on the dose distribution, i.e. to change the depth of maximum absorption for a particular energy, an air gap between bolus and applicator may not be acceptable, and special bolus to fit the contour of the patient may be required.

A setting-up difficulty occurs if the type of bolus material used is opaque, so that once in place it obscures the treatment marks. Most types of flexible bolus are opaque. The difficulty this presents is exacerbated with oblique fields, where two couch movements are involved in bringing the patient close to the applicator. To avoid inaccuracy, the light edges may be set to the marks without bolus, with the treating distance as it would be if the bolus was present, before inserting the bolus. The couch settings for the correct set-up should be noted for reuse after the bolus is in place.

The difficulty is removed if clear bolus is used, such as a flat sheet of perspex. At high energy it is acceptable to use a flat sheet, since the scatter produced by the bolus will reach the skin.

NEUTRON BEAM THERAPY

This section is an overview of the worldwide therapeutic uses of fast neutrons and their clinical trails. At present neutron beams are used only in clinical trials. They have certain theoretical radiobiological advantages (see Chs 1 and 5), but their use is restricted because of unacceptable normal tissue reactions. Further work on fractionation or their application in combined modality treatments (i.e. with photons) may lead to increased use, but this will still probably be limited to certain centres because of the cost of providing a neutron facility.

During the years 1971–1991 trials have been carried out in 10 centres in the USA using neutron beams of energy 8–66 MeV. Enhanced and sometimes irreversible normal tissue reac-

tions have limited the success gained in terms of the quality of life after local tumour control.

A clear therapeutic advantage of fast neutron treatment was seen in salivary gland tumours which were not completely resectable, and also in prostate tumours and sarcomas. For advanced tumours of other sites there appeared to be no advantage (Griffin et al 1984). Treatment of the pelvis and abdomen gave rise to bowel problems, some requiring colostomy. Surgical repair is less viable following neutron treatment. The resulting mortality caused the termination of the Clatterbridge (UK) trial for pelvic tumours (Errington et al 1991). In the prostate group, there was increased bowel morbidity but this was less for those treated at a facility employing a multileaf collimator to shield uninvolved tissue.

Typical neutron doses: head and neck, lung, prostate – 20.4 Gy TD in 12 fractions over 4 weeks.

Edinburgh clinical trials

Trials included treatment of late stage head and neck tumours, and bladder and rectal tumours.

Head and neck tumours

Better tumour control, for longer periods of time, was achieved than when photon or electron beams were used. However, serious side-effects included necrosis, including that of the temporal lobe of the brain. Neutron treatment which includes brain tissue carries serious neurological risks. Loss of the ipsilateral eye was unavoidable for sinus or salivary gland treatments.

Surgical salvage was difficult and resulted in ulcers which took a long time to heal, if they healed at all.

Bladder tumours

Treatments of advanced bladder cancer produced more morbidity than with photons. The severity of the morbidity was greater, bowel stenosis and atrophy resulted in many patients requiring colostomy, and proved a fatal complication for some patients. Mortality after neutron treatment was greater than that of patients treated with photons.

Rectal tumours

Few patients were suitable for this trial. However, those treated had severe side-effects and survival figures did not match those for photon treatments.

In conclusion, the trials in the UK have shown neutrons to be of little value in the treatment of tumours. Side-effects seem much more severe and treatment of the pelvis has led to mortalities. The side-effects and related mortality increase with time after treatment, so that the surviving fraction of patients gradually lessens.

PROTON BEAM THERAPY

Whilst neutrons seem to have no therapeutic advantage, protons have much to offer. The well defined high dose zone and low integral dose of this modality appear promising for the treatment of many tumours.

The treatment of ocular melanoma

The Clatterbridge (Finch & Bonnett 1992) proton beam energy, 62 MeV, has a maximum penetration of only 33 mm in water, which makes it ideal for the treatment of ocular melanomas more than 8 mm thick. If less than 8 mm thick these tumours would otherwise be treated with iodine plaques or seeds. (For thicker tumours, or those close to the optic nerve, conventional treatment leads to loss of sight so enucleation is then the treatment of choice.)

A clinical proton trial was conducted including:

* tumours more than 8 mm thick
* tumours less than 3 mm from the optic disc.

Treatment planning

Because of the accuracy of eye position required, this process is very complicated.

* Ultrasound scans are used for biometry measurement.
* Titanium clips are put into the eye to mark the extent of the tumour.
* The tumour dimensions and position are documented.

* The patient is immobilised in the treatment chair with mask and bite block.
* Localisation X-rays are taken at 400 cm f.s.d. to minimise beam divergence effects.
* The coordinates of the eye position are calculated so that the patient can look in exactly the correct direction during treatment.
* A three-dimensional computer plan is generated.
* The patient is realigned with the proton beam, using X-rays to verify the set-up.
* Treatment is given, monitoring the eye position throughout.

For 157 patients treated in this way, the results were much better than expected, with only one death. Useful eyesight was retained in 98% of cases even with a tumour of up to 8 mm diameter.

The treatment of chordomas

The Harvard (USA) proton beam has an energy of 160 MeV and can treat to a greater depth than the Clatterbridge (UK) beam. The main advantage of this is that much higher tumour doses can be delivered whilst sparing the local normal tissue. A typical dose is 68 Gy. The tumours treated in one trial were primarily at the base of the brain but some cervical tumours were included. The results for chordomas were very encouraging, whilst the few chondrosarcomas included in the trial showed less marked responses.

Current trials include:

* meningiomas (recurrent tumours)
* glioblastomas – moving towards higher doses, e.g. 90 Gy hyperfractionated treatments (twice per day)
* prostate
* paravertebral soft tissue sarcoma.

Clear definition of the tumour volume is obtained from thin slice high resolution CT. Planning the treatment requires a three-dimensional dose display and beam-eye views to select beam direction. Multiple noncoplanar beams (see Ch. 23) utilising table pitch and roll are used.

Automated compensators and beam shaping is employed to optimise dose delivery. Effective patient immobilisation, alignment and verification of the treatment position are used.

The Loma Linda Proton facility

The proton facility at Loma Linda, California, incorporates five treatment rooms. These include isocentric proton beams for treatment of pelvic and thoracic tumours, a horizontal beam for head and neck treatments, and a horizontal beam of lower energy for treatment of ocular melanomas.

This facility is the largest of its kind in the world, and is the result of many specialist groups joining together to devise equipment capable of supplying this type of proton beam. Clinical trials are just beginning and are to include all parts of the body. This potentially offers proton treatments at only three times the cost of conventional radiotherapy (normally much more than three-fold!).

CLINICAL USE OF UNSEALED SOURCES OF PARTICLE RADIATIONS

Various substances containing radioisotopes may be injected into the bloodstream or instilled into body cavities in sufficiently high doses to achieve a therapeutic effect for malignant or benign disease.

Suitable radioisotopes are often bound to appropriate biological compounds as radiopharmaceuticals which are metabolised to particular organs or tissue types, so that the isotope will concentrate in and selectively irradiate particular tissues. For example iodine-131 may be used in the form of an iodide ion (usually sodium iodide) to target thyroid tissue both in the thyroid gland and in secondary thyroid tumour deposits occurring elsewhere in the body. Patients require special nursing and transport arrangements, and appropriate instructions.

Low doses of radiopharmaceuticals having gamma emissions of energy 50–300 keV (iodine-131) are used for imaging physiological systems (see Ch. 11). Although it is not generally thought of as a diagnostic isotope, iodine-131 may be used to image the thyroid and thyroid secondaries prior to iodine-131 therapy.

Radioisotope therapy

Features of isotopes in use

The isotopes used have short radioactive half-lives, of the order of hours or days, so that the radiation dose is given over a discrete time interval. The radiation type is beta particle (accompanied by gamma rays) and the energy of the particle emissions and thus their range in tissue must be suitable for the size of tumours which are to be targeted. For a given isotope the cure probability is greatest for tumours whose diameter is close to an optimum value dependent on the path length of the beta particle used. Therefore a chosen isotope may not be effective in treating micrometastases, a problem analogous to a geographical miss in conventional radiotherapy (Wheldon et al 1991).

Therapeutic effect

The therapeutic effect is achieved by gauging a balance between the radiosensitivity of the tumour, the concentration and duration of radionuclide in the tumour, and the relative dose to the tumour compared to that received by the background tissue. The uptake level of radioisotope in the tumour determines the tumour dose received from a given injection. The range of penetration of the available radiation is from 0.5 mm for Copper-67 to at least 1 cm for Phosphorus-32.

Specific uses of radioisotopes

Iodine-131

A single dose of radiopharmaceutical, such as 3000 MBq giving 35–50 Gy will achieve complete remission of thyroid tumours. A similar dose may also be used for neck nodes. A higher dose, 100 Gy, may be effective in treating bone metastases. A description of the indications and issues in the radioiodine treatment of thyroid tumours is detailed elsewhere (Plowman 1986).

Thyrotoxicosis is a benign condition, commonly treated by 200–400 MBq of radioiodine. Here the volume of active thyroid tissue is reduced by the radiation dose, and artificial thyroid hormones are subsequently used to simulate normal thyroid function (Plowman 1986). Ablation of a severely toxic thyroid gland may be achieved by using a dose of up to 4000 MBq. MIBG, a pharmaceutical labelled with ^{131}I, is used to treat advanced neuroblastoma in children prior to surgery. A good and selective concentration of the agent in the tumour, and tumour sensitivity, lead to a high response rate, many inoperable tumours being rendered operable (Hoefnagel et al 1991).

Phosphorus-32

Polycythaemia rubra vera is a neoplastic condition of cell clones producing red blood cells, commonly treated by phosphorus-32 to produce symptom relief and prolong life. This treatment is described by Mair (1986).

Strontium-89

Targeted radiotherapy using strontium-89 may be used for relief of metastatic bone pain. An 80% response of partial pain relief is obtained, and 20–25% of these patients become pain-free (Lewington 1991).

REFERENCES AND FURTHER READING

Duncan W, Arnott S J, Jack W J 1986 The Edinburgh experience of treating sarcomas of soft tissues and bone with neutron irradiation. Clinical Radiology 37: 317–320

Errington R D, Ashby D, Gore S M, Abrams K R, Myint S, Bonnett D E, Blake S W, Saxton T E 1991 High energy neutron treatment for pelvic cancers: study stopped because of increased mortality. British Medical Journal 302: 1045–1051

Finch J, Bonnett E 1992 An investigation of the dose equivalent to radiographers from a high-energy neutron therapy facility. British Journal of Radiology 65: 327–333

Griffin T W, Davis R, Hendrickson F R, Maor M H, Laramore G E 1984 Fast neutron radiotherapy for unresectable squamous cancers of the head and neck: the results of a randomised RTOG study. International Journal of Radiation Oncology, Biology, Physics 10: 2217–2221

Hoefnagel C A, de Kraker J, Voute P A, Valdés Olmos R A 1991 ^{131}I MIBG therapy in the treatment of neuroblastoma. British Journal of Radiology 64: 46

Lewington V J 1991 Prostatic carcinoma: Strontium-89 therapy for metastatic bone pain. British Journal of Radiology 64: 46

Mair G 1986 Haematological malignancy in the adult. In: Hope-Stone H F (ed) Radiotherapy in clinical practice. Butterworths, London

Pickering D G, Stewart J S, Rampling R, Errington R D, Stamp G, Chia Y 1987 Fast neutron therapy for soft tissue sarcoma. International Journal of Radiation Oncology, Biology, Physics 13: 1489–1495

Plowman P N 1986 Tumours of the endocrine system In: Hope-Stone H F (ed) Radiotherapy in clinical practice. Butterworths, London

Sharp P F, Gemmell H G, Smith F 1989 Practical nuclear medicine. Oxford University Press, London

Wheldon T E, O'Donoghue J A, Barrett A, Michalowski A S 1991 The curability of tumours of differing size by targetted radiotherapy using ^{131}I or ^{90}Y. Radiotherapy and Oncology 21: 91–99.

22

Total body and half body irradiation

BACKGROUND

In this chapter we consider treatments to large areas of the body and to the body as a whole. There are certain conditions which may present as localised disease but which are essentially systemic from the outset, for example diseases of the haemopoeitic tissue such as acute lymphatic leukaemia (ALL), acute myeloid leukaemia (AML) and some related lymphomas. For these, treatment of the whole body is required, which may be achieved by chemotherapy, radiotherapy or often a combination of both.

There are three main types of whole or half body treatment:

1. High dose total body photon treatment. Radical whole body photon irradiation is described below for patients who are to receive bone marrow transplants.

2. Low dose palliation, whole or half body. Lower dose whole body irradiation may be given palliatively for widespread or systemic disease. Alternatively a high dose may be given to the half of the body giving rise to most symptoms, followed by treatment to the other half of the body a month or so later, if required.

3. Whole body electron treatment. Radical whole surface treatment by electrons is also described in this chapter, although it is not widely performed because of infrequent indications for this regime.

TOTAL BODY PHOTON IRRADIATION FOR BONE MARROW TRANSPLANT PATIENTS

High dose total body irradiation (TBI) is indicated for patients requiring total ablation of bone marrow stem cells and/or eradication of all tumour cells in the body including those in sanctuary sites such as the central nervous system, bone marrow and the testes.

TBI is used in conjunction with high dose chemotherapy to achieve tumour eradication and immunosuppression prior to bone marrow transplantation (BMT).

Indications for and expected outcome of treatment

This photon technique gives a tumoricidal whole body dose over 1–4 days, usually to treat one of the leukaemias. The patient may be in first remission but in a bad risk disease category, or in second remission after relapse following chemotherapy and local (CNS) treatment. For either category of patient, there is no suitable alternative treatment. The regime is life-threatening, but gives a 60% chance of 5-year survival for suitable patients.

A requirement of the radiation component is the reduction of the functioning of the immune system to a level where foreign tissue is not rejected, so that BMT can be performed. A drug regime using cyclosporin-A assists with immune suppression.

Bone marrow transplant

Following TBI, a transplant of healthy bone marrow cells taken either from a donor (allograft) or from the patient when in remission (autograft) is performed. Subsequent intensive care of the patient is required until the transplanted cells have established a normal blood count. An allograft is the treatment of choice for chronic granulocytic and acute myeloid leukaemias in first remission (Thomas et al 1982), but only 25% of patients have a matched related donor. Occasionally a matched unrelated donor is found via marrow banks. Patients with acute lymphoblastic leukaemia in remission, usually second remission (Clift et al 1982), may be treated using allografts. Autografts are still under investigation but the early results for poor prognostic first remission ALL patients are encouraging. A UK study for the use of autografts in AML is under way.

Techniques and equipment

There are several prerequisites for performing TBI, concerning the equipment available at a centre. There is considerable variation in the techniques used, partly dependent on machine availability.

Opposed anteroposterior fields

A simple technique is the use of two large, opposed anterior and posterior fields. For this technique, a field area large enough to cover the whole of the patient, when lying or standing, is desirable, usually from a horizontal beam.

To achieve this an f.s.d. of approximately 4.5 metres is required, for a machine with a maximum size of 40 cm × 40 cm at 100 cm f.s.d. Turning the collimators through 45° so that the patient's length is diagonally across the beam area gives more cover (Fig. 22.1). Where an ideal size/f.s.d. is not available, techniques must be modified, and are inevitably complicated, in order to give a uniform dose to a patient in a more convoluted position, e.g. with the knees bent.

Asymmetric fields

An asymmetric field setting may be used for a horizontal patient on a mobile couch, where a central field would result in the patient being at the lower edge of a very large field (Fig. 22.2). Offsetting the field ensures that the patient is central in the radiation field, so that more even scatter conditions exist. Also, the total area of the radiation beam can be reduced to minimise additional scatter.

Lateral opposed fields

For a smaller beam area, two lateral opposed fields can be used to treat a sitting (Fig. 22.2) or

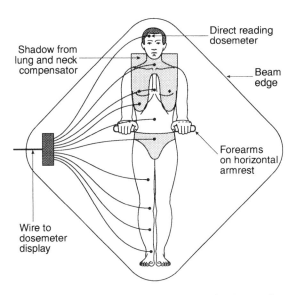

Figure 22.1 Patient supported on a saddle for the anterior TBI field using a 45° collimator angle. Direct reading electronic dosemeters are attached to the patient, so readings can be observed from the control station during exposure.

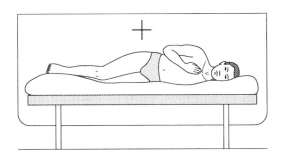

Figure 22.2 Semiprone patient positioned on an individually moulded mattress, with arm as lung compensator. The patient is central in the asymmetric beam.

semirecumbent patient, if a high beam energy such as 8 MV is used.

Beam energy considerations

The energy of the beam available is another technique-limiting factor. Cobalt beams, or megavoltage beams, up to and including 6 MV, will not give a sufficiently homogeneous dose in a large patient or a patient in a convoluted position.

Extra or boost fields may be required to top up the dose to certain areas.

If 8 MV is used, a reasonably even dose distribution may be achieved in a larger patient, even where treatment is given from lateral fields rather than anteroposterior fields. However, a patient lying supine or prone with the knees drawn up under a vertical beam, would require other top-up fields to give an adequate dose to areas which would otherwise be underdosed.

Importance of dose rate and fractionation

The dose rate used affects the tolerance of lung to radiation, especially when treatment is given as a single fraction.

Low dose rate

A very low dose rate, less than 0.05 Gy per minute, allows some recovery of lung parenchyma during treatment, so a higher dose overall can be tolerated. Low dose rate TBI may be given as a single fraction. The feasibility of low dose rate depends on the technique, since the patient has to keep fairly still for the treatment duration. Treatment then becomes more of an ordeal for the patient. Use of a low dose rate also requires the use of one machine and staff, for a whole day, for one treatment.

Higher dose rate

Above the 0.05 Gy/min threshold, a much higher dose rate is acceptable, especially where treatment is fractionated. When using high dose rate, the dose given may be lower depending on the technique and fractionation used (see Ch. 1). For a single fraction a higher dose would be tolerated at low dose rate than at high dose rate using an identical technique. A different technique using increased lung compensation or shielding would allow an increased dose to be given at high dose rate, but lung shielding also shields diseased areas.

Cobalt dose rates. The dose rate of a cobalt machine cannot be altered at will except by changing the s.s.d. used, and this restricts the available regimes.

Dose response

The order of dose used in TBI is lower than that given to cure a solid tumour, but only isolated, very radiosensitive tumour cells require destruction, so that a relatively low dose is effective. However, the dose–response curve for radiation applied to leukaemia is linear (Fig. 22.3), so the highest dose possible is applied to achieve a higher cell kill.

Technique and fractionation differences

There are many variations on techniques and dose regimes, which are largely dependent on the available resources of the participating treatment centres. However, all are designed to conform to the basic principles outlined, although in different ways, and are equally effective in outcome. A few examples are given to illustrate this:

- A midabdomen dose of 10 Gy may be given in three daily fractions at normal dose rate from an anteroposterior parallel opposed pair at 8 MV. A 7% reduction in dose over the lung fields is required to keep lung dose down in an average adult.
- A mediastinal dose of 12.0 Gy may be given in six twice-daily fractions in 3 days.
- A dose of 10.50 Gy may be given in one fraction at 0.025 Gy/min, over 6–8 hours.

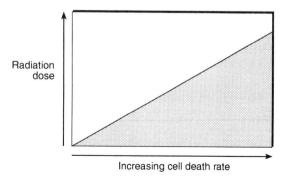

Figure 22.3 Linear dose-response curve for leukaemia.

- Increasingly, a lung dose of 14.40 Gy in eight fractions over 4 days is used, with a minimum 6-hour gap between fractions.

Machine commissioning and calculation of TBI dosimetry

Before a machine can be used for TBI, special extended commissioning tests must be performed to generate dosimetry data for the appropriate treatment conditions. Considerable time is required to gather basic output data from the machine.

Effect of walls and floor. A treating distance of 4 metres may be used, with the patient placed next to a primary beam shielding wall. Extrapolation of standard data for the machine to the extended f.s.d. is inaccurate since there may be significant scatter from the primary barrier and the floor.

Effect of patient size relative to beam size. Normal beam data are gathered by using a small beam within a large scattering medium. Here, the patient is a relatively small scattering medium within a large beam area, an entirely different situation. Therefore the beam output factor used in calculating monitor units for a given patient will incorporate a scatter component, and a representation of the cross-sectional area of the patient presented to the beam.

The treatment process as a whole

The programme which must be carried out before a patient undergoes TBI will now be described briefly, in order to demonstrate the importance of treatment conforming to the planned schedule.

Preliminaries and prerequisites

Firstly the patient is assessed against criteria designed to ensure a good chance of survival and cure. These include disease status (remission required), age and general physical and psychological fitness compatible with undergoing a rigid and unpleasant treatment programme which will result in death if it fails. A further necessity is the availability of suitable tissue for transplantation.

Where an allograft is used, there is a one-in-four chance of a sibling having compatible tissue, and outside the immediate family the chances of such tissue being available are infinitesimal. Where an autograft is to be used the patient must have had marrow harvested and cryopreserved.

Volume and processing of transplant. There must be enough marrow stem cells available in any graft tissue so that, after inevitable damage and reduction in quantity during processing, there are enough cells left to make a viable transplant. Where the donor is for example a small baby, the process may have to be delayed until the baby reaches a certain size.

For some allograft patients, the transplant tissue may be treated using monoclonal antibodies (Campath) to produce T-cell depletion, thus reducing the chance of the graft tissue setting up an allergic reaction to the patient (graft versus host disease or GVHD). This treatment process, usually used only for patients with matched unrelated donors, incidentally reduces the number of cells in the graft.

Tissue harvesting. Allograft tissue is not harvested until the day before it is to be transplanted. Autograft tissue is taken while the patient is in remission, and may undergo specialised treatment to eradicate any tumour cells present. A more detailed account of these factors is available (Griffiths 1985).

Pre- and postirradiation programme. Having fulfilled these criteria, the patient has to be allotted a space in a treatment programme, according to when resources are available. Requirements include those for radiotherapy planning and treatment, and also a special sterile room where post-TBI care will be given for a period of 6 weeks or more.

Once a treatment date is available, the patient undergoes preparation, during which a catheter (a Hickman line) is inserted through the chest wall into the right atrium. The patient will receive drugs, the graft, and have blood taken or transfused via this line. This reduces injury to the skin and thus also the chance of infections entering. However, there is a high risk of infection entering the Hickman line unless strict aseptic techniques are adhered to when the line is open.

Achieving an even dose

An effective dose is required for all the critical tissue such as bone marrow, without overdosing the lungs. A higher dose may be prescribed at midabdomen than at the midmediastinum. Where the body thickness as presented to the beam is very variable, for example the legs, missing tissue compensators may be constructed and strategically placed to even out the dose received. A sheet of bolus material is positioned near to the patient (within about 30 cm) to ensure a full skin dose.

Importance of lung dose

The lung dose is the limiting factor, since radiation pneumonitis results with an inappropriately high dose, and can cause death immediately post-TBI. The dose is higher where beams have traversed lung, because of the lower density and decreased attenuation of radiation within lung tissue.

Lung compensation methods. Partial shielding or compensators are frequently used to reduce lung dose and balance the effect of increased transmission through lung. The arms may be positioned so that they give partial compensation to the lungs, by increasing the tissue thickness presented to the beam in the lung axis, either for an anteroposterior or a lateral parallel pair (Fig. 22.4A, B). Alternatively lead lung compensators may be used. Shaped blocks 0.5 cm thick may be adhered to a standard shadow tray base for each field of an anteroposterior pair, and their alignment with the patient checked using exterior bony landmarks such as the suprasternal notch.

Treatment planning and test doses

The patient may or may not have lung compensators constructed, depending on the technique and preference of the radiotherapist. (It is doubtful whether lung compensation makes any difference to outcome.) If compensators are to be used, the patient has a CT scan of the chest about 3 weeks prior to TBI. The scan is used to assess the thickness and shape of lung in the treatment plane. An example of the compensator thickness

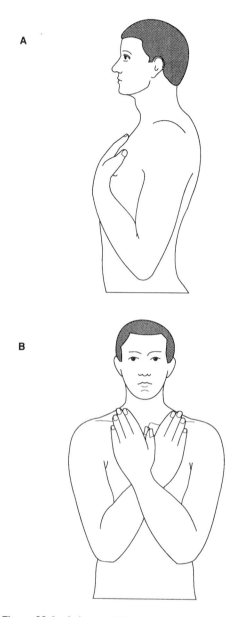

Figure 22.4 **A** Arm positioned as lung compensator for lateral field. **B** Arm as lung compensator for anterior field.

is approximately 3 mm of lead. Various measurements of the thickness and dimensions of the patient, positioned as for treatment, may be made to assist with dosimetry calculations.

Explanations about the planning and treatment are given to the patient who may also be shown the treatment unit. A week later, test doses on the treatment machine are performed to assist with the calculation of a suitable output factor for each field, and to establish whether compensation for irregular body shape or inhomogeneity is required. For the test doses, 20–25 thermoluminescent and solid state dosemeters are strategically placed on the patient, all orientated as for treatment.

Total lymphoid irradiation (TLI). TLI may be required to give a top-up dose of 6 Gy to lymphoid tissue, to increase immunosuppression in allograft patients where Campath has been used. These patients undergo planning for total nodal fields, i.e. matched mantle and an inverted-Y pair, extended to include the spleen. Planning and treatment for this is described in Chapter 19. Planning takes place at a suitable date for the patient to receive two or three consecutive daily TLI fractions of 2 Gy, completed 1 week before TBI.

The treatment schedule

The patient begins high dose cyclophosphamide at the start of the TBI week. The patient and the centre are then committed to completing the schedule. There should be a backup machine available and commissioned for TBI use in case of major breakdown.

TBI is started the day after chemotherapy stops, when the patient may still feel nauseated from both the chemotherapy and from apprehension. Vomiting during irradiation occurs occasionally, but antiemetic drugs and prior fluid infusion help most patients to avoid this. In addition to the support given by the TBI planning and treatment team, support is given by a team of BMT nurses who accompany the patient for radiotherapy. Following the last fraction, the patient is transferred to the sterile care unit and the graft administered via the Hickman line.

Radiation treatment

No sterile procedures are necessary for transfer of the patient from the ward, or in the treatment room itself, but all items used are 'socially' cleaned prior to use.

Placing of dose monitors. For one or all of the fractions, it is usually necessary to measure the doses received at strategic points on the skin. Direct reading dosemeters linked to a digital display are used, often in addition to thermoluminescent powder sachets used to give extra information after treatment. All of these must first be labelled and attached to the patient's skin or gown in such a way that there will be no confusion about which reading is for which part of the body.

Patient positioning. The patient is positioned for the first field. Patient comfort is monitored and any slight adjustments needed are made. During planning a position will have been chosen which allows the patient some freedom but where the trunk can be kept reasonably still, for the duration of the exposure.

The patient may be standing, when the use of support such as a saddle to perch on, armrests (Fig. 22.1) and a cushion behind the head are required for patient comfort and for reproducibility. When supported on a saddle, the height of the chest stays reasonably constant in relation to lung compensators attached to the accessory tray.

Irradiation, patient and dose monitoring. Irradiation is begun, and necessarily split into several exposures because of the high number of monitor units given. (Modified latch use is justifiable in this situation.) For the first exposure, readings from the dose monitor display are checked and calculated against the expected dose. Modifications to the compensators, of either their position or thickness may be made if required.

Further exposures are given and the patient carefully monitored, particularly for chest movement in relation to compensators, and for signs of distress. On completion of one field, the patient is rested briefly, reassured and repositioned for the second or subsequent fields, with the dosemeters still in place.

Dose readings are checked until acceptability is established, and irradiation is completed. Dosimetry results from the first fraction are analysed and various doses received, especially in lung, are calculated. A dose projection for the course is made and compensators modified, if necessary, for achieving the desired total dose distribution.

Post-TBI complications and processes

The major complications are now outlined since the processes designed for their prevention affect the TBI regime. More detailed accounts of post-TBI effects are available (Griffiths 1985; Mair 1986).

Three major complications are common in the immediate post-TBI phase, and the incidence of any one appears to increase susceptibility to the other two. They are:

- interstitial pneumonitis which is related in 50% of cases to the lung dose
- infection established while the blood count is low
- graft versus host disease (GVHD).

Two other major causes of failure are graft failure due to insufficient stem cells colonising in the patient's marrow, and recurrence of disease. Among the late complications are the increased incidence, over the normal population, of second tumours and various effects resulting from organ damage and hormonal changes. Cataracts and gonadal failure are very common. The risk of cataract formation is reduced by fractionation.

LOW DOSE PHOTON PALLIATION
Whole body

For conditions or patients unsuited to TBI/BMT, a gentler whole body regime giving approximately 1.5 Gy in 2 or 3 weeks is available. This regime is used for widespread non-Hodgkin's lymphoma (NHL) and is well tolerated on an outpatient basis. The median survival is 4 years for low grade NHL.

Technique

A megavoltage unit, preferably 8 MV with long lateral f.s.d., should be used to give a minimum field area of 120 cm × 120 cm to accommodate the patient sitting in the foetal position (Fig. 22.5). If a larger field is available a more comfortable position is possible. Bolus may be packed around the legs to achieve a more uniform thickness, the loss of the skin-sparing effect being irrelevant at this dose level.

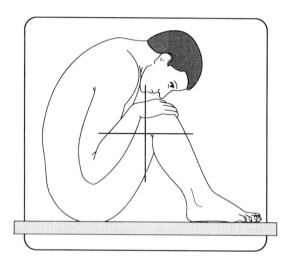

Figure 22.5 Patient in foetal position for lateral low dose field. Bolus is packed around the legs on an even shape.

One left or right lateral field is administered per fraction, alternate sides being treated on alternate fractions. Three or five fractions per week may be given. The blood count should be monitored prior to each fraction and treatment suspended if necessary.

Hemibody irradiation

An alternative to low dose TBI, especially for very poorly patients, is single fraction half body treatment. If necessary treatment to the other half of the body is given after a recovery interval of 1 month. This is a very useful treatment for multiple, widespread, painful sites and bone metastases. Again, the lung tolerance is the dose-limiting factor so a midline dose of 7.5 Gy may be given to the lower body, but only 5–6 Gy to the upper body to avoid radiation pneumonitis. A response rate of around 80% is seen using these doses. The treatment cannot be safety repeated.

The patient is treated with antiemetics and fluid infusion for 3–4 hours prior to treatment, and sedated where required. This treatment is continued during and after radiotherapy and patients are usually reasonably comfortable during treatment, which may take up to half-an-hour.

Trials have been conducted (Le Vay et al 1990) to investigate the response and toxicity using a

single dose of 4 Gy and 4–8 Gy (Hoskin et al 1992) to produce symptom relief with less toxicity, on an outpatient basis. Retreatment would be possible. Early results show that 83% of patients have good or excellent pain relief at 1 week.

Field size and technique

Parallel fields covering a wide area are used, and these may or may not be so extensive as to cover the limbs or head. The size of the field required and the equipment available will determine whether the treatment is given laterally or vertically.

Vertical fields. Linacs with maximum 40 cm × 40 cm diaphragm settings will give a 60 cm × 60 cm field at 150 cm f.s.d. assuming that:

• The couch goes low enough and high enough
• The rangefinder extends far enough or some other measuring method is devised.

However, the width for the under-couch field will be limited by the couch window size, which is usually a maximum of 45 cm in width.

It is desirable to use the smallest f.s.d. consistent with the field size needed, to minimise the treatment time. Many patients can be treated on the standard linac couch with vertical fields, where the size to be treated is consistent with the couch window size.

Horizontal fields. The isocentre height must be taken into account when choosing a supplementary couch for lateral extended f.s.d. fields. Even on a linac with a low isocentre, a minimum height of couch is required for a particular f.s.d. Limitation in couch height may result in the patient being treated by the lower half of the beam only.

A special output factor and central axis depth dose figures should be used unless asymmetric jaw settings are utilised to ensure that the patient is central within the field. Bolusing to achieve uniform patient thickness is used if required.

Field junction/borders

The field edge is often set at the level of the umbilicus for both upper body and lower body fields, but may be set to a particular vertebral level. The most divergent point of the field light edge is set at the junction level to avoid treating the same level twice, although this results in some undertreated areas around the junction. Occasionally, the whole trunk may be treated rather than upper or lower halves.

TOTAL BODY ELECTRON TREATMENT

Certain malignant cutaneous conditions such as mycosis fungoides and Kaposi's sarcoma, which involve or potentially involve the whole skin, require treatment of the whole skin. It is possible to treat the whole skin by specialised techniques using suitable electron sources, usually medical linear accelerators. (Before electrically produced beta ray beams were widely available, special high output strontium-90 units were used.) A dose of 36 Gy in 6 weeks, at three fractions per week, is typical. Other regimes such as 24 Gy in 12 fractions over 18 days have been successfully used.

Beam energy and dosimetry

The beam energy used is commonly 2–6 MeV, because of the unique depth–dose characteristics exhibited, i.e. a high surface dose with a rapid build-up to a maximum dose, then a fast dose fall-off. This effect allows the surface to be treated to a high dose, whilst sparing critical structures such as the central nervous system, haemopoeitic systems and the gastrointestinal tract. These systems are only spared if contamination of the beam by Bremsstrahlung (X-rays produced by electron interactions with matter in the beam) is low.

At a depth of 2 cm the dose is 10% or less. A lesion up to 1 cm thick can be treated with a 3 MeV beam. Clinically uninvolved areas are shielded by 2 mm lead sheet. There are various techniques in use.

Techniques

Whole body field

The patient sometimes has to stand at a consid-

erable distance (e.g. up to 7 metres) from the source so that the field size is large enough to cover the whole length of the patient. The patient must present different aspects of the body surface to the beam so that the entire surface is exposed. It is not possible to obtain a homogeneous dose over the entire skin surface, and areas where the dose is low may be later sites of recurrence.

Sanctuary sites and top-up fields. Recognised sanctuary sites are the scalp, shoulders, infra-mammary folds, soles of the feet, genitalia and perineum, which the wide fields cannot reach, and any residual patches of disease may have separate fields to top up the dose. These fields can be treated using superficial X-rays.

Dose rate and field size. A large treating distance results in a low dose rate and unless this can be enhanced, for example by alteration of the beam-scattering foil arrangements, treatment times are protracted. In addition to increasing the output to shorten treatment times, it is necessary to de-grade the energy of the beam to scatter it over a larger area. This is achieved by introducing a scattering medium into the beam, which unfor-tunately increases the amount of Bremsstrahlung X-ray contamination.

Patient rotated in beam

The most usual technique is to rotate the patient in the beam so that all aspects are equally irradiated, giving a relatively uniform dose distri-bution. The patient support may be rotated in order to achieve this (Fig. 22.6). Use of the rotational technique increases the dose to internal structures from Bremsstrahlung, but otherwise gives an optimal dose distribution.

A platform rotating at 5 rpm is used at the appropriate distance to produce the required beam size. For example, a distance of 2.85 metres on a modified linac described by Kim et al (1984), is used where a dose rate at the patient of 0.25 Gy/min results in a treatment time of 10 minutes per fraction to give a 2.50 Gy skin total dose. The patient stands on the platform and is supported by holding an overhead handgrip with alternate arms, which also helps to ensure the axillae are irradiated.

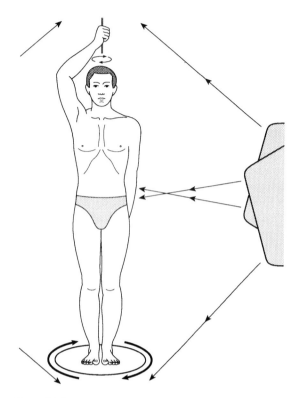

Figure 22.6   Patient rotating in electron beam, positioned on turntable and holding overhead support. The field may cover the whole patient, as on the left of the diagram, or two matched fields, using the gantry angled slightly to either side of the horizontal position, may produce the required cover.

Dose and fractionation. Two fractions per week are given for a total skin dose of 30–35 Gy. Small electron fields may be used to boost underdosed areas and bulky disease, at 3.0 Gy per fraction for 4–8 fractions, concurrently with or after large field radiotherapy. The patient may be rested for 2–3 weeks if acute reactions such as oedematous swelling of the lower extremities occur during the course.

Shielding. The eyes may be protected by lead spectacles, in patients with no periorbital involvement. Intraconjunctival lead shields may be used in patients with periorbital involvement. The hair and nails in irradiated areas may be shed, and in some techniques the whole head and the nails are shielded to avoid this. Nails may be shielded by the use of lead thimbles.

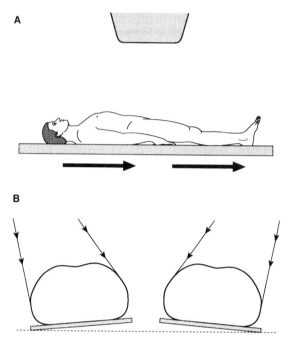

Figure 22.7   **A** Patient on couch moving through overhead stationary beam. **B** Patient on couch tilted to one side then the other for exposure to oblique beams. The tilt reduces the obliquity of incidence of the beams at the patient's extremities.

Half body matched fields

If the field area is insufficiently large to treat the total body, the gantry may be angled to either side of the horizontal in order to treat the upper and lower halves of the body separately (Fig. 22.6). The upper and lower fields are matched in a way which gives no serious under- or overdosage at the junction. Over such a small depth, the geometry of matching beams is simplified, and the 'exit' dose is irrelevant as it is low.

Four-field technique

A technique for a patient lying on a suitably modified standard treatment couch has been developed (Williams et al 1979) using a standard linac. In this technique the table top moves longitudinally through the electron beam thus exposing the whole length of the patient to each of four beams. The patient is treated supine and then prone (Fig. 22.7A, B).

Field arrangement and set-up. Two anterior and two posterior fields are used. The patient is centred 2.5 cm on either side of the midline for each field. No applicator is used and an even distribution over a 50 cm wide patient can be achieved from two fields applied obliquely from either side. For any field the patient is tilted laterally towards the beam by 5° in order to present each body surface more normally to the beam and even out oblique incidence to the sides of the body. This tilted positioning helps to obtain a more even dose distribution to the curved lateral aspects of the body, since the dose at a given depth is reduced when the beam is applied tangentially.

All techniques are complicated and time-consuming, and should only be performed in specialist, suitably equipped centres to ensure quality. The limited description we have given may be supplemented by reading the material listed below.

REFERENCES AND FURTHER READING

Clift R A, Buckner C D, Thomas E D et al 1982 Allogenic marrow transplantation for acute lymphoblastic leukaemia in remission using fractionated total body irradiation. Leukaemia Research 6: 509

Dobbs J, Barrett A, Ash D 1992 Practical radiotherapy planning, 2nd edn. Arnold, London, Chs 34, 35

Freeman C R, Suissa S, Shenouda G et al 1992 Clinical experience with a simple field rotational total skin electron irradiation technique for cutaneous T-cell lymphoma. Radiotherapy and Oncology 24: 155–162

Griffiths S E 1985 Lymphatic, haemopoietic and locomotor systems. Therapeutic radiography. Postrad Unit Seven, Lancaster, p 11–18.

Hoskin P J, Price P, Easton D et al 1992 A prospective randomised trial of 4 Gy or 8 Gy single doses in the treatment of metastatic bone pain. Radiotherapy and Oncology 23: 65–136

Kim T H, Pla C, Podgorsak E B Pla M 1984 Clinical aspects of a rotational total skin electron irradiation. British Journal of Radiology 57: 501–506

Lanzkowsky P 1989 Manual of paediatric haematology and oncology. Churchill Livingstone, Edinburgh

Le Vay J, Keen C, McKinna F 1990 Low dose 'hemi-body' radiotherapy for metastatic bone pain. Work in progress. Radiology and Oncology, British Institute of Radiology Congress 1990

Mair G 1986 Haematological malignancy in the adult. In: Hope-Stone H F (ed) Radiotherapy in clinical practice. Butterworths, London

Thomas E D, Clift R A, Hersman J et al 1982 Marrow transplantation for acute nonlymphoblastic leukaemia in first remission using fractionated or single dose irradiation. International Journal of Radiation Oncology Biology, Physics 8: 817

Trump J G, Wright K A, Evans W W et al 1953 High energy electrons for the treatment of extensive superficial malignant disease. American Journal of Roentgenology 69: 623–629

Williams P C, Hunter R D, Jackson J M 1979 Whole body electron therapy in mycosis fungoides – A successful technique achieved by modification of an established linear accelerator. British Journal of Radiology 52: 302–307

23

Sophisticated techniques

CONFORMAL THERAPY

Concepts and rationale

The 'ideal' treatment would give a lethal dose to the tumour without giving any dose to the rest of the patient. This cannot be completely achieved with photon beams, but is possible with proton treatments (see Chs 5 and 21). Conformal planning and treatment techniques have been developed to reduce the treated volume and thus achieve something closer to this ideal than when using conventional techniques.

In conformal therapy the treatment volume is shaped in three dimensions so that it conforms to the shape of the tumour. The effect of this is to reduce the total volume of tissue treated, so that adjacent tissue damage is reduced and a higher dose can be given to the tumour, increasing the chance of cure with fewer long-term complications. Any site where the tissue requiring treatment is of an irregular shape is suitable for this type of approach. Conformal therapy may be achieved using brachytherapy (see Ch. 20).

Volume treated relative to tumour size

In conventional radiotherapy, a volume of tissue with uniform cross-section, such as a cylinder, containing the irregularly shaped tumour (Fig. 23.1) is treated by three or four regularly shaped crossfiring fields. A larger volume of tissue than is optimal is treated by virtue of the shape of the high dose zone and the related morbidity is greater because adjacent normal tissue is inevitably included. Examples of the relative volumes of target tissue to treated tissue are shown in Figure 23.2A for a spherical tumour within a cubic

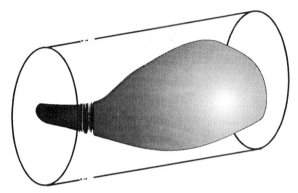

Figure 23.1 The irregularly shaped tumour contained in a treatment volume or isodose envelope of regular cross-section, as in conventional techniques.

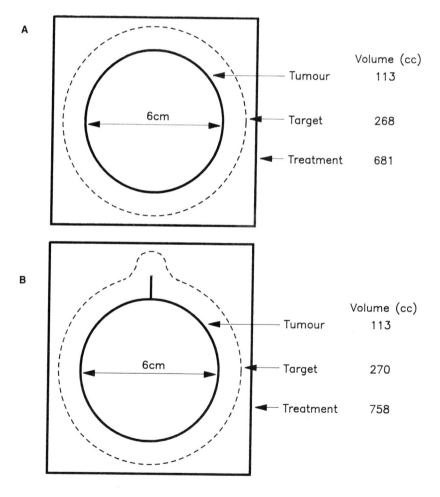

	Volume (cc)
Tumour	113
Target	268
Treatment	681

	Volume (cc)
Tumour	113
Target	270
Treatment	758

Figure 23.2 The relationship between tumour volume and treated volume in cc for **A** a regularly shaped tumour, **B** an irregularly shaped tumour. (Courtesy of P Williams, Christie Hospital, Manchester.)

treatment volume, and in Figure 23.2B for an irregular tumour.

Conformal planning and treatment allows reductions in the treated volume (Fig. 23.3) of the order of 20–30% compared with the same tumour using a conventional plan (Fig. 23.1). With high precision treatment delivery, smaller safety margins can be used and a further volume reduction is possible. In addition, if new technological facilities allow the required tumour dose to be delivered from fewer or smaller portals, then the volume of normal tissue in the entry or exit path of the beams will be reduced, so that the integral dose to the patient will be lower. A volume reduction of 50% would allow a significant increase (approximately 8%) in the dose prescribed without an increase in morbidity. However, there is an alternative view that the clinical tumour volume cannot be defined precisely enough to warrant this resource-consuming approach; three different clinicians will mark three different volumes for the same tumour.

Planning and shaping the treated volume

This requires an imaging facility to localise an accurate target volume shaped in three dimensions and a treatment planning facility which can optimise and display dose distribution in three dimensions. For conformal therapy the normal (conventional) coplanar or noncoplanar beam arrangements may be used, but each field is shaped to fit the tumour (Figs 23.4 and 23.5).

Alternatively a high number of small adjacent fields (Fig. 23.6) or a scanning beam may be used to achieve irregular beam/high dose volume shapes.

To plan and perform dynamic conformal therapy, where fields are shaped by more complex methods, requires more sophisticated modes or facilities on both the linac and planning system.

The 'beam's-eye view' approach

Serial CT or MRI slices (obtained with the patient in the treatment position) may be summated by three-dimensional reconstruction software to allow planning using a 'beam's-eye view' approach (i.e. viewed along the beam axes or potential beam axes).

This approach requires a clinician skilled in delineating target volumes in anatomy viewed

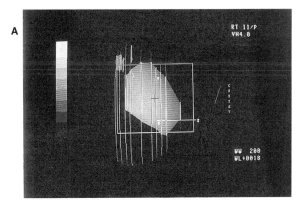

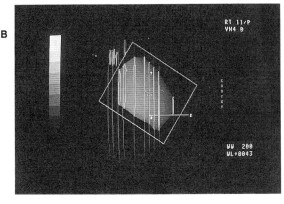

Figure 23.4 **A** Field selected by beam's-eye view, and **B** orientated to contain the tumour and avoid other organs. (Courtesy of S McNee, Beatson Oncology Centre, Glasgow.)

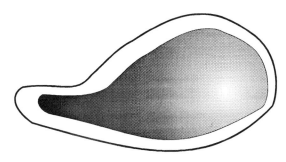

Figure 23.3. The tumour contained in a conformal volume or isodose envelope.

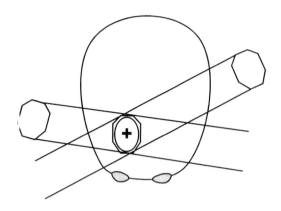

Figure 23.5 Noncoplanar fields with paths selected to avoid other organs.

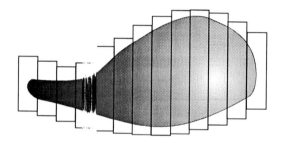

Figure 23.6 The treatment volume divided into sections for the planning and application of multiple small fields.

from unconventional angles. The method allows visualisation of the tumour in relation to its surroundings, in order to optimise the beam shape, size and orientations required to treat the tumour and miss critical organs in the tumour vicinity and along the beam paths (Figs 23.4 and 23.5). This may result in a coplanar or noncoplanar (McNee 1992) combination of beams, each individually shaped and directed. The plan for achieving the desired dose distribution may then be devised.

Beam-shaping methods and equipment

Once the beams are identified, there are various methods of physically shaping the volume treated, each requiring suitable equipment both for planning and treatment.

Static field-shaping systems. If the number of fields is few and the field arrangement is suitable, shaping may be achieved by using manual shielding for each field (static conformal therapy). The use of multileaf collimators is a less physically demanding method, especially where there are multiple beams.

Beam shaping via dynamic machine/collimator movements. Dynamic movement of the linac gantry and collimators together with suitable couch movements and changes in beam energy or mode are employed so that many (e.g., up to 90) rectangular fields effectively shape the high dose volume in the patient.

Dynamic movement of a slit beam over the patient. Here the treatment volume is divided up into segments (Fig. 23.6). Each of the segments has an approximately constant cross-section along its length. The smaller the section length, the better the fit of the fields to the target volume. A single rectangular beam or crossfire beams of appropriate size are applied to each section. This effect may be accomplished by means of a sweeping movement of the asymmetric collimators along the length of the volume, while dynamically altering the width of the collimator aperture to fit each segment traversed (Fig. 23.7 A–C). This is in essence a slit beam of varying width which moves along the treatment volume length. Independent or asymmetric movement of one or both pairs of collimators may be used.

Dynamic couch motion. Alternatively, a tracking unit may be used in which the couch moves the patient (Davy 1987) so that the planned movement of the isocentre along the tumour is achieved, together with dynamic collimator movements to alter the beam shape or size. Where multileaf collimators are available, fewer segments or less couch movement may be required, reducing treatment complexity and time, and therefore cost, for the same quality. A quality assurance programme to verify the couch movements and position in relation to the isocentre is required (Morgan 1992), under treatment conditions, i.e. with a humanoid phantom on the couch.

Equipment requirements

To plan and perform dynamic conformal therapy requires sophisticated facilities. Computer-controlled accelerator and/or couch movements are required, together with a powerful and intelligent treatment planning system which can au-tomatically prepare a plan, taking into account the linac characteristics, and which is capable of choreographing the linac (Davy 1987) to perform the treatment sequence.

The CT or MRI scanner, the treatment planning system and the linac must be compatible (e.g. compatible definition of parameters, scales

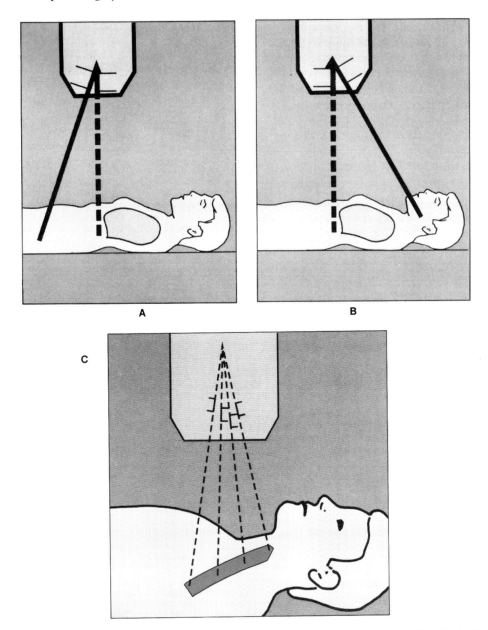

Figure 23.7   A–C The use of sweeping collimator movements to produce dynamic beam movement along the treatment volume. (Courtesy of Philips Medical Systems.)

or readouts) and must be able to communicate with each other in order to transfer accurate data from one unit to the others. An on-line portal imaging system is required.

Quality assurance

The technique is not recommended where there is a lack of technical ability to perform three-dimensional planning or to monitor day-to-day treatment reproducibility (Soffen et al 1991). Good communication and cooperation between radiotherapists, planning and treatment staff is essential in the design, execution and verification of these techniques (Mijnheer 1992).

Pretreatment verification processes

Simulation of treatment cannot be performed with conventional simulators, although a unit fitted with multileaf collimators can simulate field shape. Therefore special software programs on the treatment planning system, using the three-dimensional volume shape, are used to verify the parameters. Calibration to ensure that the linac receives and interprets the plan, and carries out the treatment program as intended is required. Verification that the high dose volume is accurately located at the tumour-bearing tissue in the patient is almost impossible, but may be partially indicated via portal imaging systems.

Accuracy and monitoring of treatment delivery. Complex field shapes have more error potential than rectangular shapes, as discussed in Chapter 18. With conformal techniques where multiple shaped fields are applied, there is an even greater potential for missing part of, or many parts of, an irregularly shaped volume. Where field dimensions vary, a set-up variation or patient movement may lead to a small field or fields being applied to a larger cross-section of the target than was intended, and a general misfit of the treatment to the target volume (Fig. 23.8). Treatment using computer-controlled machine movements requires greater skill levels in radiographers, both in accurately positioning the patient (Davy 1987), and in understanding the special needs involved in checking and monitoring of treatment delivery.

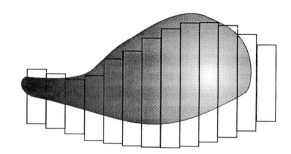

Figure 23.8 Misfit of the treated volume to the tumour caused by a small set-up variation/shift.

Staff performing techniques using dynamic machine movements must develop and use safe systems of work which incorporate checks on beam and dose parameters, wherever possible. Immobilisation devices and proven set-up methods, which have a predictable degree of accuracy, are necessary both for treatment and for allowing appropriate safety margins during the planning process.

Treatment field checking and verification processes

The placement accuracy of a limited number of beams can be checked from portal or verification films, but this is an impractical way of checking up to 90 beams! It is desirable to be able to view the anatomy treated using online digital imaging systems. Intratreatment movement should be monitored. Feedback links between, and compatibility of, megavoltage imaging systems and the treatment planning system may provide facilities for verification of the treatment field placement in the future.

Monitoring the dose

For such high dose, high precision techniques, an accurate knowledge of the dose delivered is also required. In vivo dosimetry measurement is therefore useful. The positions of diode detectors in the patient can be verified on portal images (Heukelom et al 1992).

Communication with the patient

Appropriate communication with the patient is

required to ensure that the importance of keeping still for the treatment duration is understood. He or she must not watch machine movements since movement of the head from side to side has been seen to rotate the chest/trunk, and this is likely to cause movement of the target anatomy. The patient must expect to hear collimator movement etc. and not be worried by it.

CONCOMITANT BOOST

The concomitant boost technique allows a higher dose to be given to a 'boost' volume within the gross treated volume, during the treatment course for the gross volume. Suitable dose and fractionation schedules are used for both the gross volume and the boost, for example the fraction dose for both the basic treatment and the boost may be reduced to achieve the same dose in the same overall time. There may be some advantages related to the greater ease of monitoring the accuracy of the boost fields when these can be imaged within the larger field areas which contain more landmarks (Keus & Lebesque 1991). This is basically an experimental regime to establish whether there is any radiobiological advantage. The technique is likely to use rather more machine time because of the extra fields or complexity of each fraction.

The concomitant boost may be achieved by adding the boost fields to the basic treatment fields for some or all of the treatment course. The method may alternatively require an irregular dose intensity across the beams used.

Inverse planning techniques

This is a method under development where the intensities at different points in the beam cross-section are matched to the dose requirements at points in the patient. This may be achieved in the future by using technology such as scanning beams, or, more simply, using a 'compensator'. This is the reverse of the process employed when using tissue compensation to restore the dose distribution across the beam to a uniform status at a given depth in the patient.

A simple example of the use of this process is

the concomitant boost technique where a thin shield of low melting point alloy, similar to that used for shaping electron fields, is used in the beam. This reduces the dose delivered to areas under the shield. Some bony landmarks in the tissue under the shield can be seen on a portal image (Keus & Lebesque 1991).

Another example of this process is the use of concomitant brachytherapy and external beam fields in treating the cervix. Here a cone-shaped compensator (Fig. 23.9A, B) may be planned for use within external beam fields, to alter the external beam intensity through the tissue which receives intermittent (e.g. once-weekly) intracavitary treatment. The compensator design allows the summated dose distribution from external beam and brachytherapy to be manipulated so as to give a higher dose at the high risk site with a lower dose to the remaining tissue, without unacceptable hot spots. The brachytherapy is used as a concomitant boost, the compensator aligned with the clips placed in the cervix at the brachytherapy insertion. The external beam central axis coincides with the centre of the compensator. An asymmetric field setting may then be required.

Quality assurance

Wherever a varying intensity across the field is used, any field misalignment has dosimetric consequences within the field area, in addition to those at the field margins. Treatment methods giving high field placement accuracy are required, as is monitoring by portal images.

Summated varied intensity treatments. Summating two treatments of varying intensity has a potential for even greater dosimetry consequences if there is a mismatch (Fig. 23.9C). For example when using a compensator, to balance a brachytherapy dose, as in treatment of the cervix, misalignment of the field or compensator changes the summated dose pattern across the tissue receiving significant dose from the brachytherapy. Similarly, if there is uncertainty as to the day-to-day position of the cervix relative to its position during brachytherapy, the expected dose distribution will not be obtained. Imaging of the brachytherapy applicators in situ is required.

A

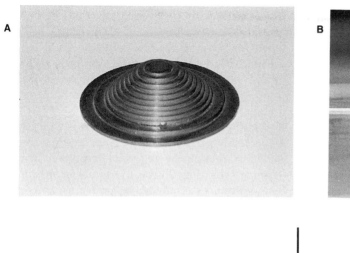

B

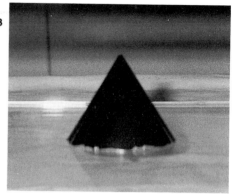

C

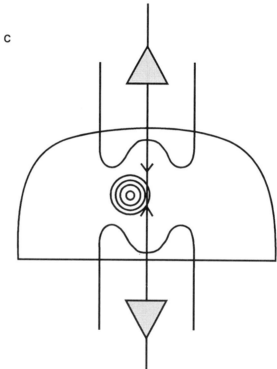

Figure 23.9 **A** Stepped brass filter to compensate for a brachytherapy dose to the cervix. **B** Cone-shaped brachytherapy compensator (lead). **C** Mismatch of brachytherapy zone and compensated areas of external beam treatment.

Metal clips attached to the cervix are helpful in localising its position when planning external beam fields.

Similar principles apply to other sites where two modalities are combined to effect a concomitant boost.

STEREOTACTIC RADIOTHERAPY

Stereotactic radiotherapy, or radiosurgery, is an extended form of arc therapy which uses a conformational therapy approach to achieve an extremely high concentration of absorbed dose, in an intracranial target of diameter ranging from 2 mm to 5 cm. Originally small volumes such as a 2 mm sphere were treated, using proton beams from a cyclotron or a special cobalt unit with multiple small sources. Up to 201 sources or fields were used, so treatment planning and delivery were very time-consuming and the method was pioneered by few centres.

Accessory systems to enable the technique to be used with a standard linac have now been developed. Stereotactic radiotherapy may be performed using brachytherapy (see Ch. 20).

Conditions treated

Treatment by 'stereotactic radiosurgery' using high dose single fractions eliminated the need for major surgery. Primarily, arteriovenous malformations (AVM) within the brain have been treated and 50–72% obliteration rates (at 2–3 years after treatment), are reported. The technique is now extended to larger volumes of 1–5 cm, which is potentially useful for small tumours including metastases, gliomas, pineal tumours and a range of benign tumours in the cranium. These require fractionated treatment because of the larger treatment volume.

The availability of linear accelerator stereotactic systems and relocatable frames will increase the availability and therefore the range of clinical applications of the technique.

Patient positioning and set-up

Special methods of immobilising the patient reproducibly enough to plan treatment, and to treat a volume which is 2 mm in diameter are required, and usually involve the use of a stereotactic frame fixed both to the skull and the treatment couch. The halo-type frame can be surgically attached to the patient before CT or MRI scans. The frame is used both to position and immobilise the patient, and also various localisation devices are integral with or attached to it.

Stereotaxy

Stereotaxy is the use of a three-dimensional system of X, Y and Z coordinates for spatial definition of the target centre position to points on the stereotactic frame. The target position, relative to the localisation points on the frame, is pinpointed via the three-dimensional coordinate system. The coordinates are used with conventional three-dimensional cross lasers and table movements to position the target centre at the isocentre in imaging, planning and treatment.

Types of stereotactic frame

If the treatment is to be given in one fraction, use of an invasive frame (Fig. 23.10), indented into the skull with steel-tipped screws, which stays on the patient from imaging to treatment, may be used. For fractionated treatment, a detachable, noninvasive, reproducible frame is used so that

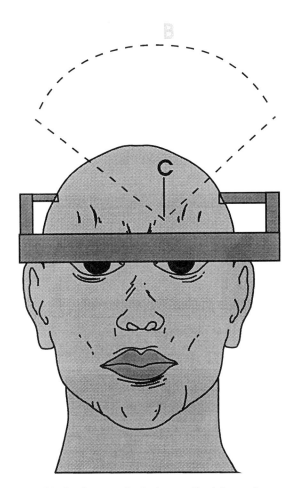

Figure 23.10 Stereotactic single arc with static couch.

the patient can be freed from it and travel home between treatments. One such frame has a dental fixation plate which allows it to be accurately clamped into position. A detachable plate also has the advantage of allowing ample time to plan and prepare treatment after imaging.

Localisation

The target tissue is localised from CT or MRI scans or a combination of these and cerebral angiography, and the subsequent accuracy of treatment is largely determined by slice thickness. Angiography is required to localise an AVM and the digitised image is transferred to the planning computer for analysis and correction for distortions etc. From these, the X, Y and Z coordinates of the target centre are determined.

Simulation

Simulation is performed using orthogonal films to verify the reproducibility of the frame position, preferably with a long f.s.d. such as 400 cm so that divergence is minimised.

Dosimetry considerations and beam arrangements

Dosimetry requirements

Radiosurgery results in necrosis of the target volume, after a single fraction, and therefore requires a sharply defined high dose volume. Such a regime can only be used for a very limited volume size, e.g. of 3 cm^3.

Doses, volumes and CNS tolerance. The dose limitations stem from limits in normal brain and cranial nerve tolerance:

- The maximum dose tolerated at the optic chiasma is 10 Gy.
- A single dose of 50 Gy gives an integral dose of 1 kg gray, which is below the tolerance limit for brain tissue.
- A dose of 20–38 Gy is given/tolerated for a small brain metastasis or AVM.

For a 3 cm diameter volume the maximum recommended dose in a single fraction is 20 Gy.

With this dose level, later reirradiation is possible. For volumes larger than 5 cm in diameter, even with fractionated regimes, there is little or no dosimetric advantage over conventional treatment using multiple fields.

Dose distribution and beams used. The centre of the target volume is placed at the isocentre and the dose should be normalised to the isocentre. There should be no cold spots, but hot spots within the tumour are acceptable. For the dose distribution to be acceptable and to minimise the dose to normal tissue, a steep dose gradient at the periphery of the target volume is required. Proton beams are ideal since they have small penumbrae and the dose absorption characteristics (Chs 5 and 21) result in a steep fall in dose outside the target area. Photon beams require complex beam arrangements to achieve this.

Some couch rotation is required to achieve the required rapid fall-off of dose in several planes. This may be achieved by couch rotation during a single gantry arc (Fig. 23.11). Alternatively four or five (or up to nine) noncoplanar, converging arcs, with a different fixed table angle for each, may be used. Oblique coronal arcs are used for a patient in the sitting position (Fig. 23.12), oblique sagittal arcs for a patient lying supine (Fig. 23.13).

Limitations. Multiple isocentres may be required for multiple lesions. The method is inevitably technically complex, and the effect of the position, size or shape of the tumour may preclude the production of a viable plan. For example, the tumour may lie close to the eyes, the skull, the headrest system or frame, or the exit paths of beams may pass through the orbit.

Treatment planning software

A special programme to compute the three-dimensional dosimetry of the noncoplanar beams is used on a standard treatment planning system, and does not require excessive computing power or time.

Quality assurance

Validation of the planning software and the treatment should be performed by calibration of

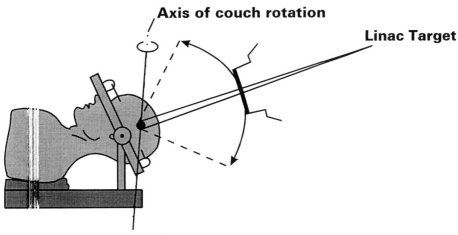

Figure 23.11 Stereotactic arc with couch rotation.

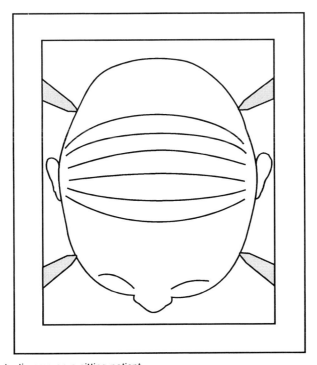

Figure 23.12 Coronal stereotactic arcs on a sitting patient.

the treatment performed on a phantom, using combinations of densitometry and semiconductors and cross-checking results.

Requirements for accuracy in treatment delivery

An isocentric linac is rotated round a single target site to achieve the optimal dose distribution. One or more arcs or planes may be used.

Remotely controlled couch and gantry movements. Remotely controlled or computer-controlled couch and/or gantry rotation, with minimal inaccuracy arising during rotation, is necessary to achieve the required dose gradient at the volume edge.

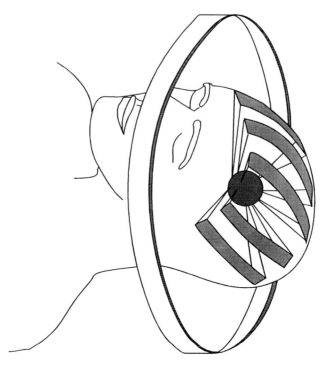

Figure 23.13 Sagittal stereotactic arcs on a supine patient.

Collimation systems. In order to accurately treat very small volumes, extra collimation systems are required so that very small field sizes, without penumbrae, can be produced. Systems consist of a range of applicators with different-sized inserts to give a range of circular field sizes. Circular beams are suitable for the spherical volumes treated. The special collimator assemblies are designed both to give a sharp penumbra and to ensure reproducibility of beam size and position-ing. These effects result from the collimators' extending towards the vicinity of the isocentre.

Head support systems and movement accuracy. The frame is designed to attach to any treatment or imaging couch used in the process. In some cases it is fixed to a special stand, attached directly to the rotating bearing of the couch assembly to overcome any possibility of play in the couch, which would compromise accuracy during rotations. The system may provide move-ment in all three axes, providing pitch and roll to allow correct beam direction, and allowing precise positioning of the beams by means of

docking points for the special collimator attach-ments. The geometrical accuracy obtained under treatment conditions is ±1 mm, with a dosimetric accuracy of ±3%.

The irradiation takes around 20 minutes, but extra treatment room time is required to set up the various special attachments.

Special patient care

There is some risk of airway blockage since the patient's head is totally immobilised for a consid-erable time. Suction apparatus should be avail-able. Also there is some likelihood of acute reaction including vomiting (Smith et al 1990), so staff must be instructed regarding the fast release of the patient in an emergency. Close monitoring of the patient is required throughout.

INTRAOPERATIVE THERAPY

In order to treat the tumour directly, intraoperative techniques are being developed which allow several fractions of radiation to be applied through a surgical wound, which exposes the tumour and allows other organs to be moved aside. This geographical selectivity allows accurate application of radiation to the tumour, removing many of the uncertainties associated with treatment beams directed from outside the body. Brachytherapy techniques lend themselves to intraoperative applications, both at low and high dose rate (see Ch. 20). The technique may be used for primary or locally recurrent gross disease or for subclinical disease. Promising results are reported for the stomach, pancreas and rectum, but the technique is not yet clinically proven.

Regimes and dosimetry issues

The technique may be used alone or as a boost to external beam treatment. A single fraction, usually of 15–30 Gy may be used but is inappropriate if normal tissue receives a similar dose to the tumour. Postoperative complications are not increased by the treatment but radiation complications can occur according to the site treated. Fractionation improves the therapeutic ratio.

The dose is specified at the 90% isodose. For a boost in the case of subclinical disease, 10–15 Gy is used; for gross disease, 15–25 Gy. The use of electron beams of 9–20 MeV is ideal since the 90% isodose falls within 4.5 cm with a sharp cut-off beyond this (see Ch. 5).

External beam intraoperative therapy

Some departments have dedicated treatment units, such as 50–100 kV X-ray contact units or electron units, located within or adjacent to an operating theatre. However, this ideally requires a dedicated linac, with surgery taking place in the treatment room, which limits the use of the machine. Patients may alternatively be transferred to the treatment room using aseptic procedures, such as sealing over a surgically positioned applicator and the wound with a thin transparent film during patient transportation and treatment. External applicator cones 'dock' via an adaptor, with the applicator in the tissue, with the seal intact. For fractionated treatment, the wound is temporarily sealed between fractions, the patient being housed on a surgical care ward for the duration of the intraoperative treatment phase. Applicators of 5–12 cm diameter are used, each specially commissioned.

An electron applicator system has been developed (Huss et al 1990) which provides contact-free intraoperative electron irradiation using a wide range of applicators, and permits continuous observation of the alignment and treatment area by means of a special camera.

REFERENCES AND FURTHER READING

Bijhold J, Lebesque J V, Hart A A M, Vijlbrief R E 1992 Maximising set-up accuracy using portal images as applied to a conformal boost technique for prostatic cancer. Radiotherapy and Oncology 24: 261–272

Brahme A 1988 Optimisation of stationary and moving beam radiotherapy techniques. Radiotherapy and Oncology 12: 129–140

Davy T J 1988 Conformation therapy methods and systems. Proceedings of International Symposium on Dosimetry in Radiotherapy. Vol 2. International Atomic Energy Authority, Vienna

Heukelom S, Lanson J H, Mijnheer B J 1992 In vivo dosimetry measurements during pelvic treatment. Radiotherapy and Oncology 25: 111–120

Hounsell A R, Sharrock P J, Moore C J, Shaw A J, Wilkinson J M, Williams P C 1992 Computer assisted generation of multi-leaf collimator settings for conformation therapy. British Journal of Radiology 65: 321–326

Huss A, Krull A, Block T, Ihlow C, Hubener K -H 1990 Contact free electron applicator with surveillance of the radiation field for intraoperative radiotherapy. RAD 16 (184): 25–27

Keus R, Noach P, De Boer R, Lebesque J 1991 The effect of customised beam shaping on normal tissue complications in radiotherapy of parotid gland tumours. Radiotherapy and Oncology 21: 211–217

Leksell L 1949. A stereotactic apparatus for intracerebral surgery. Acta Chirurgica Scandinavica 99: 229–233

McNee S G 1992 Non-coplanar radiotherapy planning. 50th Annual Congress of British Institute of Radiology. Abstract

Mijnheer B J 1992 Conformal radiotherapy. (Presentation at ESTRO postgraduate teaching course for radiographers.)

Morgan H M 1992 Quality assurance of computer controlled radiotherapy treatments. British Journal of Radiology 65: 409–416

Podgorsak E, Pike G B, Olivier A, Pla M, Souhami L 1989

Radiosurgery with high energy photon beams: a comparison among techniques. International Journal of Radiation Oncology, Biology, Physics 16: 857–865

Ryan-Kidd S 1992 A comparison between two computer systems for planning stereotactic brain implants. Radiography Today 58: 24–26

Smith V, Larson A L, Schell M C 1990 Linac-based stereotactic irradiation – a brief survey. Radiotherapy Applications and Developments. Centerline

Soffen E M, Hanks G E, Chang Hwang C, Chu J C H 1991 Conformal static field therapy for low volume low grade prostate cancer with rigid immobilisation. International Journal of Radiation Oncology, Biology, Physics 20: 141–146

Tait D, Nahum A, Southall C, Chow M, Yarnold J R 1988 Benefits expected from simple conformal therapy in the treatment of pelvic tumours. Radiotherapy and Oncology 13: 23–30

Thomson E S, Gill S S, Doughty D 1990 Stereotactic multiple arc radiotherapy. British Journal of Radiology 63: 745–751

Working Group on the Evaluation of Treatment Planning for External Photon Beam Radiotherapy 1991 Report. International Journal of Radiation Oncology, Biology, Physics 21(1): 1–258

Managing and shaping the service environment

24

Choosing equipment and costing treatment

The equipment available in a department either facilitates a high quality service, with flexibility to allow developments, or limits the service provision and imposes organisational constraints. Evaluating equipment currently on the market and working with a team to select an appropriate treatment machine (or simulator) is one of the most important roles of the radiographer. The official lifespan of a treatment unit is 15 years, that of a simulator 10 years, so the consequences of the choice made are long-standing. Ease of use of the equipment affects the daily fatigue levels and safety of the radiographers and the achievable throughput rate for a particular type of work, and therefore influences the daily treatment capacity and relative cost per patient.

CHOOSING EQUIPMENT FOR SIMULATION AND TREATMENT

The choice of machine should be appropriate to the technical service requirements, with ergonomic features allowing easy, fast and accurate use. Ease of use and shorter treatment times benefit the patient, whose time on the treatment table should be minimised.

Where a new model or new accessories or features are offered, a system which has undergone trial and been proven reliable by routine clinical use should be chosen, unless there is an acknowledged wish to assist the manufacturer with an evaluation and development phase. It is unwise to purchase a system with promised but untried new basic features if the unit is urgently required to perform well for a high patient workload, unless reliable routine use of the machine can be made by bypassing the new feature.

Long-term planning considerations

The choice of an individual linac should be considered as part of a long-term strategy for the overall service requirements, rather than as an isolated event. The strategy should ensure that, where possible, technically compatible machines are paired. This simplifies patient scheduling and allows multiple patient transfer during breakdowns, without the need for replanning and the associated safety hazards and staff time usage. (The more complex the treatments and the technology, the greater the difficulty in transferring patients.) However, it should be possible to modify the long-term plan in the light of changing requirements, i.e. the plan should be flexible.

Beam energy

The first major decision concerns the energy/ energies of treatment beam required. So-called 'baby' linacs have a single energy X-ray beam of 4–6 MV only. Linacs with an energy of 8 MV or above also have electron facilities and usually a choice from which to select two X-ray energies, e.g. 6 MV plus 10 MV. These higher energy, dual-modality linacs cost approximately one-third as much again as a baby linac; however, most departments have at least one high energy machine. There are many advantages to having twinned machines at any energy and, in the current climate of development towards conformal techniques, there are considerable advantages in having twinned multienergy facilities, even in a relatively small department (Blue Blook 1991). Thus the choice of energy should take wider factors into account than a current or projected demand level for a particular energy.

Managerial and organisational advantages of twinned multienergy treatment units. The range of available energies and/or features of a proposed treatment unit, when considered in relation to existing units, affects the departmental flexibility in both delivering a wide range of treatments,

and offering compatible backup during machine breakdown.

The operation of all of the current generation of linacs is complex and specific to each manufacturer. The features which make the linacs complex to operate are essential for, and facilitate, current technical practice. It is prudent to ensure that these features can be provided by and are compatible on more than one machine for the following reasons.

1. Management of workload.

• Patient waiting times may be reduced, either when waiting to start treatment requiring a particular mode or facility, or from day to day when holdups cause a backlog on one machine.
• Patients may be transferred from one unit to the other during breakdown or servicing (where time allows), without the need for a backup treatment plan etc.
• Greater choice of treatment energy and machine availability.
• Simplification of the patient booking system, for booking staff, radiographers, physicists, doctors.

2. Management of staff.

• More flexibility in the staffing rota as there will be less workload specialisation on individual machines.
• Standardised set-up procedures (these necessarily differ with linac design).
• Reduced staff training load.
• Faster staff induction and less error potential when staff change machines.
• Less staff stress, higher quality of treatment and service.

Features and design factors

Many technological features, such as dual asymmetric collimators and computer control and laser backpointers, are integral to most new simulators and linacs. Other features such as record and verify systems, multileaf collimators and megavoltage imaging are extras. Yet other features, such as autowedges, may be integral to one make of equipment and unavailable for another. Accessories such as electron applicators and lead trays are also extras. One fact prevails, that all systems differ in construction and mode of operation from one manufacturer to another, and to some extent from one model to another. This extends to basic features of the machine, such as the range and speed of movements and the hand controls for these. Therefore, with each purchase, unless twinned, an extra staff training load arises, not only at the start of clinical use, but each time a member of staff moves from one unit to another (see Ch 26). The need may range from a quick refresher following a 6-month rota elsewhere, to a complete training for a newcomer to the unit. With four different machines there will be four routines for achieving the same technique, as opposed to one with four identical machines. In addition, the workload on each unit may become specialised if a particular facility or extended range of movements is limited to one unit only. This presents a higher student training load also, and placement complications with regard to the syllabus. It also presents numerous complications to patient booking and scheduling systems.

The convenience of the systems varies. Design factors which should be assessed include the ease of use of features such as the wedges, lead tray etc. and the following limitations of their use:

- The range of wedges and the available wedged field sizes vary, and affect flexibility and treatment complexity (an inadequate system generates an extra workload, see Ch. 8).
- The field size, clearance and visibility available with multileaf collimators may be reduced.
- The working dose rate affects treatment times and throughput.
- The dimensions of the machine affect the working height and thus radiographer safety (isocentre and accessory or wedge mount height, Fig. 24.1).
- The dimensions and shape of the treatment head affect the visibility of set-up, and also isocentre-to-accessory clearances, which influence flexibility of set-up.
- Clearances and treatment head design also affect the equipment-generated scatter component and contamination of the treatment beam.
- The clarity of optical systems affects the accuracy of set-up.

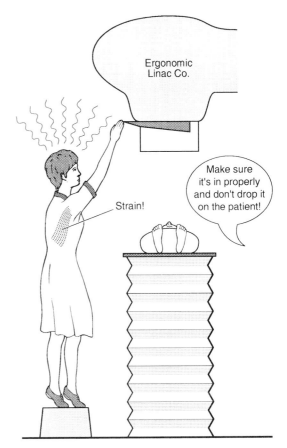

Figure 24.1 The dimensions of the machine affect the working height and radiographer safety.

- The stability and rigidity of the couch top when locked affect the accuracy of use (Fig. 24.2).
- The construction of the couch top affects accuracy and flexibility of machine use.

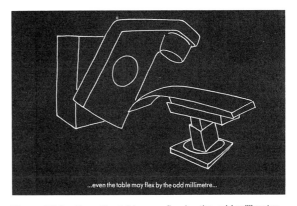

Figure 24.2 Even the table may flex by the odd millimetre.

• The fine movement control and the speed and range of movements of the couch respectively affect accuracy, throughput and flexibility of use of the machine.

• The weight and mode of attachment of wedges and accessories affect the physical effort required to use them. Such factors are now subject to assessment for the new EC manual handling directive, one of seven areas of additional health and safety legislation effective from 1993. Equipment will have to conform to fit with the guidelines by 1997.

The details of variations and their effects on treatment methods are interwoven in the foregoing text, particularly Chapters 2, 7, 8, 9, 10, 14 and 15.

Other factors affecting purchase choice

• Model and feature availability and reliability record.

• Professional backgrounds and knowledge of evaluation team making the choice.

• Multidisciplinary views and perceptions of priority features and specifications required.

• Compatibility with existing units.

• Perceived customer relations and aftersales service record of manufacturers.

• Availability of a good, fast spare parts delivery and breakdown assistance service (Fig. 24.3).

• Price and/or a good case for purchasing a highly priced unit. For a treatment unit with an official life of 15 years in the UK, the effect on unit costs of a small annual capacity advantage should outweigh the effect of a higher initial purchase price.

A good case can be made for purchasing particular features, using various organisational considerations, for example the potential advantages of purchasing multileaf collimators include:

• increase in flexibility for shaping volume during planning: quality gain
• shorter treatment preparation time: no blocks to make
• flexibility for block changes during treatment
• health and safety gain for radiographers and patient-risk management gain
• health, safety and efficiency gain for mould room and workshop staff
• increased sophistication in planning work: resources required released by efficiency gains in the planning process
• simplified delivery of complex treatments
• potential for increasing throughput on linac compared with conventionally shielded beams
• increased machine capacity gives better utilisation of capital with equal revenue costs, leading to reduced unit costs.

Estimating costs for an additional or replacement machine

Replacement machine costings should always include a building element, as well as a revised revenue requirement. (The replacement unit may need altered staffing levels, because of additional workload or technical features.) There may be other consequences or prerequisites, such as additional treatment planning software or hardware requirements.

Usually a building plan is required simultaneously, so that tenders for this as a turnkey or separate process can be made, even for a machine replacement in an existing chamber.

Linac suite design

The more compact the layout, the greater the efficiency potential and reduction in distance walked daily by staff and patients. For example, the machine chambers may be arranged in a

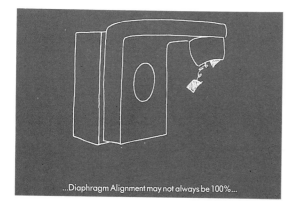

...Diaphragm Alignment may not always be 100%...

Figure 24.3 Diaphragm alignment may not always be 100%.

circle with a central reception and waiting area. Intercom systems can reduce the number of telephone calls and thus noise in the treatment and control areas.

Linac chambers and associated areas

Where the equipment is to be installed in a new building, a 'standard' all-purpose linac chamber may be designed and the building begun before a machine is chosen. The maximum X-ray or electron energy envisaged for the room determines the construction. A room will last longer than a machine, so the layout should be designed to accommodate possible future needs. The room should be tastefully decorated, avoiding the use of wall or ceiling pictures since these can attract the attention of the patient during treatment and cause movement.

Shelving should be carefully sited for minimum walking and lifting by staff using accessories and shielding blocks stored there.

Control area. The layout of the room and associated control and waiting areas should be compatible with patient care needs, while providing a private, undisturbed control area. The control area should have sufficient space to accommodate staff switching on the linac, staff undertaking patient administration and student training. There should be ample desk space for computer systems and for writing and checking activities, with extra capacity to take additional equipment such as multileaf collimator controls.

There should be a linked but separate area where data input at a remote workstation can be performed, out of earshot of the activity associated with treating patients.

Changing facilities. Patient changing facilities should be situated close to the machine control area and designed so that patients, including those in wheelchairs can:

- enter a cubicle from the waiting area, with an accompanying relative, and lock the door for privacy
- have plenty of room to undress
- enter the treatment room from a second cubicle door, on being invited by the treatment staff (who control patient access at this second door)

- leave belongings in the cubicle knowing that it can only be entered by staff
- have time to dress at leisure with access to a sink and a mirror.

Thus a bank of three cubicles is required for each machine so that one is occupied by a patient undressing, one 'belonging' to the patient on the treatment table and one occupied by a patient dressing. This arrangement allows dignified changing conditions for the patients and assists efficiency of patient throughput for the treatment unit. It also provides privacy for a member of the treatment team to talk with and reassure any patient prior to their treatment.

The purchasing process

After planning, and the approval of funds to go ahead, the purchasing process is carried out as follows:

1. Write specification which desired machine must meet, including special features and operational ease. This requires some research and is best undertaken during the planning phase so that the purchasing process is not delayed by it.
2. Submit advertisement, in the European trade journal for a minimum number of weeks, for expressions of interest to tender.
3. Supply details of specification to respondents.
4. Allow 6 weeks for them to submit tenders.
5. Assess tenders against specification and make a choice.
6. The purchase is made by a purchasing body.
7. Pre-site and site meetings are held to establish protocols and iron out problems as the building and installation processes proceed.

COSTING TREATMENT

The cost of a treatment depends on a number of interrelated factors.

Basic costs integral to service provision

1. The capital cost of the equipment, the treatment rooms, and the capital charges

arising from these, and the square footage of space used to manage and deliver the service.

2. Revenue costs of running the units for a fixed working day length, including radiographer, physicist and medical time.
3. The overheads, such as power, water, building maintenance costs.
4. Overhead costs for planning treatment (unless charged separately).
5. Overhead costs for managing the service, within the department and within the hospital or functional unit.
6. Overhead costs for patient support services.
7. Inpatient hotel costs.
8. Outpatient transport costs.

Costs which vary with working day length

Extra revenue costs are accrued when the working day is lengthened, either on an ad hoc basis, or on a planned basis. This will involve overtime for radiographers, physicists, physics technicians and support services staff. Depending on the type of hospital in which the service is run, these costs will vary. For example, a department in a general hospital where portering and catering services, medical and nursing cover are available in the evening, extra costs will be restricted to staff involved with treatment delivery and patient transportation. In a specialist centre operating on a mainly outpatient basis, such backup services are unavailable after 5.00 pm and costs accrue for a much wider group of staff.

Costs related to individual treatments

From the cost factors above, a cost per treatment room-minute can be derived, inclusive or not inclusive of planning or overheads. The cost of delivery of a treatment can ideally be calculated as a multiple of the room-minute costs, for the time used. However, such sophistication is dependent on the quality of information available about time taken for individual treatments or patients. A more general, simplified costing can be derived related to the average cost of a treatment exposure.

Cost of an exposure

The average number of exposures per fixed day length can be derived from annual workload statistics. This can be related to the cost per day of providing the treatment, so that an exposure cost is defined, equal to the cost of a number of machine-minutes. Again, overheads and planning costs may be included or not. However, the higher the exposure rate or daily throughput achievable, the lower the cost of an exposure, and the lower the relative costs of overheads etc. per patient treated.

Basic costs of running a single machine per annum:

Some of these include:

- radiographer salaries and overheads plus appropriate portion of superintendent cost
- proportion of consultant costs (no consultants – no patients, no machine – no need for consultant radiotherapists!)
- proportion of physicist and technician costs
- portering and transportation costs
- proportion of support service costs (reception, secretarial, dietitian, nursing etc.)
- capital cost of machine divided by life in years, plus associated capital costs
- capital cost of building divided by life in years, plus associated capital costs
- machine servicing and maintenance costs
- the cost implications for contingency plans which may be imposed during major breakdown
- power, water, rates etc.
- building maintenance costs
- domestic servicing costs
- consumables
- hospital/department-wide overheads.

From this list it can be seen that a 10–20% difference in the purchase price of a machine is not the overriding factor, and since all the revenue costs are unavoidable, it makes sound economic sense to maximise the throughput during the standard, funded working day length. Any long-term commitment to extended hours to achieve a higher workload, not only increases the revenue costs disproportionately as overtime or the creation of extra posts in a number of disciplines, but also results in higher servicing costs and ultimately in a shortening of the machine lifetime. The higher the number of patients, the greater the difficulty in accommodating them on other units in the event of major breakdown. Unless extra posts are available, it is therefore prudent to work efficiently with an adequate number of staff during a standard day, rather than to split the staff team into two inadequate teams who work less efficiently over a longer (more expensive) day but achieve no significantly higher overall output (see Ch. 25).

REFERENCES AND FURTHER READING

Greene D 1983 The cost of radiotherapy treatments on a linear accelerator. British Journal of Radiology 56: 189–191
Blue Book 1991 Radiation oncology in integrated cancer management. Report of the Inter-Society Council for Radiation Oncology (USA)

25

Workload management

Workload management is an increasingly important task since the level of demand for patient treatment and associated care exceeds the available resources for many departments. The resource requirement is for both machines and radiographers, the two being completely interdependent in determining the treatment capacity available in a department.

Any statement of the treatment capacity of a linac or group of linacs should be qualified by the number of radiographers required to achieve that capacity, the number of operational hours per day and by the workload type or complexity. Any change in the caseload mix, treatment patterns, or number of radiographers available will change the output, i.e. the capacity of a particular machine (including a treatment simulator) for a given number of operational hours. The motivation and skills of staff also influence the achievable and safe level of output. Similarly, the make or model of machine and the features it incorporates, affect the capacity, interlinking with the workload and staffing factors. The actual capacity is therefore related to the circumstances in a particular department. It is complex and subject to change.

The management of workload involves analysis of and planned manipulation of elements of the referred case-mix and of the available staff time, teams and skills (see Ch. 26), and optimising their distribution across the available equipment. The use of workload statistics is invaluable in this process, both for planning and monitoring trends and outputs. The use of a booking system for efficiently scheduling patients in advance, according to clinical criteria and priorities, technical requirements and available capacity, is a necessity for waiting list management.

TREATMENT CAPACITY, WORKLOADS AND STAFFING LEVELS

The authors have much experience in utilising available staff and equipment to maximise the throughput of patients, whilst allowing for the highest quality of treatment to be given. This experience includes the monitoring of workload achieved, related to equipment factors, staffing levels and type of work and is drawn on for both crisis management and future planning.

Working day length, radiographer time, machine life

Because of the present shortage of treatment machines, common to many centres, a high number of patients must be treated each day in order to minimise or avoid waiting lists. Most centres use a 7- or 8-hour day and try to maximise throughput. The new range of computer-controlled and verified linacs tend to have more breakdowns, some of which are associated with computerisation and complex technology. Heavily utilised machines break down or need replacing in a shorter time span.

Optimising the use of radiographer time

Predicted skills shortages may limit the number of radiographers available, in spite of efforts to retain and re-recruit staff (see Ch. 26). If the limiting factor on whether or not the workload demand can be met is radiographer availability, the primary consideration must be to increase the treatment productivity for each radiographer.

The radiographer time available for carrying out radiation treatments and ensuring accuracy, which are the primary functions of radiographers, should be maximised, while allowing reasonable scope for nontechnical patient care needs to be met. There are various options available to maximise the treatment workload achievable by a given number of radiographers.

Reducing the range of tasks undertaken by radiographers

The taskload of radiographers can be reduced by performing nontechnical tasks with the assistance of computerised patient management systems (see Ch. 10), and employing support staff to help with patient care and reception. However, allowing the available radiographer time to be utilised entirely for the treatment of patients will not in itself result in achievement of the same workload by fewer radiographers.

Making the appropriate equipment available

The availability of ergonomically good machines, capable of easy use for a fast throughput for a wide range of treatments, and an increased number and greater compatibility of treatment machines available allows maximum use of the available radiographer time.

Local analysis shows that more than three-quarters of all treatment exposures are complex, and therefore require more staff and machine time and skills to achieve safely. The complexity of treatment is related to the fundamental aims and desired outcome, and is likely to increase rather than decrease. However, the associated workload for radiographers can be minimised by choice of appropriate equipment and development of standardised working systems and treatment techniques.

Efficiency model for simple work

A convenient model based on recorded daily exposure averages, for simple work on a cobalt machine with two different staffing levels, is used to demonstrate the relationship of the staff to machine ratio and its effect on output:

- Four radiographers achieve 60 exposures per day on one machine (30 exposures each).
- Two radiographers achieve 40 exposures per day on the same machine (40 exposures each).

Therefore four radiographers can achieve 80 exposures on two machines, and productivity per person rises by one-third. A higher overall workload demand could then be met by fewer radiographers per machine by increasing the number of treatment machines available (assuming non-treatment tasks are reduced to the minimum).

Practical drawbacks. *A minimum of two radiographers must work together for reasons connected with radiation safety. When operating with only two staff, if one is off sick or on leave, the unit cannot operate at all,* especially if the whole department is planned on this type of staffing level so that no one can be found to supply cover. Changing the rostered staff is very problematical if one of them requires training on the unit. There is little time available to train students. Daily machine quality assurance, normally undertaken by one or two radiographers starting early and leaving early, must now be undertaken during the treatment hours.

There is no possibility for either of the two staff to attend meetings, lectures etc. When only two radiographers are available for a machine, work must stop for break periods. (The work is both mentally and physically demanding so breaks are essential if fatigue-related errors are to be avoided.) Treatment must also cease during administrative work such as treatment card checks and preparation of diary lists. The number of machine-hours available for treatment each day therefore falls from 8 to approximately 5, and the treatment of patients is slowed as telephone enquiries and other tasks still have to be handled by the two radiographers.

Where the treatment work is relatively simple and there are few related tasks, two staff can achieve two-thirds the work of four, but where the work is complex, two staff can achieve little more than half the work of four. Thus the workload achieved depends on the complexity of treatments and the related tasks.

Adaptation of the efficiency model for complex linac work

This model needs adaptation for more complex work carried out on linacs, where a minimum of three staff are required to work together to keep up with checking, computer verification and organisational work at the same time as treating patients. Routinely, four radiographers run a linac, which can only be used continuously from 9.00 am to 5.00 pm if staff go in relays for breaks. This reduces the number of staff available to work to two for half the day, with many of the drawbacks described above. During the rest of the time there are many card-checking tasks to undertake. Ideally at least five staff per linac are required to achieve an optimum throughput over a continuous 8-hour day. When considering the work that six staff could achieve on one machine in contrast to that using three on each of two machines, the concept applied for simple work is valid and the drawbacks somewhat reduced.

Planning and organisation to optimise the use of resources

Planning the achievement of a particular workload then depends on which resource is most limited, equipment or staff. If adequate numbers of linacs are available but staff numbers are limited, it is better to spread the available staff over as many linacs as can be manned with three staff each. The choice may be between working a 10-hour day on one machine, using six staff, or using three staff working a normal day on each of two machines, which, even after stopping for breaks, generates 12 treating hours. Using two machines allows:

- a gain in total treatment time per day
  less stress on the individual as three staff are available to work together the whole time
- fewer patients per machine
- saving in overtime costs or time for other staff groups/superintendents providing backup outside the normal day
- potential reduction in frequency of machine breakdown; there is some evidence that machine life in years is shorter when longer days are used, and also parts replacement intervals are related to usage
- potential throughput gain per day
- flexibility to cope during breakdown or servicing

Example:

Normal 8-hour load achieved with 4 staff on one user-friendly linac = 105 exposures.

130 exposures are performed in 10 hours on this linac (average 13 per hour), by 6 staff.

If 2 identical linacs operate at 13 fields per hour for 6 hours each, then the output is:

156 exposures per day
78 exposures per machine.

This provides a net gain of 26 fields per day over the single machine 10-hour day.

This is achievable because slightly more useful radiographer time is available per day per machine. (The average number of staff available per hour is less than three over the longer 'flexiday' because of breaks; which does not allow all tasks to be completed together with an optimum patient throughput. See Ch. 26.)

Spreading the work over more hours is logistically difficult with six staff, if the throughput level is to be kept high and some continuity (for quality, safety and throughput reasons) is to be achieved. Two of the team work a normal day, but others start early or finish late, working over a marginally shorter overall time period and having fewer breaks. This allows them to gain sufficient time at one end of the day to compensate for the inconvenience at the other, and a consequently altered lifestyle. Even so, staff find that they get more tired so the system can only be used for a limited period, or throughput drops, which negates the capacity gain.

The authors' experience shows that staggering starts and finishes with a team of four achieves the same workload over a longer (more expensive!) day. We have anecdotal evidence that where it is routine practice to run a machine for 12-hours with two overlapping shifts of two staff, a similar number of patients (or less) are treated per machine per day than when using four staff over an 8-hour day.

Costs and support available. For similar reasons a minimum of eight staff per machine and a two-shift system are required to cover a 12-hour day, but here the costs rise astronomically because of the number of extra hours or posts required for both radiographers and many other staff groups. These costs will vary according to the support services normally locally available in

the evening (see Ch. 24). Depending on the location of the hospital, the distances travelled by patients, and the proportion using ambulances or staying as inpatients, it may be difficult to organise patient attendances and review in the evening. This factor must be borne in mind when considering how to meet workloads if a machine is down.

Contingency plans for machine breakdown or replacement periods

Machine replacement periods of 12–18 months are likely to occur every few years in a major centre, and workload management systems and contracting levels should build in an allowance to ensure that workloads can be safely met during breakdown and replacement periods.

Any workload management system should have some flexibility to allow patients to continue their treatment during a major machine breakdown. For example, where a 9.00 am to 5.00 pm day is the norm on four machines, during breakdown of one machine an extended day is necessary on the other three units to accommodate the shortfall.

Compatibility of machines, time and safety factors for planned treatments. This solution depends on the staff available, and is not simple, becoming more complex and risk-laden where machines are technically incompatible so that replanning of transferred patients is necessary. The radiographer time required to reorganise patients and recalculate treatments reduces that available to help with extended hours of work on the remaining units.

Where units are technically incompatible, there are high risks when the patients have been replanned (so have more than one plan), and are transferred to a different machine where there are different staff working under high pressure. There are also risks where staff transfer to a different machine which they may not have operated for months or years, under high pressure conditions, with unfamiliar patients and technical methods. A study by Probst (1992) showed significantly decreased set-up accuracy when staff worked under time-stressed conditions, compared with the accuracy achieved under relaxed conditions. The study involved a complex cranial set-up (part of a whole neuraxis treatment) and the inaccuracies were at critical points, i.e. at the matchline and eye shielding, so that treatment safety and outcome were both at risk.

Extension of hours provides a partial solution, but when departments are routinely working a longer day, this option is lost as further significant extension of the day becomes impractical. Patients having radical therapy who miss several treatments may have a 20% lower chance of cure owing to regrowth of the tumour (see Ch. 1). Delays have a knock-on effect on patient schedules and waiting list management.

Staffing, continuity and skill factors. The length of day worked, and the efficiency of machine utilisation throughout the whole working period, are critically dependent on the number of radiographers available, and on their skills (see Ch. 26). To routinely achieve a high patient throughput with complex treatments, with some degree of safety and throughout an extended day, requires a minimum of eight highly skilled radiographers per unit. Even so lack of staff continuity (see Ch. 26), and the sheer volume of patients and associated data, create safety hazards as no one person can be in control of all the treatments. This represents suboptimal usage of a scarce staff group, who could provide a safer, higher quality service for more patients if using more machines for a normal day (the machines would breakdown or need replacing less often too!).

WORKLOAD STATISTICS AND THEIR IMPORTANCE

The number of megavoltage machines (normally linacs) available for each million head of population varies with geographical region and country. The recommended number is a minimum of three, but a need for up to nine has been forecast, to accommodate developing treatment trends and future referral numbers (Blue Book 1991). The incidence of cancer is over 4000 cases per million head of population, and it is recommended that radiotherapy be available for 45% of these. This generates around 2000 referrals per million per annum, requiring a number of linacs (and radiographers) dependent on the relative mix of palliative and curative treatments, the average treatment patterns and complexity involved.

On average locally, each patient referred will receive 1.5 treatment courses in a year, be they concurrent courses using two modalities such as afterloading plus external beam, two or more consecutive phases, or treatment to more than one primary (e.g. two basal cell carcinomas or bilateral breast), or treatment to recurrences or secondary tumours.

It is increasingly important that data may be collected which is detailed enough to be used in different ways for service planning for the population served.

Korner statistics

Korner-type statistics are used for providing basic activity levels, particularly exposures, fractions and courses and constituent parts thereof (e.g. multiphase or multimodality).

Time-consuming procedures and exposures. This data should allow estimation of the relative exposure levels for treatments which take much longer than the norm. For example TBI should be counted at 20 exposures for every hour used, as specified by Korner. There are now additional categories not as yet recognised by the Korner system as being more time-consuming, such as complex electron work, afterloading work and conformal therapy. Hyperfractionated treatments should also be identified, and, for budgeting purposes, patients treated using overtime or as emergency call-out work. It is useful also to record quality assurance check exposures, portal film exposures, and any extra exposures occurring during the normal day. Data entry and editing time should also be recorded as it represents a workload.

Use of machine time. Details of breakdown time (and treatments cancelled or postponed related to this), planned maintenance time and machine hours used for routine or special treatment outside the normal working day are important cost factors.

Billing information

Activity data is required in a form which allows billing for a service, which the 'customer' can understand but which also reflects the actual work involved rather than a number of exposures. Many centres 'band' treatments into one of 5 or 6 charge categories, each of which reflect a quantity of planning time in addition to treatment time factors. It is possible to use software programs which allocate a patient to the appropriate band by summating basic data incorporating key words such as 'shell' plus a number of exposures.

Information for service management and planning

Regular reports are required which identify trends in referrals or treatment patterns, for management use in service planning, budgeting etc. These cannot necessarily be generated from Korner or billing data, and must be understandable to the lay person, i.e. a manager unfamiliar with terms and data which are used. For example, for a given number of referrals, has the number of fractions changed and produced a work overload, or was it the fields or exposures per fraction, and for which type of diagnosis? Such information can be simply expressed, e.g. 'Over the last 2 years, the average number of treatments for a head and neck patient has increased from 25 to 30, so that treatment takes 6 full weeks rather than 5, giving a workload increase of 20% for each'. This sounds simple, but is difficult to achieve without appropriate data or software, or weeks of manual investigation.

Other activities, such as simulation, use of computer verification systems, treatment card preparation and checks, patient care and organisation and staff and student training, affect the taskload of a department. Statistics on numbers of, and time used in, these activities should also be available where possible.

The above information allows a good assessment of workload and use of available resources. The importance of matching workload to resources in ensuring quality in radiotherapy was stressed by a Working Party (Bleehen et al 1991) which investigated and reported on the issues contributing to a major radiation incident.

REFERENCES AND FURTHER READING

Bleehen N M et al 1991 Quality assurance in radiotherapy. Report of a Working Party. Standing Subcommittee on Cancer of the Standing Medical Advisory Committee
Blue Book 1991 Radiation oncology in integrated cancer management. Report of the Inter-Society Council for Radiation Oncology (USA)
Horiot J C, Johansson K A, Gonzalez D G, Van der Scheuren E, Van den Bogaert W, Notter G 1986 Quality assurance control in the EORTC cooperative group of Radiotherapy 1. Assessment of radiotherapy staff and equipment. Radiotherapy and Oncology 6: 275–284
Probst H 1992 An experiment to test the effect on the accuracy of a set-up for whole cranial irradiation with lead shielding when the work pace for radiographers is increased, BSc project, University of Teesside (copy held at Cookridge Hospital, Leeds)

26

Staffing for an effective treatment service

The quality of the treatment delivery and the effective use of high cost equipment (see Chs 24 and 25) are both dependent on the skills of the radiographer. Treatment is planned and prescribed on paper to the satisfaction of local standards, but whether the plan is achieved depends on details of the equipment and setting-up processes. Treatment failure has been linked to inadequate technical practice resulting in geographical miss of the tumour (Kinzie et al 1983).

Additional factors such as workload, treatment complexity, equipment availability and compatibility, continuity of staffing, organisational factors, time-stress conditions, skills, training and training loads influence the quality with which treatment can be delivered. Inadequacy in treatment delivery reduces the value of providing state-of-the-art equipment and sophisticated treatment planning techniques.

In this chapter, some of the current issues in staffing, such as skill mix, are discussed against the background set out by this book. A summary of the processes used to treat each patient and each treatment field, if considered in conjunction with the foregoing text, will show the complexity of the task and the organisational factors, and set the scene against which radiographers work and train others.

SKILLS REQUIRED FOR TREATMENT DELIVERY

Technical skills, knowledge and prerequisites

• Assurance from checks that all equipment is functioning within specified limits.

• Radiographer familiarity and competence with all local techniques, and with individual consultants' requirements.
    • Familiarity with numerous equipment controls, features and their functions.

Summary of processes used in each set-up

Most of the processes below are essential to the correct alignment of the patient with the radiation beam, i.e. to the correct treatment being given. All settings etc. are checked by two qualified therapeutic radiographers for radiation safety reasons. The setting-up processes are completed concurrently, within a total time of 2–3 minutes plus 2 minutes irradiation time during which monitoring and other tasks are undertaken. Most of the processes relate to the majority of set-ups. Computer tasks related to set-up, administrative and organisational processes are concurrently carried out. Because of the technical and professional care aspects of the work, together with the continually mixed caseload encountered, only the tasks marked* could be carried out by an unqualified person. Professional decision-making skills are used throughout:

Escort* the patient to the treatment room:

• Check identity.
• Establish rapport and see how the patient is feeling.
• Check whether the patient has followed instructions, e.g. emptied bladder.
• Give appropriate instructions.
• Make decisions if the patient describes reactions etc.
• Make suitable arrangements with the patient.
• Liaise with other departments or staff as appropriate.
• Help patient to remove clothes or gown*.
• Help patient onto couch when couch arrangement ready as below*.

Prepare couch:

• Remove items used for previous patient (unless needed again)*.

• Clean couch top*.
• Turn couch to required position, change slat arrangement if appropriate.
• Select prescribed patient support or immobilisation devices.
• Check and adjust setting of support devices and check name.
• Add hygiene tissues*.

Position patient on couch in prescribed position:

• Check settings of immobilisation devices and set patient accordingly.
• Check patient is straight using laser where appropriate.
• Check arm, leg, head position, check hands safely above couch top.
• Correct patient rotation using lateral lasers where appropriate.
• Adjust patient position until correct.
• Move couch vertically to required height, check with prescription.
• Move couch horizontally and longitudinally to centre patient.
• Check/measure treatment centring position.
• Re-mark centre or other marks as necessary.
• Check rangefinder reading and make decision on acceptability.

Prepare machine:

• Add or remove accessories as appropriate.
• Set/check gantry angle.
• Set/check size on each diaphragm.
• Check/set symmetric or asymmetric diaphragms, both X and Y.
• Check field orientation (and symmetry) on patient.
• Set/check collimator rotation (even if zero).
• Set/check couch rotation (even if zero).
• Check light field on patient or shell and make decision on acceptability.
• Position lead shielding if appropriate and check prescription.
• Check no obstacles in beam, including other parts of patient in exit beam, e.g. eye.
• Add bolus if appropriate and check prescription.

- Check field cover is appropriate and make decision.
- Insert wedge if appropriate (unless autowedge) and check orientation.
- Insert compensator if appropriate and check orientation.
- Check prescription to make sure all items complied with.
- Set check film up if required, and label.
- Check centre cross on patient.
- Select energy or mode if appropriate.
- Turn up lights and turn off optical devices (switches integral with machine controls).
- Reassure patient.
- Latch room door when only the patient remains in the room.

Set machine to give treatment:

- Check dose and time and machine units for field, set or check these on machine.
- Select and confirm energy and mode.
- Select and confirm wedge requirement for field (even when no wedge).
- Switch on radiation beam.
- Watch all beam monitoring devices/dose channels/timers.
- Be ready to react to possible machine malfunction.
- Watch to detect any patient movement or distress (second radiographer to do this).
- Take decisions if patient moves.
- Watch for persons approaching the treatment room entrance*.
- Record radiation given on treatment card and check against verification record.

Help patient from room:

- Take down set-up.
- Help patient off table*.
- Reassure and confirm arrangements for next attendance*.

All of the above processes apply for each field treated, except for getting the patient to and from the table. (The patient's position is always rechecked before treating another field and sometimes must be adjusted.) The list is not exhaustive.

Other daily procedures

Some of the concurrent tasks performed through the day are:

- new patient treatment card calculations
- subsequent checks on treatment card calculations
- data entry to record and verify systems
- vericord checks and file handling
- diary, check cards for treatment and care messages
- interdepartmental communication regarding treatments
- organisation of patient flow to unit
- patient support and referral to other services
- staff training on the unit
- student training on the unit.

Normally four radiographers run a linac, working together to ensure an optimum patient throughput. Two radiographers work together to set up the patients, a third interacts with their activities and ensures a continual flow of patients and data on the unit, greets and makes professional judgements about patients, and continually liaises with other staff groups. The fourth member of staff is occupied with routine treatment and data checks and document preparation. One person carries overall responsibility for quality.

Training, skills and skill mix

An ability to spot flaws in treatments, make technical judgements and decisions, adapt quickly to new concepts and to critically evaluate practice, rather than operating by rote, are required of therapy radiographers, in addition to organisational and caring skills. A substantial specialist education with a pronounced practical content is necessary for the development of these qualities and those skills required to manage the service.

The adequacy of basic training programmes

The pre-practice training programme is currently under review in Europe, with a view to a common core standard being reached. Many European programmes have utilised training courses designed for diagnostic radiographers or other professions. However, these are perceived as inadequate for the therapy radiographer or 'radiation therapist' who must be responsible for his/her own safe practice, especially when using the newer technology. For example, an anatomy or radiation physics syllabus designed for diagnostic radiographers addresses few of the issues which are important in radiotherapy. Equipment, use of equipment, technical practice, radiobiology and radiation safety of the patient have negligible common features between the two professions.

Following qualification, continual updating is required, in a culture where the need to continue to acquire knowledge and undertake development work is understood.

Skill mix issues

For demographic and political reasons, there is a need to analyse work processes and identify areas where unqualified support staff can be used. The authors have addressed this issue and found that, although there are undoubtedly areas where suitable staff can be utilised, such as in reception, clinic and administrative functions, these staff support the radiographers rather than substantially reduce the number required to deliver the treatment service. Because of the volume of required knowledge, only a few of the processes involved in treatment are suitable for an unqualified person. These do not make up a significant portion of the whole, so a full complement of qualified staff is required in order to operate efficiently.

A few disadvantages accrue from bringing in unqualified staff, apart from the need to give basic training. These disadvantages include some loss of flexibility within the staffing, so that it becomes more difficult to usefully occupy any radiographers who are pregnant or suffering some temporary disability and cannot work on a treatment unit. Also cover must be provided when the support staff are absent, which can be problematical when the organisational knowledge to undertake their tasks efficiently has been lost by the qualified staff. Conversely, there is no

possibility for the support staff to cover for the absence of a radiographer.

Skills related to departmental equipment and staffing organisation

Most departments have different units within them. Where technical methods related to the equipment and its features (see Ch. 23) differ, different skills are required from unit to unit. In addition, good staff continuity is required on each unit for reasons of treatment safety, efficiency, and patient confidence. Thus staff rostering and organisation influence the effectiveness of the service.

Equipment complexity, computerisation and staff specialisation

The increasing complexity and computerisation of equipment give rise to a need for specialist staff with high profile training and technical development roles. Ideally a specialist should develop expertise with each specialised treatment unit, and with each computer system, as each has its own user problems which require a troubleshooter. Computerisation may pose efficiency and safety problems if appropriately skilled staff are not available.

These specialist roles require individuals who are suitably skilled and perceived by their peers and by juniors to be competent and to contribute to the work effort. The need for competent specialist staff to achieve the best quality of treatment is related to the probability of cure in the 1984 Report of the International Commission on Radiological Protection (Report 1984). Specialist staff have the opportunity to undertake research and development work to widen their role and benefit the profession and the service. Specialist roles affect the organisation and the development of the staff group.

Staff organisation systems and related issues

There are two main approaches to staff organisation: radiographers are either recruited to and work on one unit, or they move from one unit to another at intervals. Retaining staff on one unit has the advantages that a high level of expertise on the unit is gained and induction training is simplified to a general introductory period. Continuity can be good using this system, but it is more difficult to provide competent cover during staff absences etc. because of the narrow experience of each staff member. Junior staff may feel disadvantaged and demotivated by lack of challenge in their role, and the flexibility and transferability of staff is very limited. It is desirable for new staff to gain an all-round basic level of expertise, so that they have a broad knowledge of departmental activity. However, it is not possible for staff to gain the highest level of expertise in any area while continually moving round.

Quality management related to continuing training

The 'Quality Assurance in Radiotherapy' report (Bleehen et al 1991) sets out a framework for formally managing quality, which includes a requirement for identifying and meeting the ongoing training needs of staff to ensure their continued competence in their areas of practice, which is also recognised by the College of Radiographers (1993). Given the current climate of rapid development of technology and practice, these training needs apply to all staff using each piece of equipment. This is further supported by the World Health Organisation (WHO 1988). Thus specially designed equipment-specific training programmes are necessary.

Linac training programmes

The current generation of linacs are all complex to operate and thus a structured approach to staff training is required. Initially a number of staff should undergo a relevant training course provided by the manufacturer. Depending on the number of features new to the staff, a period of several months should then be designated for training, developing safe systems of work and gradually increasing the patient throughput. A normal patient load cannot safely be accommodated until a significant number of staff are familiar with all features and functions. Following this, staff subsequently rostered to the unit must undergo the same training, facilitated by a clinical specialist who remains on the unit to ensure consistency in the training process. The clinical specialist would devise an appropriate schedule, including some form of assessment for each trainee.

Effect of training on patient throughput

On handover of a new piece of equipment for clinical use, there may be an assumption that a full workload can be achieved immediately. However, for a linac, this will not be the case unless an identical machine is already in use in the department.

The authors have analysed the throughput on a newly commissioned computer-controlled linac over a period of 4 years. This showed that initially there was a definite learning period during which the activity increase was rapid. This is because the initial period of familiarisation is relatively short and it is possible to gain sufficient knowledge to operate the linac at a very basic level, providing there are no unfamiliar technical difficulties.

The throughput increased over 6 months. Following this, each time a new team leader was assigned to the unit, activity tended to drop. This type of staff change and ad hoc 'sitting by Nellie' approach to training had seemed relatively unproblematical on older, simpler equipment, but was found to be inappropriate for the new technology in terms of throughput, morale, and treatment safety. Four years later, with established systems of work on the unit, plus more appropriate training and staff rotation, the throughput greatly exceeds that using conventional machines, even though there is an online record and verify system which is in routine use. There is also an extremely low parameter 'error' rate, compared with that before these systems were established, when programming errors remained undetected owing to an inappropriate reliance on the computer to set parameters correctly (Short 1992). A similar machine with an off-line programming workstation could presumably yield an even higher output, given an appropriate staff skill level.

Systems of work and training should also address and seek to minimise the health and safety problems associated with use of the equipment, such as the risk of back injury (College of Radiographers 1993), and stress associated with work demands (Lightfoot 1993).

Training and induction of new staff

Induction courses should be provided, covering general organisational policy and prescribing practices. The current technical protocol sheets should be available to assist in speedy understanding of the details of technical practice of the centre.

A settling-in period of at least 6 months, for learning the intricacies of critical practices, should be allowed before the radiographer is expected to carry full responsibility for practice on a treatment unit. In a large department, a 12-month period is required for a full-time radiographer to gain broader familiarity with the organisation and its practice, and longer than this on taking up a more senior post.

Recruitment and retention issues

Factors influencing recruitment and whether or not qualified staff stay in the profession must include the career structure offered. The level of recognition of the abilities and skills of individual radiographers is an important factor, reflected in the structure and culture of a department. It is also important, for staff commitment, to establish shared individual and organisation values and goals.

The perceived significance of collective or individual roles and of the responsibilities of radiographers to the organisation is important. The perception of each person, or peer group, of their value to the organisation is a demotivating or stress factor if they feel that they are undervalued (College of Radiographers 1993), or that they would be valued more highly in another organisation.

Part-time and job-sharing staff

Those wishing to return to regular practice after career breaks or maternity leave often want only part-time work. The use of part-time staff in radiotherapy has been limited and is acknowledged to be particularly difficult (College of Radiographers 1988). The use of part-time staff at a senior level is impracticable because of the need for continuity of senior staff from one day to the next, partly because of their responsibility for correctly reproducing each patient's treatment on each day of a course, and partly because of the need for one person to be team leader. There is a grading and responsibility conflict where junior staff have to provide the continuity and make the related treatment decisions, whilst being accountable to a different senior person each day.

Two part-time or job-sharing staff, sharing a week, take at least twice as many weeks to gain competence on a particular unit as does one full-time person, because there are two people learning and because of the intermittent nature of their work.

In the future it is possible that a substantial refresher course, with a clinical practice content, will be a mandatory preregistration requirement following a break, as is the case for most professionals already. It was suggested in the Manpower Advisory Group report (College of Radiographers 1988) that returners be retrained as supernumerary members of staff. However, there are logistical problems where there is already a heavy staff and student training load. One possibility is to retrain staff for one particular unit, but this limits the flexibility to move other staff through that unit.

Training logistics

Given this ongoing need to train and update all staff in clinical practice, a problem arises in accommodating this together with training students, new staff, and refresher training for staff having had a career break. The number of persons undergoing training on a unit must be limited, for the dignity of the patient and his or her confidence in the treatment staff, for throughput reasons, and for the quality and effectiveness of the training. The taskload of the staff, carrying out treatment and concurrently training peers and students, must also be taken into account. Having regard also to the length of training experience required by each trainee on each unit, a practicable number of trainees should be determined, and not exceeded. Training commitments should be balanced against clinical demands and the quality of patient care.

The skill mix of the future

The general trend towards increasingly diverse and complex treatment techniques and technology requires higher levels of skill and responsibility, and a more specialist role, for radiographers undertaking 'routine' treatments. An 11% increase in the number of therapy radiographers working the UK was noted between 1984–1986, with a relatively higher increase in senior staff.

This was related to increasing treatment complexity (White 1993). A second phase of this trend must be imminent, and is certainly required, if it can be resourced. The technical ability and stage of development of newly qualified staff must allow them to cope with complex practice on qualifying, and also give them the potential to move rapidly to positions of greater responsibility, since there may be a reduced need for less senior staff. The move towards degree training in this country should address these needs. Meanwhile, the challenge and interest that new developments have added to the practice provide a greater incentive for radiographers to stay in the profession and take on an ever-widening role in the planning, provision and delivery of radiotherapy services.

REFERENCES AND FURTHER READING

Bleehen N M et al 1991 Quality assurance in radiotherapy. Report of Working Party. Standing Subcommittee on Cancer of the Standing Medical Advisory Committee

College of Radiographers 1988 Staffing for the 1990s. Radiography News, September

College of Radiographers 1993 Networking radiotherapy. Radiography Today 59: 28–31

Drummond A 1987 The maintenance of post-diplomate competence. Radiography 52: 75–78

International Commission on Radiological Protection 1984 Report, p 39

Kinzie J J, Hanks G E, Maclean C J, Kramer S 1983 Patterns of care study: Hodgkin's disease relapse rates and the adequacy of portals. Cancer 52: 2223–2226

Lightfoot J 1993 Stress – its incidence and effect on radiographers. Radiography Today 59: 12–15

Short C S 1992 The safe use of computers in radiotherapy treatment delivery. Radiography Today 58: 19

White E 1993 Radiotherapy helpers – where do we go from here? Radiography Today 59: 16–19

World Health Organization 1988 Quality assurance in radiotherapy. WHO, Geneva

INDEX